"Packed with eighty delicious recipes and realistic nutrition tips, this cookbook makes eating simple, satisfying, and full of flavor. Just as nutrition was intended: uncomplicated and delicious."

—Sarah Williams, MS, RDN,
@NutritionalSarah

"Great recipes but also meal prep tips, how to shop on a budget, and evidence-based nutrition education—this is so much more than just a cookbook!"

—Zach Coen, RD, LN

"I've admired Steph's work since the day we connected. She has a rare gift for making nutrition feel supportive, grounded, and easy to understand. *Crave, Cook, Nourish* captures all of that. It's packed with balanced, flavorful recipes and the kind of evidence-based guidance people can truly trust!"

—Kylie Sakaida, MS, RD,
author of *The New York Times* bestseller *So Easy So Good*

CRAVE, COOK, NOURISH

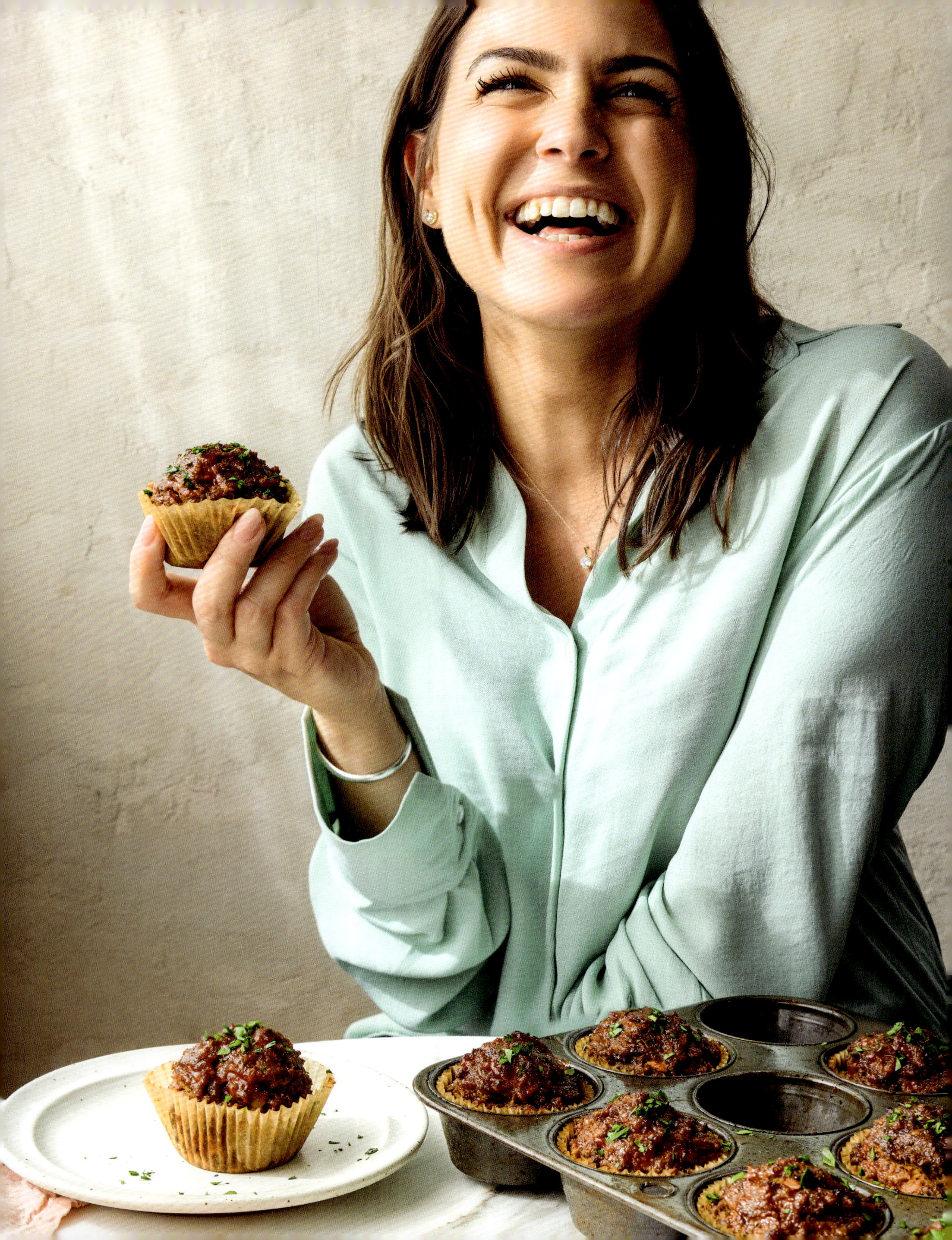

Steph Grasso, MS, RD
with Liz Crain

CRAVE, COOK, NOURISH

80+ Recipes and Expert Guidance for Healthy, Happy Nutrition

Photographs by Erin Scott

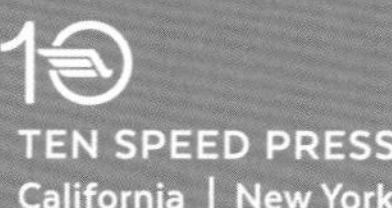

TEN SPEED PRESS
California | New York

CONTENTS

Nourishing Mains

Nutrition-Boosting Sides

Doctored-Up Comfort Classics

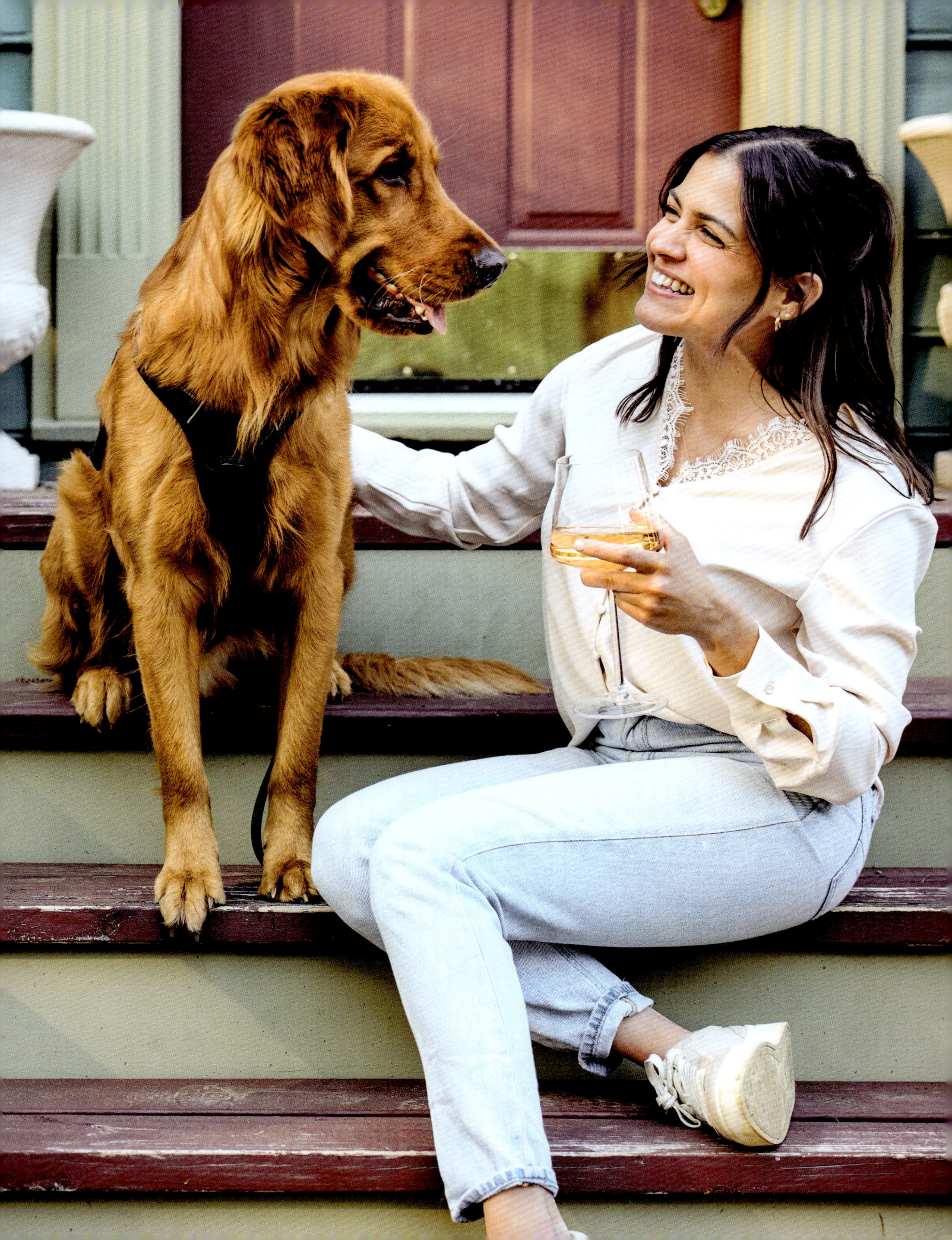

My Story

When I was growing up in Northern Virginia, I often had a digital camera in my hands. From a young age I was very creative, and for years, videography was my number one creative outlet. I loved it so much that in high school, I even bussed to a different school, several miles away, for a TV production class. My teenage dream: become a TV or movie director.

My dad has a heart of gold, *and* he's always been incredibly strict with my two sisters and me. I'm the youngest. He wanted me to get a college degree in the sciences because he thought that would lead to a more stable job than an arts degree, so that's what I did.

During those early premed months in college, I was most engaged in my nutrition classes. Unfortunately, the same time that I was hitting the books, I personally got tangled up in toxic diet culture. After quickly gaining my Freshman 15, I set my sights on one restrictive diet and weight-loss tactic after another. I went from vegetarian to vegan (the horror—I *LOVE* cheese!), to Whole30, to obsessing over detox teas. Not only did these diets and tactics not work, they also really negatively affected my relationship with food and with myself.

I wanted to dig deeper into food and nutrition, so I switched from premed to nutrition in the dietetic field. Through my education and studying evidence-based research, I learned that the diets and weight-loss tactics I was trying were not, in fact, good nutrition. I learned that cutting good from-the-earth foods out of my diet—and essentially starving myself—was also not good nutrition. I began to look critically at all the ever-changing, and often quite harmful, current and historic nutrition myths, fads, and diets. Through education, I slowly but surely got to a better place.

I graduated from Virginia Tech in 2018 with my Master of Science degree in nutrition and dietetics, and in 2019 I became a clinical dietitian at a hospital in Haymarket, Virginia. This was around the same time that TikTok was gaining traction and rising in popularity, especially with millennials like me. At first, I didn't see the appeal. It seemed like a never-ending supply of short, silly videos of kids dancing. I didn't get it.

When the Covid pandemic hit several months later, our hospital became a different place overnight. It's still hard for me to properly convey what those early pandemic hospital shifts were like. With all the long nerve-wracking days and incredible stress, I gave in and downloaded TikTok. I wanted to distract myself when I wasn't masked up and helping patients. It worked. Once it was on my phone, I was hooked. I needed that escapism.

While watching TikTok, I'd get nutrition video ideas from the lyrics of a song or from a certain beat. I decided to use my expertise as a dietitian and try my hand at teaching some of the nutrition lessons I'd learned in grad school. I featured songs that were trending and posted videos every few days. I had fun making them, but they didn't seem all that impactful.

That is, until my magnesium video came out. I wanted to show people how important magnesium is, especially for managing stress and overall well-being. It felt like a very important and timely PSA for myself and my coworkers (we definitely needed to manage our stress!) and I wanted to share that intel with my TikTok followers.

I posted my magnesium video early in the morning, before arriving at the hospital. At some point midday, while charting a patient, my phone started to blow up. I mean, BLOW UP. I got thousands upon thousands of views on that video, and they kept coming. All day.

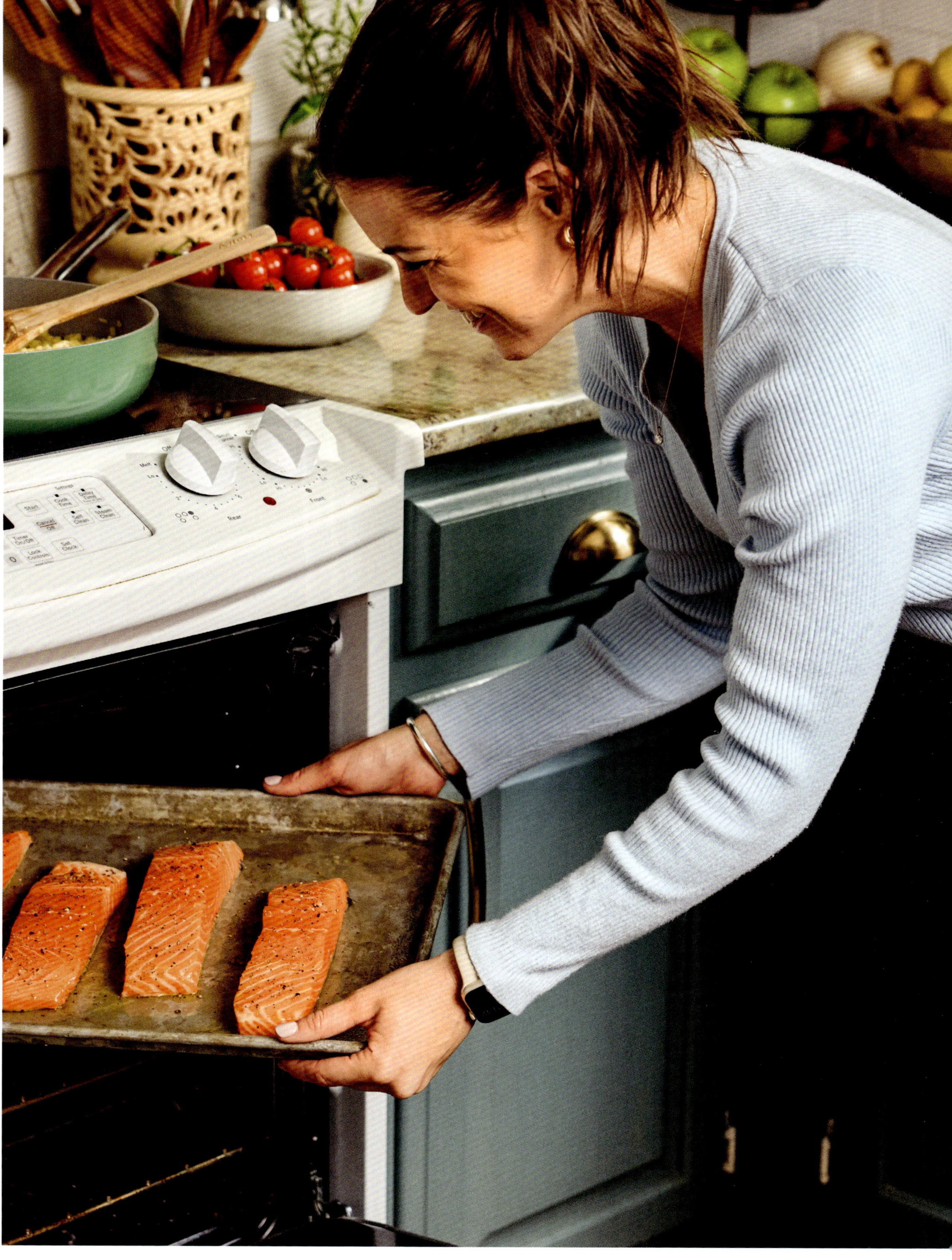
Start
Cook Time
Delay Time
Cancel Off
Self Clean
Steam Clean
Timer On/Off
Set Clock
Lock Controls
Rear
Front

All night. And ultimately, all week. The fact that people were interested in nutrition on TikTok completely caught me by surprise. From that day on, I posted something nutrition-based almost every day.

From 2020 to 2021, I gained millions of followers. It was all so exciting. Little, fresh-out-of-university me suddenly had an audience. And it wasn't small! There was this huge group of people all around the world interested in what I had to say about nutrition. And they were *really* interested. In the beginning, that seemingly overnight success was a bit overwhelming, for sure, but I also loved it. I was helping people. And I was having fun while doing so. I'd sort of become the director younger me had dreamed of becoming. Sure, it looked a little different from what I'd imagined, but I was filming and editing and widely sharing impactful information.

My life completely changed in the following years. I quit my job and became a full-time content creator making nutrition-related posts and videos. Along the way, I've shared so much helpful nutrition info and guidance, developed all sorts of delicious and nutritious recipes, gained amazing social media friends, and partnered with dream brands that I admire. I still think it's wild how two of my primary passions, videography and nutrition, just naturally came together.

And the very best part? What I do doesn't feel like a job. It really doesn't. I'm living my dream. I get to help millions of people develop an informed understanding of nutrition and intuitive eating in large part through my favorite medium, videography. I love my life.

Navigating Nutrition via Social Media

I am, of course, incredibly grateful for social media. I would not be where I am today without it. That said, I've learned a few things about safely navigating it and using it to your advantage versus falling into its many all-too-common pitfalls.

Since we do not prioritize preventive care when it comes to health and wellness in the US, most of us simply treat health problems as they arise. That's understandable since, for the most part, health insurance doesn't cover preventive services. If you seek nutrition and diet services for yourself or a loved one, you're likely going to pay out of pocket, and dietitians are not cheap. This is in large part why so many people turn to social media for nutrition guidance. It's free! But, of course, there are strings attached.

There is so much harmful misinformation out there about what you should and shouldn't be eating. Repeated exposure to this misinformation trains your brain to believe it's the norm. Social media giants and their algorithms don't care about your mental health; they care about your watch time.

Let me explain. On your feed, you might see beautiful, aesthetically pleasing videos: restocks of pristine refrigerators or someone showing off a gorgeous equipped-with-every-expensive-gadget kitchen. Everything looks perfect . . . the person, the fridge, its contents. These videos get a lot of attention, and the algorithm takes note. It starts feeding you more and more of the same.

Soon, your feed is full of unattainable lifestyle content. You keep watching and watching, and inevitably you start to feel the pressure to be more like what you see. You think, is this what good health looks like? Is this what my kitchen and the foods in it should look like? Is this how my body should be? These videos create unrealistic expectations. Social media has a way of making you feel like whatever you're doing isn't enough. It's exhausting and harmful, especially when the nutrition focus is largely on weight and weight loss rather than overall health and nutrition. I do my very best to counter *all of that* in various ways.

Food Access & Food Scarcity

While living in Georgetown in Washington, D.C., I started dating my fiancé, Miles. We'd known each other since 2015, when we became friends at Virginia Tech. When our worlds collided post-college, it felt like something straight out of a Hallmark movie, except for one barrier: the distance. Because of his work, Miles lived in a rural area more than three hours away from me. I didn't care. I was head over heels, so I kept my place in Georgetown but spent most of my time with Miles. While living in what felt to me like the middle of nowhere, I began to think more deeply about food access and food scarcity.

There was only one grocery store in the area, and its produce section was often nearly empty or stocked with poor-quality items. Most of the time, I had to buy whatever was available. I also frequently shopped at Dollar General, my only other option. That's the reality for so many Americans. Some people don't even have access to the transportation needed—public or otherwise—to get to a Dollar General.

Most viral videos about food and wellness come from big cities, but millions of Americans live in suburban or rural areas without access to the same resources. Nutrition advice should be realistic, flexible, and rooted in compassion. For many, living a healthier lifestyle doesn't even feel like a viable choice due to lack of access. Since I first lived rurally with Miles, I've worked hard to create content that cuts through all that unrelatable noise, that's helpful for a much larger sector of society. I'm all about shopping on a budget and choosing and celebrating affordable and accessible.

My Crave, Cook, Nourish Mission

I've built my life around sharing my nutrition knowledge and nourishing meal inspiration. You won't find anyone more passionate about or driven by what they do. I want to empower *you* to make your own delicious and nutritious choices. My recipes are all extremely accessible. They call for easy-to-source ingredients, include simple steps with minimal time commitment, and require zero fancy kitchen tools or equipment. Life is hard. Eating well shouldn't be.

My book offers up healthful and satisfying food and the basic nutrition behind it. There is nothing bougie here. I repeatedly walk you through the freezer aisle (I love my frozen fruits and veggies, page 44) and I celebrate canned foods. I promote adding rather than restricting. I want to help you nourish yourself.

I wholeheartedly believe that if you understand the basics of nutrition, you'll be more inclined to make healthier choices in your life. You'll also be able to move past a restrictive mindset, and stop obsessing over calories. I've included calorie counts for my recipes because that's useful information when you think positively of calories (they are your body's energy!) and eat intuitively. I give you the median calorie count, by the way, when a recipe has a serving range.

Diet culture is still the big, ugly, scary monster that I fight head-on every day through my work. Diet culture is about money, power, and control. No one is doing you any favors in the wide world of diets, whether it's a social media influencer trying to sell you on their favorite "nature's cereal" (it's just fruit and water, people! As if cereal is unnatural and bad for you . . .) or a national diet company's campaign trying to hook you. I go deeper into the history of diet culture in the next section of the book (see The Evolution of Diet Culture, page 14).

Whether you're most interested in my Pantry Power & Ingredients section (page 38); my Grocery Shopping & Meal Prep Tips & Hacks (page 49); or Mastering the Art of Balance (page 34), where I give you an easy and fun template for building a balanced plate, I think you'll find a lot of inspiration in these pages. And when it comes to recipes, my killer Cheesy Kielbasa Skillet (page 185) that Katie Couric loves, my vegan Lizzo Salad (page 125), or any of my delicious and accessible recipes, including my Doctored-Up Comfort Classics (hello, Healthy Hamburger Helper, page 244, and Doctored Instant Ramen, page 243!), I want you to please, please be kind to yourself and have fun.

I hope that my cookbook sometimes lives in your kitchen (when you're cooking from it!), other times in your bedroom (when you've got your feet up and are flipping through for meal inspo), other times in your car (when you're off to the grocery store for a stock-up and need some guidance), and not in a way-back, dark, dusty corner of some closet. I want to be there for you at each and every one of those times because guess what . . .

I've got you. I'm 100 percent here for you. Now let's go have some kitchen fun, okay?!

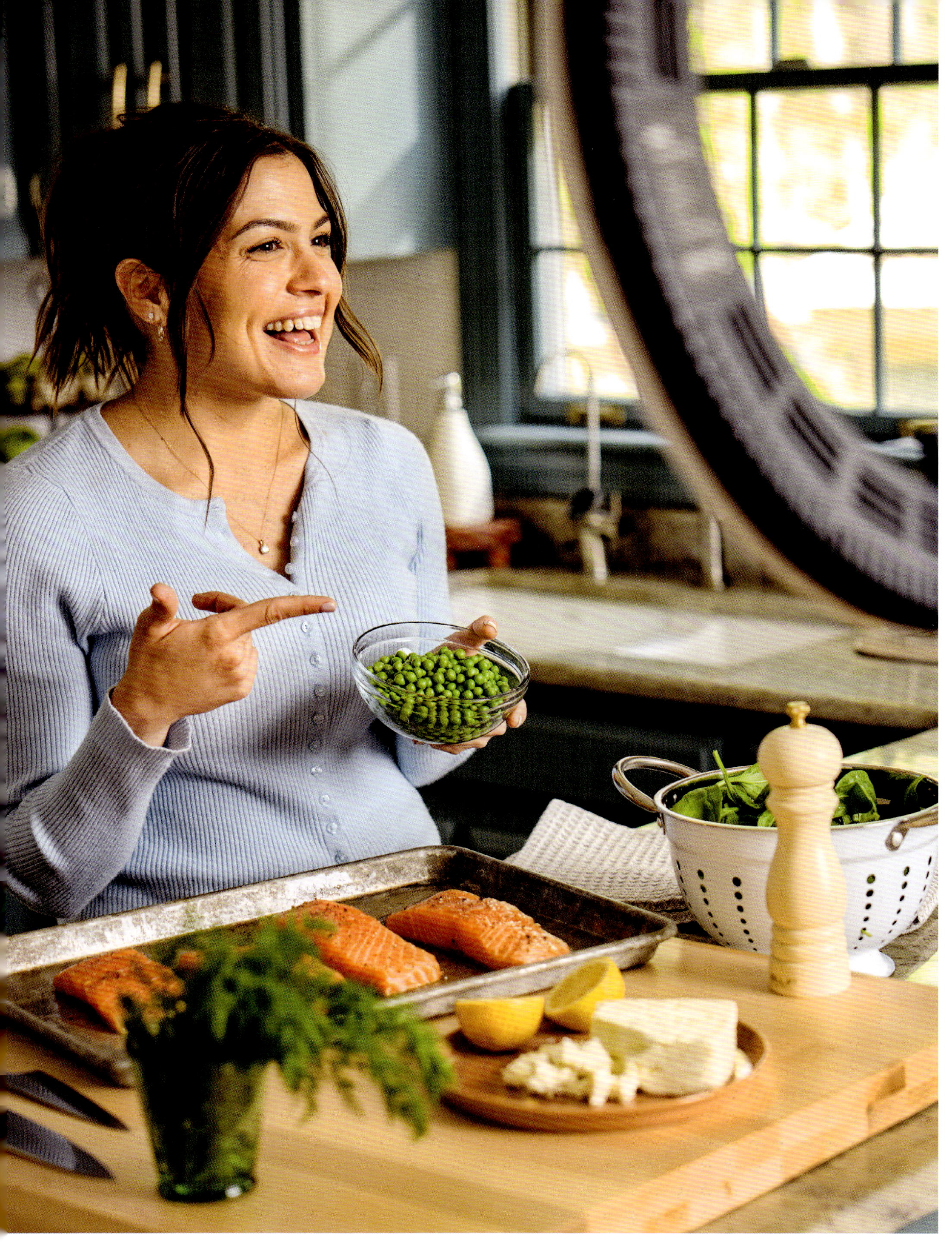

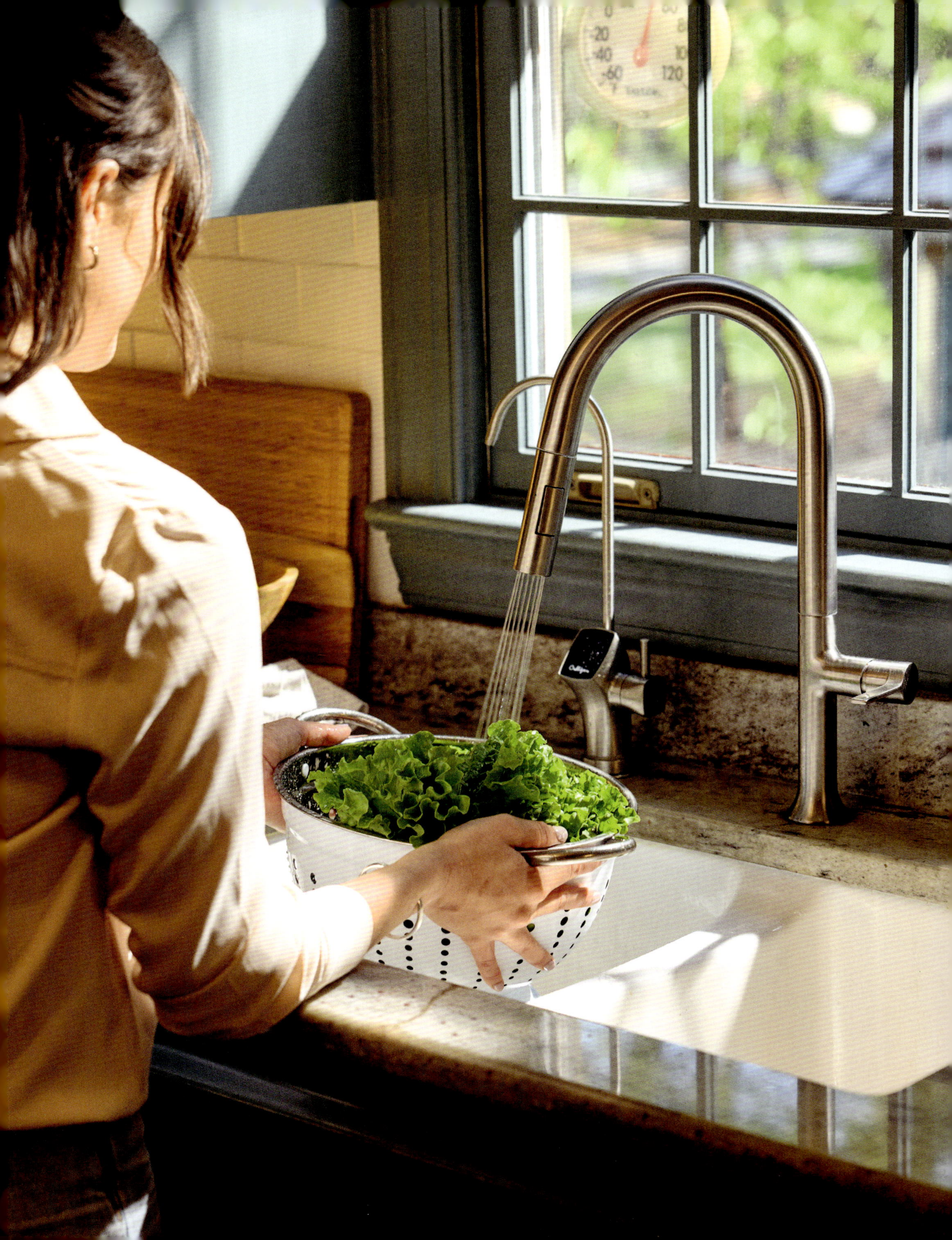

Nutrition Basics

The Evolution of Diet Culture

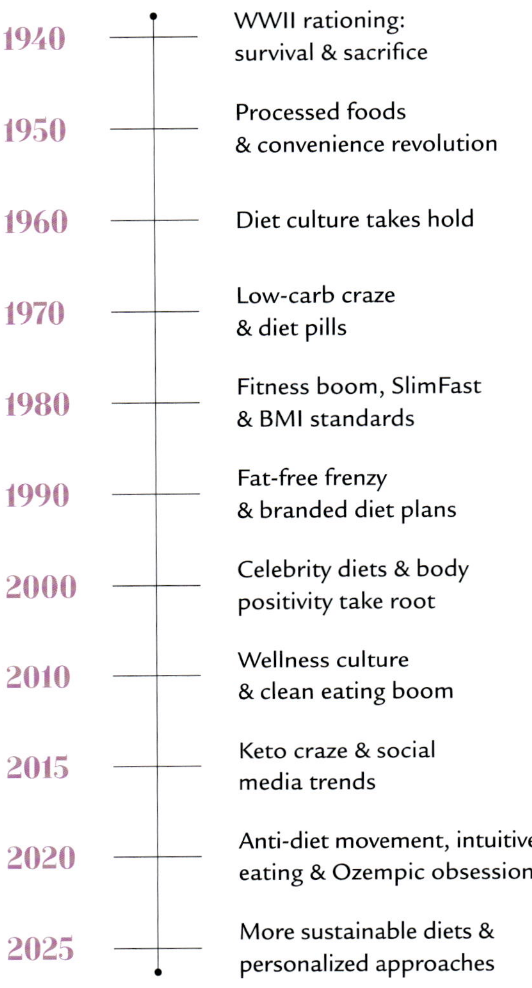

It's always helpful to have at least a basic understanding of the past—including historic milestones—for anything that you deeply value in the present. In this section, I give you a clearer idea of the cultural shifts in dieting and nutrition in the US during the past eighty years: from the 1940s and World War II era, to the rise of processed foods and slim ideals of the 1950s, all the way up to today. It's by no means comprehensive, but it's a solid overview that connects some dots between our current health, wellness, and dieting trends and those of previous generations. Norms and values around eating, dieting, and health have significantly evolved since the 1940s but history does still repeat itself.

Today, the US diet industry rakes in $70-plus BILLION annually. It's devastating to see who determines and sets our mainstream diet and nutrition standards—basically companies looking to take your money. I want you to recognize and understand harmful patterns and extreme dieting trends when it comes to things such as starvation diets, diet pills, and the glorification of thinness through the decades. The hope: You'll be better able to evaluate harmful products and tactics disguised as "wellness" or "clean," especially if you don't have the best relationship with food. I want you to stop blaming food, to stop seeing certain foods as "bad," and, most important, to stop blaming yourself.

Big-money media, corporate marketing, and advertising machines have perpetuated body image and diet insecurities and influenced cultural standards, from the early diet product ads of the 1950s to the highly curated social media trends of the 2000s and beyond. My aim with this historical context is to help you navigate all this noise more mindfully. If you understand how trends have shifted (again, often repeating themselves), you'll likely be able to make more informed, intentional choices that align with your values and needs. Okay, let's educate ourselves!

1940s: World War II & Food Rationing

The world was deep in World War II, and food symbolized sacrifice and survival. With so many resources going to support our soldiers, regular folks had to get by with *a lot* less. Food rationing kicked in, and families were only allowed small amounts of ingredients such as sugar, butter, canned milk, and canned meats and fish. You couldn't just stroll into a store and grab what you wanted. Ration books were filled with coupons that you used for limited supplies.

Meal planning wasn't about feeding a craving for a favorite dish, it was about stretching what little you had. The focus was certainly not on being thin or dieting—it was about staying healthy and strong amid the scarcity. More and more women were stepping into tough factory jobs, working long, physically demanding shifts. Eating enough food wasn't judged or frowned upon, it was an essential part of powering through the day.

1950s: Postwar Boom & Rise of Processed Foods

The economic boom of the 1950s completely changed the way people ate. With more money to spend, convenience became the name of the game. Kitchen appliances such as refrigerators and freezers became a fixture in most homes and all sorts of advances in food technology came on the market. Processed foods like TV dinners, canned soups, and boxed cake mixes lined grocery store shelves. Their promise: make cooking quicker and easier for busy families. Ahem, for moms. Ads aimed at housewives pitched these new products as time-savers that still delivered that "home-cooked" feel.

But it wasn't just about saving time. These factory-produced foods also signified progress and prosperity. Ingredients like powdered milk, dehydrated potatoes (see Instant Spuds Made Right, page 231!), and canned veggies, originally developed to feed wartime soldiers, were now kitchen staples. Brands like Swanson and Betty Crocker turned into household names while frozen dinners became the modern solution for getting dinner onto the table with ease. While all these foods definitely saved time, they were also heavily processed and loaded with sugar, salt, and preservatives. They drastically changed the nutritional makeup of at-home meals.

Cultural attitudes were shifting. With so much affordable high-caloric food available after years of wartime scarcity, diet culture began to take hold. Thinness became synonymous with beauty and self-control. Convenience was a relief to many, but there were trade-offs when it came to health and societal expectations.

1960s: Weight Watchers & Twiggy

The 1960s were a big turning point for diet culture. First, Jean Nidetch launched Weight Watchers in 1963, creating a structured, group-based way to diet. The program focused on calorie control, low-fat meal plans, and weekly accountability meetings. It caught on fast, making dieting mainstream and also a social activity. At the same time, Twiggy, the British model, actress, and singer, became a global icon. Her ultrathin physique set a new beauty standard almost overnight. Magazines and ads capitalized on Twiggy's look, driving home the idea that being thin was the key to beauty and success. Together, Weight Watchers and Twiggy sparked a growing obsession with weight loss. The message: Being thin wasn't just desirable, it was expected. Dieting was no longer something you did; it was a way of life.

1970s: The Atkins Diet & Diet Pill Craze

Two major diet trends that left a big mark on weight loss culture came to be in the 1970s. The Atkins Diet created by Dr. Robert C. Atkins flipped the script on the low-fat craze. Instead of cutting fat, Atkins told people to drop carbs, and load up on meats and fats. His diet promised speedy results that wouldn't leave you feeling hungry, which made it super popular. At the same time, diet pills, like Fen-Phen, were having a moment. Marketed as a miracle solution for quickly slimming and trimming, they were packed with amphetamines and appetite suppressants, and had very scary side effects, including heart problems and addiction. The beauty and thinness ideal was becoming harder and harder to reach.

1980s: The Fitness Boom, SlimFast & BMI

Dieting and fitness joined forces in the 1980s, sparking a full-on obsession with the "perfect" body. The fitness craze, led by icons like Jane Fonda with her famous aerobics videos, made exercise a must for weight loss. Gyms and fitness classes skyrocketed in popularity, and catchy phrases like "No pain, no gain" pushed the idea that to be thin meant constantly working out. On the dieting side, SlimFast's "shake for breakfast, shake for lunch, and a sensible dinner" promised a quick, convenient way to lose weight. It was heavily advertised across the country.

Around this time, the Body Mass Index (BMI) became the go-to for measuring health. Originally developed for population studies, it took hold with the general public. This is when categorizing people as "underweight," "normal," or "obese" based on their height and weight alone became normalized. Being thin meant being healthy. The BMI system, inherently flawed, is not an accurate measure of one's health.

1990s: Fat-Free Foods, The Zone & South Beach Diets

The fat-free craze dominated the 1990s. Grocery store shelves were packed with low-fat and fat-free products, and brands like SnackWell's skyrocketed by promising "guilt-free" snacks. However, in order to replace all that flavor lost from cutting out the fat, these foods were loaded up with sugar and artificial ingredients, which led to many unexpected health issues. People were eating more processed food than ever. At the same time, diets like The Zone Diet and The South Beach Diet took off. The Zone focused on tracking a specific percentage of carbs, protein, and fat, while South Beach zeroed in on controlling "good" and "bad" carbs. Both promised weight loss without feeling hungry, which again attracted millions. All these trends fueled an even bigger obsession with controlling what and how people ate. By now diet culture was just another part of daily life.

2000s: Celebrity Diets & the Rise of Body Positivity

The 2000s were all about celebrity diets as stars shared their weight-loss secrets in magazines and interviews. From Beyoncé touting the Master Cleanse to Jennifer Aniston praising the Zone Diet, celebrities set the bar for what the "perfect" body should look like. Fad diets like the Cabbage Soup Diet and myriad juice cleanses blew up, promising quick fixes for anyone chasing that Hollywood look. This was also the era of diet-focused reality shows like *The Biggest Loser,* which glorified extreme weight loss and pushed a good deal of toxic ideas about health and body image.

Not everyone was on board. The Body Positivity Movement started to take hold, especially online. It challenged these narrow beauty standards and called for acceptance of all body types. Instead of focusing solely on weight loss, the movement encouraged self-love and shifted the conversation toward a more inclusive and empowering view of body image. While diet culture still ruled the 2000s, the seeds for a healthier, more accepting approach to health and beauty were in the ground.

2010s: Wellness Culture & Clean Eating

Dieting got a makeover and was rebranded as "wellness" in the 2010s. Instead of a discussion about weight loss, the focus shifted to aiming for a "healthier" lifestyle. This brought on trends like "clean eating," which celebrated whole, unprocessed foods and demonized anything "artificial" or "unclean." Grocery store products were emblazoned with buzzwords like "gluten-free" and "sugar-free." Cutting out certain foods was seen as virtuous, rather than restrictive. Social media added fuel to the fire. Influencers and celebrities posted picture-perfect meals (kale smoothies, quinoa bowls, avocado toast), setting often unrealistic standards for what a "healthy" life should look like. Gluten-free diets, which were originally devised for people with celiac disease, went mainstream, anti-inflammatory foods became synonymous with healthy, and going sugar-free was marketed as a way to "detox" from toxins. At first glance, wellness culture seemed like it might be a positive shift, but it often cloaked the same appearance-driven, restrictive goals of old-school dieting.

2015–2019: The Keto Craze & Social Media's Weight-Loss Trends

Between 2015 and 2019, the Keto Diet reemerged as a prominent dietary trend. By significantly reducing carbohydrate intake and favoring high-fat foods, the diet promised rapid weight loss and increased energy through a metabolic state known as ketosis. Endorsed by celebrities and influencers, the diet led to a thriving industry complete with keto-friendly snacks, supplements, and cookbooks. While some individuals reported health benefits, many found the diet's restrictive nature challenging, often resulting in cycles of adherence and relapse.

Simultaneously, social media influencers began reshaping diet culture. Platforms became inundated with posts promoting products like "detox teas," flat tummy shakes, and other quick-fix weight-loss solutions. Trends such as waist trainers and extreme calorie restriction gained popularity, further normalizing unattainable and harmful beauty standards. Intermittent fasting, which is rooted in cultural and religious norms and has been practiced for centuries, also gained significant traction as an influencer health trend and weight-loss tactic.

2020s: The Anti-Diet Movement, Intuitive Eating & the Ozempic Obsession

And where are we now? The 2020s have generated a significant pushback against traditional diet culture, marked by the growing influence of the anti-diet movement. This movement rejects the idea that thinness equals health and encourages intuitive eating—listening to your hunger and fullness cues instead of following rigid diet plans. Its advocates, from influencers to authors, promote self-acceptance and prioritize overall well-being over weight loss.

At the same time, the weight-loss industry has adapted and evolved, with pharmaceutical interventions like Ozempic and other GLP-1 receptor agonists gaining ground. These pharmaceuticals, initially developed for managing diabetes, have become popular for their weight-loss effects. Endorsed by celebrities and influencers, this has sparked debates about societal pressure to be thin and the ethics of using medication solely for appearance-focused goals.

The anti-diet movement empowers individuals to embrace food freedom and to cultivate body neutrality, while the rising demand for weight-loss medications shows how mainstream cultural ideals remain firmly rooted in thinness. Society continues to navigate ever-shifting attitudes toward food, health, and body image.

Health will never be a one-size-fits-all thing, and health absolutely does not mean weight loss. It all depends on what your goals are. I do not shame weight loss. I applaud you, if it is one of your many health-improving nutrition goals and you work toward it. But if you are trying to lose weight because you've been told you will only look better and be better if you do, that's a problem. There is so much commercial interest, now and historically, in selling quick fixes, cleanses, and try-and-fail weight loss products and programs.

In the next few sections of the book, I guide you through various fun and easy ways to understand the building blocks of nutrition. After that, I give you the tools needed to take nutrition matters into your own hands by shopping and cooking smart and eating well. I want you to listen to your cravings, nourish yourself 24/7, and ultimately build a healthy relationship with your body and what you eat. Let's do it!

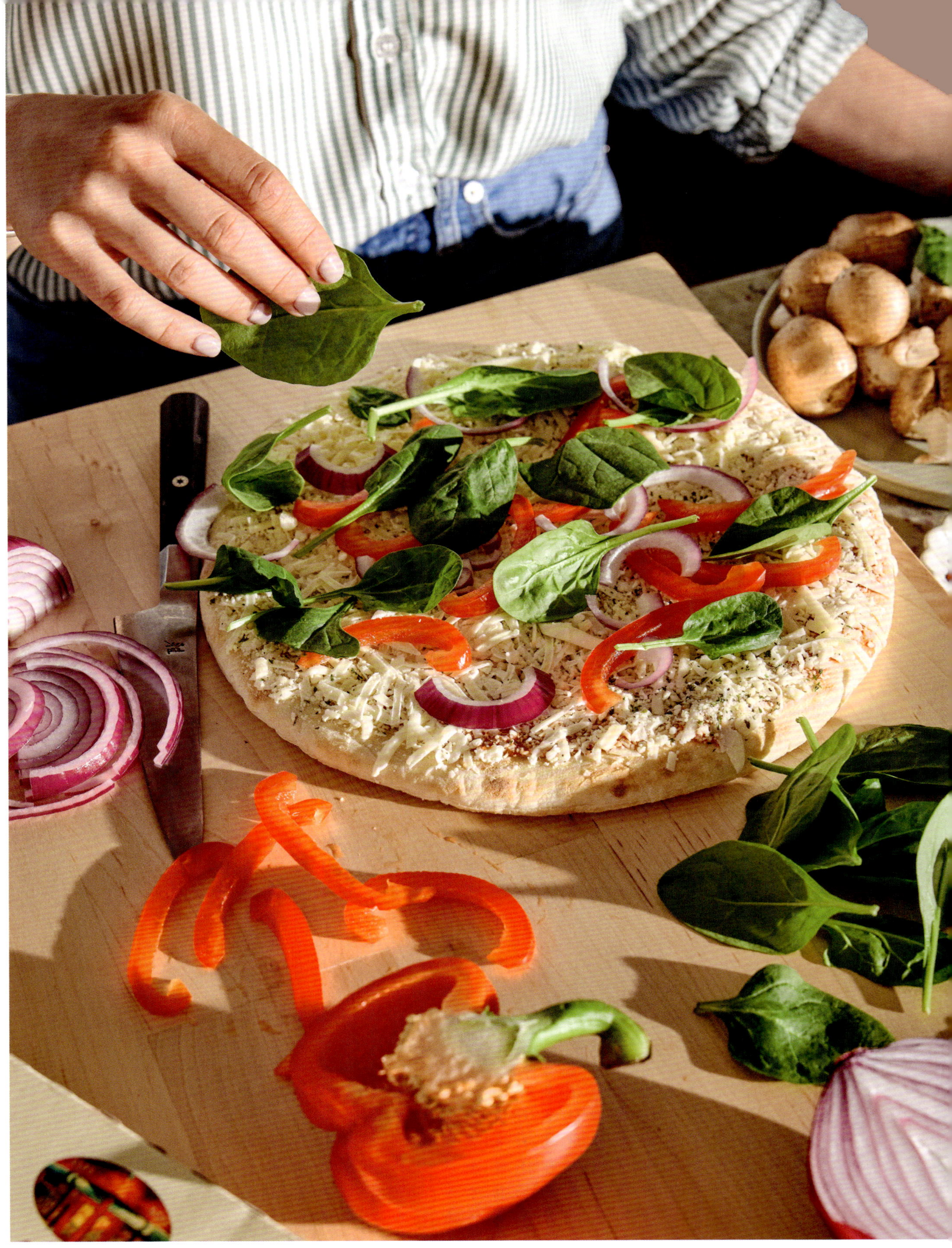

Understanding Your Unique Nutrition Needs

In order to explain energy intake and nutritional balance I'm going to use a familiar analogy: tending a garden. In 2024, I bought my first house. One of my favorite parts of being a homeowner has been dreaming up, digging up, and tending my home garden. In the past couple of years, I've planted edibles, ornamentals, perennials, and annuals, and *you know* I love growing a rainbow of summer veggies.

Along the way, I've learned that a garden needs the proper amount of water, sunlight, and nutrients (and care!) to fuel it, just as our bodies need the right balance of energy to function at their best and to thrive. When we frame calories as simple, natural, and much-needed energy rather than demonize them or hyper-focus on their numeric value, we move away from calorie-counting and focus instead on nourishing our bodies intuitively.

I want to help you make mindful, balanced food choices without obsessing over the numbers. I want you to feed your body with care and confidence, and to feel bright, strong, and full of life as a result. Like my beautiful sunflowers!

Energy Balance

Instead of solely counting calories and demonizing them, I focus on an energy balance approach. Energy balance is the relationship between the energy you take in from food and drink and the energy your body uses for daily functions and physical activities.

Achieving energy balance isn't just about maintaining weight, it's about ensuring that your body has the energy it needs to thrive, recover, and function at its best. When you strike this balance with an array of nutrient-rich and nutrient-diverse foods that I detail in the next section, you feel energized, healthy, and ready to meet the demands of day-to-day life.

By tuning into your body's signals and focusing on energy balance, you can nourish yourself without meticulous calorie counting or dietary tracking. You listen to your body so that you can properly fuel it and keep it aligned.

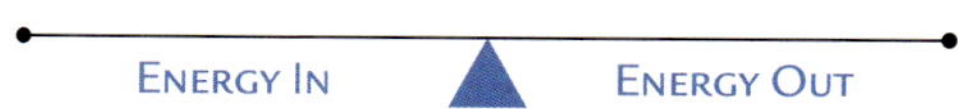

MAINTENANCE: THE FOOD AND DRINK ENERGY YOU CONSUME *EQUALS* THE ENERGY YOUR BODY NEEDS FOR DAILY FUNCTIONS AND ACTIVITIES.

Positive Energy Balance

A positive energy balance means you're consuming more energy (calories) than your body utilizes, which results in energy being stored in adipose (fat) tissue. Over time, this can lead to increased body fat and weight gain and related health challenges. Consistently consuming more energy than your body needs can disrupt its balance and create fat storage that your body doesn't require.

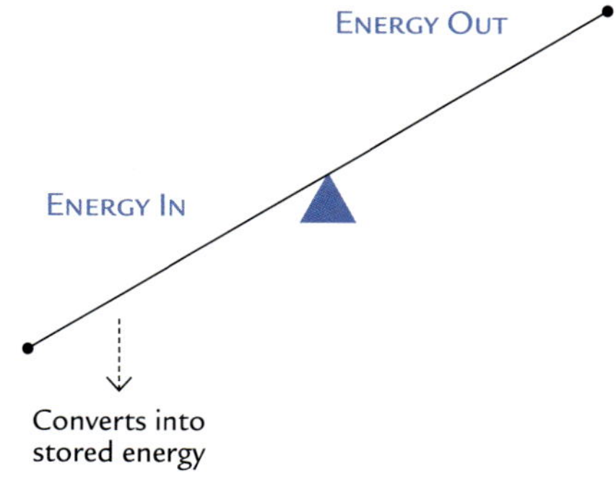

SURPLUS: THE FOOD AND DRINK ENERGY YOU CONSUME *EXCEEDS* THE ENERGY YOUR BODY NEEDS FOR DAILY FUNCTIONS AND ACTIVITIES.

Negative Energy Balance

A negative energy balance happens when you consume fewer calories than your body needs to function. In order to keep running during a negative energy balance, your body taps into its energy reserves, breaking down stored fat and sometimes muscle, for fuel. If the deficit is extreme and consistent over time, it can lead to muscle loss and nutrient deficiencies. Prolonged extreme energy deficits put unnecessary stress on your body and can negatively impact your overall health. Over time this sort of deficit can take a toll on hormonal balance and immune function, as well as your mental well-being.

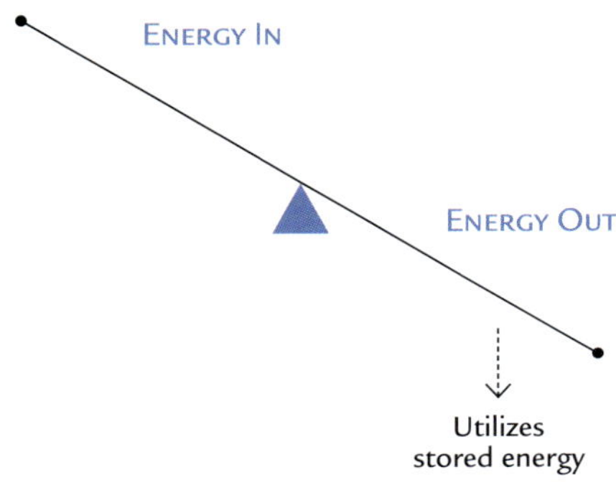

DEFICIT: THE FOOD AND DRINK ENERGY YOU CONSUME IS *LESS THAN* THE ENERGY YOUR BODY NEEDS FOR DAILY FUNCTIONS AND ACTIVITIES.

Calories

Calories are a measure of energy. Essentially, they tell you how much energy your body will get from the food and drink you consume. Everything you consume contains calories, and your body converts that energy into fuel to power you. From the basic functions that keep you alive, like breathing, digesting, and circulating blood, to more active pursuits such as walking, exercising, and even thinking—calories are the driving force. I want you to appreciate calories rather than fear them. They are essential to your health, energy, and overall well-being.

Our bodies need the right balance of calories to function optimally. If you don't consume enough calories, you may feel sluggish, tired, and unable to perform at your best. Consuming too many calories consistently, on the other hand, can lead to excess energy storage, and if you do this regularly, to unwelcome health conditions. Calories are not the enemy—your body needs them! It's about balance and nourishing yourself in a way that fits your needs and lifestyle.

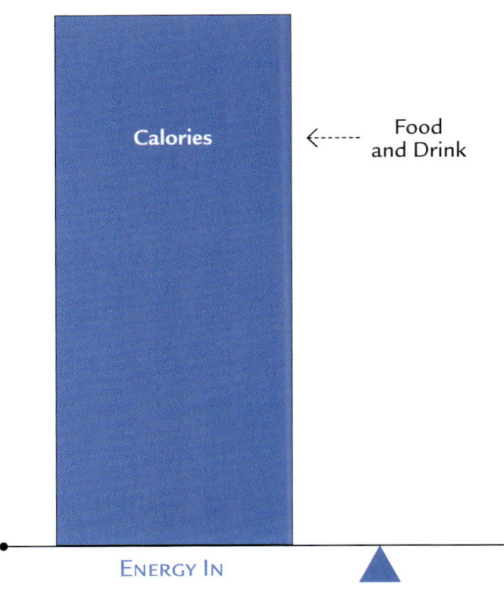

CALORIES = JUST ANOTHER WORD FOR ENERGY. FOOD AND DRINK CALORIES POWER EVERYTHING YOU DO.

Everyone's Needs Are Different

There is no one-size-fits-all when it comes to nutrition. Our nutritional needs are incredibly diverse and influenced by all sorts of factors like age, gender, genetics, lifestyle, and body composition. Understanding your unique nutritional needs is a lot like learning what makes a garden grow. It's important to take a personalized approach to nutrition.

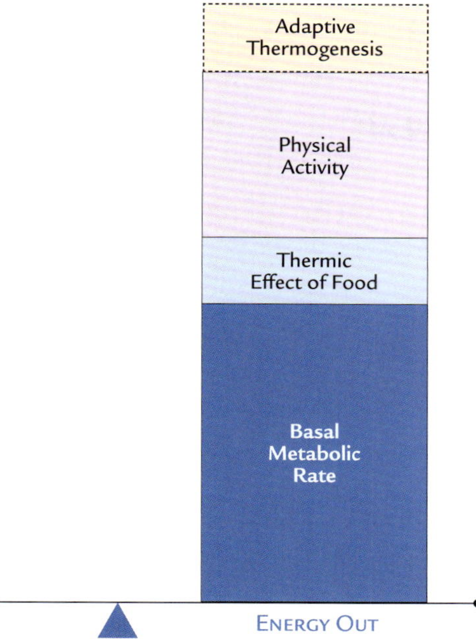

THERE IS NO ONE-SIZE-FITS-ALL WHEN IT COMES TO NUTRITION. ALL OF THESE FACTORS INFLUENCE TOTAL ENERGY EXPENDITURE.

Basal Metabolic Rate

Your Basal Metabolic Rate (BMR) accounts for 60% to 75% of your total energy expenditure and is the number of calories your body requires to perform its essential functions while you are at rest—breathing, circulating blood, producing cells. Essentially, it's the energy needed to sustain life when you're not active and moving around.

BMR varies from person to person due to several factors. Muscle mass plays a key role—the more muscle you have, the higher your BMR, as muscle requires more energy to maintain. Age also impacts BMR, as it naturally declines over time, starting after childhood. Genetics plays a part, too. We inherit various metabolic attributes that affect how efficiently we burn energy. Additionally, body size and composition matter, since larger bodies require more energy to function. Hormones, including thyroid hormones, insulin, and sex hormones, also influence metabolic rate, regulating how efficiently our bodies use energy. Understanding these factors can help explain why BMR differs between individuals and why energy needs shift over time.

Influencing Factors of BMR

Age
Assigned sex at birth
Body composition
Genetics
Health status
Hormones

Online BMR calculators can be fairly accurate, but they certainly have limitations. They typically use the Mifflin-St. Jeor Equation, which is one of the best formulas available. I used it while working at the hospital. Keep in mind, though, that BMR calculators provide a rough estimate since most do not account for all of the influencing factors mentioned above, plus your activity levels. You will need to consult with a health professional or registered dietitian for a finely tuned BMR.

Mifflin-St. Jeor Equation

Women

BMR = (10 × weight in kg) + (6.25 × height in cm) − (5 × age in years) − 161

Men

BMR = (10 × weight in kg) + (6.25 × height in cm) − (5 × age in years) + 5

Physical Activity Level

Physical activity makes up 15% to 30% of your total energy expenditure and includes everything from intentional exercise to everyday movements and exertion. The more active you are, the more calories your body requires as fuel. Athletes or individuals with physically demanding jobs often need significantly more calories than those with more sedentary work or lifestyles.

Intentional exercise and workouts, such as strength training, cardio, and sports, require substantial energy and help improve overall fitness. However, everyday non-exercise movements also play a role in energy balance. Walking, standing, fidgeting, and doing household chores all contribute to daily calorie burn. Additionally, job-related activity influences energy needs, with sedentary jobs requiring much less movement than physically demanding work like construction, nursing, or warehouse labor.

Activity levels are often grouped into categories such as sedentary, lightly active, moderately active, and very active. Recognizing where you fall on this spectrum will help you understand your caloric needs better and ensure that you sufficiently fuel your body.

Thermic Effect of Food (TEF)

The Thermic Effect of Food (TEF) makes up 5% to 10% of your total energy expenditure and is the energy your body uses to digest, absorb, and process nutrients from the food you eat. Think of it as the metabolic effort required to break down meals into usable fuel. Every time you eat, your body uses energy just to process what you've consumed, and different macronutrients require different amounts of energy. Protein has the highest thermic effect, meaning your body works harder to digest it, while fats require the least energy. Understanding TEF helps shift the focus toward how food fuels your metabolism, making balanced eating about more than monitoring energy intake, but also about how efficiently your body processes what you consume.

TEF %
(calories burned during digestion)

Protein: 20%–30%
Carbohydrates: 5%–10%
Fats: 0%–3%

PROTEIN REQUIRES THE MOST ENERGY TO BREAK DOWN. YOUR BODY USES ABOUT 20 TO 30 PERCENT OF PROTEIN'S CALORIES TO DIGEST IT, IN COMPARISON TO ABOUT 5 TO 10 PERCENT FOR CARBOHYDRATES AND 0 TO 3 PERCENT FOR FATS.

Adaptive Thermogenesis

Adaptive Thermogenesis is a flexible component and is your body's way of adjusting energy expenditure in response to changes in environment, diet, and lifestyle. When you eat less or burn more energy than usual, your metabolism doesn't stay static, it adapts. If you're in a prolonged calorie deficit, your body may slow down its metabolic rate to conserve energy. On the flip side, during periods of overfeeding, your metabolism can temporarily speed up to burn off excess energy. Factors like stress, sleep, hormones, and extreme dieting can all influence these metabolic shifts. Metabolism isn't fixed; it's a dynamic system that responds to your habits and environment.

Tracking Energy Intake

Understanding your body's energy needs helps you maintain balance, ensuring you're neither overly full nor running on empty. Tracking energy intake doesn't mean obsessing over every calorie, it's about being mindful of and flexible in responding to your body's cues, while considering factors like meal composition, activity levels, and overall energy.

For instance, if you have a lighter, low-energy breakfast, you can adjust by eating a more substantial lunch and dinner to stay balanced. Conversely, if you know you'll be enjoying a rich, energy-dense dinner, it might be wise to keep breakfast and lunch more moderate. Activity level also plays a role. On days with higher physical activity, your body may require more fuel, while on less active days, energy needs may be lower. It's not about restriction; it's about listening to your body and its hunger and fullness cues—what it feels like when you've eaten too much of something, or not enough of another thing. By doing so, you can then make simple adjustments, without judgment, to maintain steady energy throughout the day.

Eat What You Crave

Food is energy, but it's also meant to be enjoyed and appreciated, so please feed your body what it wants and needs. It's nourishment. When you respect and listen to your body, you ultimately take care of yourself. The more you restrict, the more likely you are to obsess over certain foods, which often leads to overeating or overindulgence.

Denying yourself certain foods often causes you to hyperfocus, launching an endless cycle of wanting, avoiding, and then ultimately overindulging. When you listen to your body and satisfy your cravings, you're less likely to obsess over a particular food. If you allow yourself pizza when you want it, you remove the forbidden aspect that makes it feel almost irresistible. Over time, pizza becomes just another of many options, not something you feel you must have all the time.

It's not the pizza itself that's the issue. It's the fear and restriction built up around it. When you give yourself unconditional permission to eat *all* foods, the intense desire for "off-limit" foods diminishes, and you can enjoy that cheesy saucy yummy pizza (ummm, see page 239) in a way that feels good and nourishing for your body and mind. I want that for you.

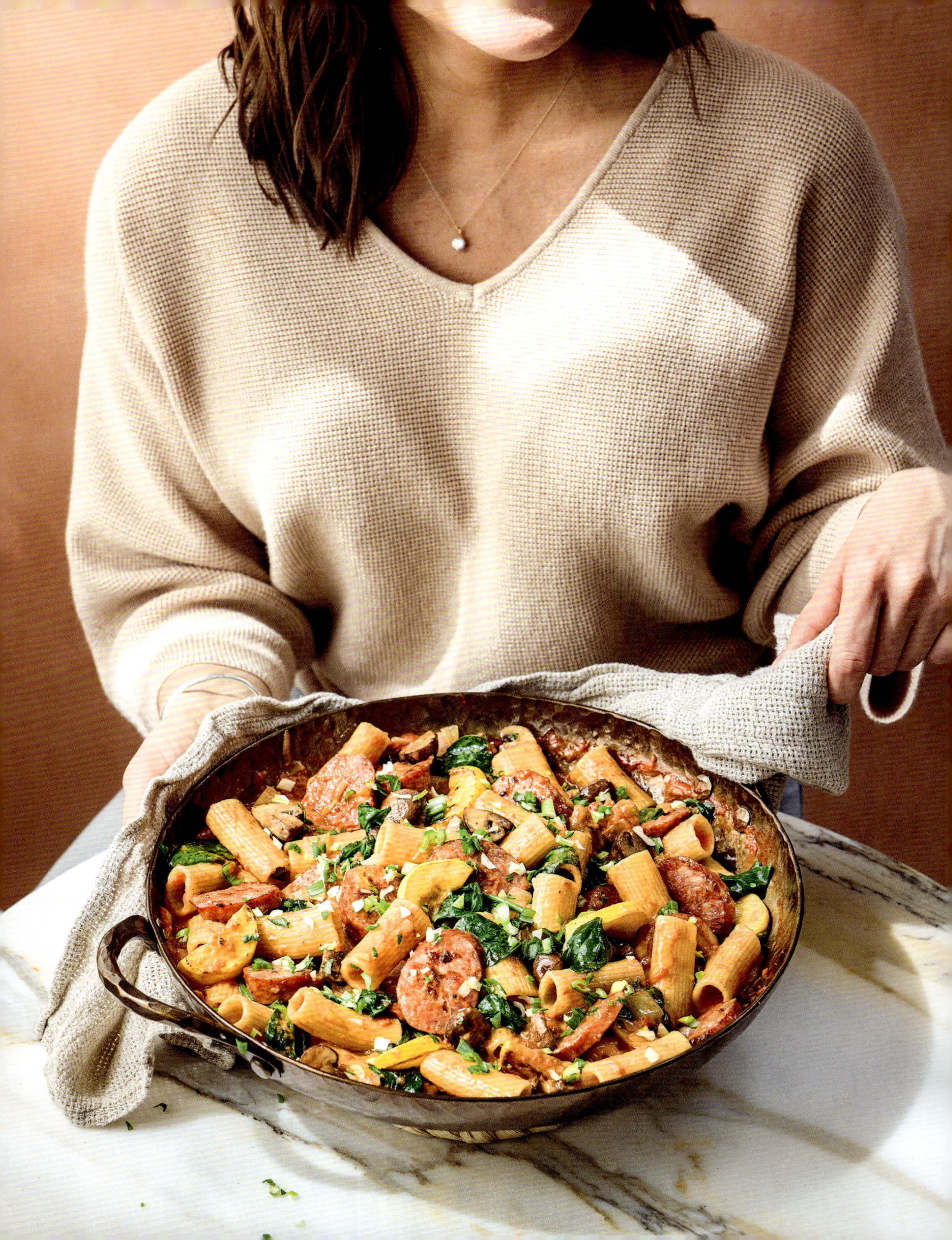

Nourish Your Needs with Nutrition

Now that you have a better understanding of how to fuel your body's caloric needs—and how those needs are so wildly different for all of us and are always changing—let's take it a step further. In the next several pages, I'm going to introduce you to the building blocks of nutrition.

Please don't feel like you need to memorize all of this! *Any* of it. I don't ever look at my meal and think, hmm, I need a larger serving of vitamin D. That's not how I live my life and that's certainly not how I want you to live yours, unless you have specific health needs. If you are diabetic, for instance, you'll need to monitor your carb intake. In cases like that, please consult with a dietitian to tailor to your unique nutrition needs.

For the rest of us, the focus is on adding, not restricting. I want you to ask yourself, what can I add to make my meals more balanced? A balanced plate means filling it with a variety of nutrient-dense foods that work together to fuel your body and support overall health. What follows are the core nutritional components that I want to introduce you to—to slap nametags on so you recognize them. I want you to get up close and personal with this group. You need each and every one to survive and thrive.

A well-balanced plate brings all of these components together in the right proportions. Carbohydrates, proteins, and fats (the three key macronutrients) all play a vital role in your health and wellness. When combined properly, they provide steady energy, support essential bodily functions, and leave you feeling satisfied and nourished.

Carbohydrates

Carbohydrates are your body's primary source of energy. Yes, you read that correctly. When you consume carbs, your body breaks them down into glucose (sugar), which is then absorbed into your bloodstream and used by cells to fuel everything from brain function to physical activity. Your brain, muscles, and organs all depend on glucose to function at their best.

Why Carbs Matter

Primary Energy Source: Carbs are your body's preferred fuel. Glucose, derived from carbs, powers everything from your brain and its deepest thoughts to your workouts.

Stored Energy: Excess carbohydrates are stored in the liver and muscles as glycogen, which can be tapped into for energy during exercise or between meals.

Brain Function Support: The brain relies heavily on glucose, which is why extremely low-carb diets often lead to mental fatigue or brain fog.

Types of Carbs

Complex Carbohydrates: These carbohydrates, which are often high in fiber, are generally better for sustained energy and overall health. They are made up of longer chains of sugar molecules, which take more time for the body to break down and digest. They also provide essential vitamins, minerals, and antioxidants.

> **Some Sources:** Whole grains (like brown rice, oats, and whole-wheat bread), legumes, starchy vegetables like potatoes.
>
> **Effects on the Body:** Complex carbs provide a more sustained energy release, are often rich in fiber, and keep you full for longer while supporting stable blood sugar levels.

Simple Carbohydrates: These carbohydrates are made up of one or two sugar molecules, which means they are quickly digested and absorbed by the body.

> **Some Sources:** Fruit, milk, honey, refined or added sugar sources (soda/sugary drinks, candy, baked goods, cereals, white bread, white rice).
>
> **Effects on the Body:** Simple carbs provide quick energy, but excess simple carbs can cause blood sugar spikes and crashes if consumed without fiber or protein to slow absorption.

Fiber is a type of carbohydrate that the body can't digest. It passes through the digestive system mostly intact, helping to regulate blood sugar and promote healthy digestion. There are two types of fiber: soluble fiber and insoluble fiber. Soluble fiber dissolves in water and forms a gel-like substance, which helps lower cholesterol and manage blood sugar. Insoluble fiber doesn't dissolve—it adds bulk to your stool, which helps prevent constipation and supports regularity.

Some Sources: Soluble: oats, beans, lentils, fruit; insoluble: whole wheat, vegetables, nuts, seeds.

Effects on Body: Fiber supports digestive health, lowers cholesterol levels, feeds your gut microbiome, helps maintain stable blood sugar levels, and can aid in weight management by promoting satiety.

Carbohydrates are an absolutely essential part of a balanced diet. Instead of fixating on counting every gram, focus on consuming whole-food sources like whole grains, vegetables, and fruits. These options provide long-lasting energy and a range of nutrients to keep your body thriving. Embrace carbs, they fuel you!

Protein

Proteins are the body's structural and functional workhorses, made up of smaller building blocks called amino acids. There are twenty different amino acids that make up proteins in humans, nine of which are considered essential. Essential amino acids must come from your diet since your body can't produce them on its own.

Protein is the key to feeling full, stabilizing blood sugar, and supporting muscle maintenance and recovery. That's why it is very important to include it in every meal. Lean meats, eggs, dairy, legumes, nuts, and seeds are all excellent protein sources that provide your body with the essential amino acids it needs to thrive.

Why Protein Matters

Tissue Growth & Repair: Protein is necessary for the growth and repair of body tissues, including muscles, skin, hair, nails, and organs. It's especially important for muscle recovery and growth after exercise.

Immune Function Support: Protein is vital for producing antibodies and other immune system components that help fight off infections and diseases.

Enzyme & Hormone Production: Many hormones and enzymes, which regulate various bodily processes, are made from protein. Enzymes, for example, help speed up chemical reactions in the body that are essential for respiration, digestion, and muscle function, while hormones regulate functions such as metabolism, growth, and mood.

Energy Provider: Protein is less efficient as an energy source compared to carbohydrates and fat, as it is spared for structural roles. Each gram of protein provides 4 calories, the same as carbohydrates.

Types of Protein

Complete Proteins: Amino acids are the building blocks of protein. Complete proteins contain all nine essential amino acids.

Some Sources: Meat, poultry, fish, eggs, dairy, and some plant-based sources, such as quinoa, soy, and chia seeds.

Incomplete Proteins: Lack one or more of the nine essential amino acids.

Some Sources: Most plant-based foods, like grains, legumes, nuts, and seeds.

Combine for Completeness: Eating a variety of plant-based protein sources, such as beans and rice, throughout the day can provide all the essential amino acids.

Protein isn't just about building muscle, it's an essential nutrient for every system in your body. By incorporating a variety of protein-rich foods into your meals, you're not just meeting your daily needs, you're giving your body the tools it needs to grow, repair, and flourish.

Fats

Fats, along with carbohydrates and proteins, are one of the three essential macronutrients. They play a critical role in your body's functions, from energy storage and hormone production to brain health and vitamin absorption. Fats have a higher calorie content (9 calories per gram compared to 4 per gram for protein and carbohydrates), but as you'll remember, calories aren't the enemy! Healthy fats are vital for maintaining a balanced diet and supporting overall well-being. Not all fats are created equal, though. Understanding the different types will help you make healthier dietary choices.

Why Fats Matter

Energy Storage & Fuel: Fats provide a concentrated source of energy, stored in the body for use when carbohydrates are unavailable. They're particularly important during prolonged activity or fasting.

Cell Structure & Function: Fats form the building blocks of cell membranes, helping to maintain their structure and flexibility. They're crucial for brain and nerve cell function.

Vitamin Absorption: Fats enable the absorption of fat-soluble vitamins (A, D, E, and K), which are essential for various bodily functions.

Hormone Production: Fats are key in producing hormones like estrogen and testosterone, which regulate many body processes.

Insulation & Protection: Fats help maintain body temperature and protect vital organs by acting as a cushion.

Types of Fats

Unsaturated Fats: These are generally considered to be healthy fats, beneficial for heart health and reducing inflammation. There are two types: monounsaturated fats and polyunsaturated fats.

Monounsaturated Fats: These fats may help lower LDL (bad) cholesterol and support heart health.

Some Sources: Olive oil, avocados, almonds, peanuts, and seeds.

Polyunsaturated Fats: These include omega-3 and omega-6 fatty acids, which are essential because your body can't produce them. Omega-3s, found in fatty fish, walnuts, and flaxseeds, are especially important for brain and heart health.

Some Sources: Salmon, trout, walnuts, chia seeds, and sunflower oil.

Saturated Fats: These fats, which should be consumed in moderation, are easy to spot because they are solid at room temperature and found in animal products and tropical oils. While not as harmful as once thought, consuming too much saturated fat may raise LDL cholesterol levels, increasing the risk of heart disease.

Some Sources: Fatty meats, butter, cheese, coconut oil, and palm oil.

Effect on Health: Limit intake to protect heart health.

Trans Fats: Trans fats, also known as partially hydrogenated oils, are artificial fats made by adding hydrogen to vegetable oils to make them more solid and extend shelf life. They are the most harmful type of fat and should be avoided where possible. The FDA banned trans fats from foods made and/or sold in the U.S. in 2018 (many other countries ban them), although trace amounts are permitted. Margarine sold in the U.S. historically contained high levels of trans fats but now consists of varying amounts of saturated fat.

Some Sources: Processed foods, baked goods, fried foods.

Effects on Health: Increases LDL (bad) cholesterol, decreases HDL (good) cholesterol, and raises the risk of heart disease, stroke, and inflammation.

Fats are essential to balanced diets. By focusing on healthy fats, moderating saturated fats, and avoiding trans fats, you support your heart, brain, and overall health.

Vitamins & Minerals

We've covered the three essential macronutrients, now it's time to dig into our micronutrients—vitamins and minerals. Incorporating a healthy and varied dose of both is essential to a balanced diet since they support everything from immune health and muscle synthesis to bone health and brain development.

Fat-Soluble Vitamins

Fat-soluble vitamins dissolve in fat and are stored in your fatty tissues and liver. Unlike water-soluble vitamins, which are excreted through urine if consumed in excess, fat-soluble vitamins can accumulate in the body over time. Because of that, it's important to consume them in moderation, as overconsumption may lead to toxicity.

These vitamins require dietary fat for proper absorption. Pairing them with a source of healthy fats, like olive oil, avocado, or nuts, can significantly enhance their uptake and ensure your body makes the most of them. Fat-soluble vitamins play essential roles in bodily processes like vision, bone health, and immune function, making them a crucial part of a balanced diet.

Water-Soluble Vitamins

Water-soluble vitamins dissolve in water and are not stored in the body. Any excess amounts that you consume are excreted through urine. Unlike fat-soluble vitamins, they don't accumulate in the body, making consistent intake vital for maintaining optimal health.

These vitamins are key players in essential bodily functions, including energy production, immune system support, and maintaining healthy skin, nerves, and cells. By including a variety of fat- and water-soluble vitamin-rich foods in your diet, you ensure that your body has a steady supply of these crucial nutrients.

FAT-SOLUBLE VITAMINS

Vitamin	Functions	Some Sources	Deficiency Symptoms
A	Supports vision, immune function, and cell growth	Carrots, sweet potatoes, spinach, liver, and eggs	Night blindness, dry eyes, and weakened immunity
D	Promotes calcium absorption, supports bone health and immunity	Sun exposure, fortified milk, fatty fish (salmon, mackerel), and egg yolks	Rickets (soft bones in children), osteoporosis, and fatigue
E	Acts as an antioxidant, protects cells from damage, and supports skin and eye health	Nuts, seeds, vegetable oils, spinach, and avocado	A deficiency is rare, but can lead to muscle weakness and vision problems
K	Essential for blood clotting and bone health	Leafy greens, broccoli, and Brussels sprouts	Excessive bleeding or easy bruising

Water-Soluble Vitamins

Vitamin	Functions	Some Sources	Deficiency Symptoms
B_1 (Thiamine)	Helps convert food into energy and supports nerve function	Whole grains, pork, sunflower seeds, and legumes	Fatigue, weakness, and in severe cases, beriberi
B_2 (Riboflavin)	Produces energy and supports healthy skin and eyes	Dairy products, eggs, leafy greens, and almonds	Cracks at the corners of the mouth, sore throat
B_3 (Niacin)	Aids in energy production and DNA repair	Chicken, fish, peanuts, and fortified cereals	Pellagra (diarrhea, dermatitis, and dementia)
B_5 (Pantothenic Acid)	Helps with fat and carbohydrate metabolism	Meat, avocados, broccoli, and whole grains	A deficiency is rare, but can lead to fatigue and irritability
B_6 (Pyridoxine)	Supports brain development, red blood cell production, and metabolism of amino acids	Bananas, potatoes, poultry, and fortified cereals	Anemia, depression, and confusion
B_7 (Biotin)	Essential for healthy hair, skin, nails, and energy metabolism	Eggs, nuts, seeds, and sweet potatoes	A deficiency is rare, but can lead to hair loss and brittle nails
B_9 (Folate/ Folic Acid)	Key for cell growth and DNA formation, especially important during pregnancy	Leafy greens, citrus fruits, beans, eggs, and fortified cereals	Anemia, fatigue, and birth defects (during pregnancy)
B_{12} (Cobalamin)	Crucial for nerve function, red blood cell production, and DNA synthesis	Meat, fish, eggs, and dairy products (vegans may require supplementation)	Anemia, nerve damage, and fatigue
C	Antioxidant that supports immune health, collagen formation, wound healing, and iron absorption	Oranges, strawberries, bell peppers, broccoli, and kiwi	Gum disease, fatigue, bruising, and in severe cases, scurvy

Minerals

Minerals are essential nutrients that your body requires to function properly. Unlike vitamins, minerals are inorganic compounds derived from the earth, water, and soil. They play a crucial role in maintaining your overall health and well-being. From building strong bones and teeth to supporting proper nerve function, minerals are involved in countless bodily processes. They regulate critical functions like muscle contraction, hydration, and maintaining a healthy balance of fluids, making them indispensable for your body's daily operations. By incorporating a variety of mineral-rich foods into your diet, you ensure that your body gets the foundational support it needs.

MINERALS

Mineral	Functions	Some Sources	Deficiency Symptoms
Calcium	Builds strong bones and teeth, supports muscle function, and helps with blood clotting	Dairy products, leafy greens, tofu, and fortified plant milks	Osteoporosis, muscle cramps, and weak bones
Chloride	Works with sodium to maintain fluid balance and produce stomach acid	Table salt, seaweed, and tomatoes	A deficiency is rare, but can lead to dehydration
Copper	Helps form red blood cells and supports iron absorption	Shellfish, nuts, seeds, and whole grains	Fatigue, anemia, and weakened immune function
Fluoride	Strengthens tooth enamel and supports bone health	Fluoridated water, in black, green, and some herbal tea, and fish	Increased risk of cavities
Iodine	Essential for thyroid hormone production, which regulates metabolism	Iodized salt, seafood, and seaweed	Goiter (enlarged thyroid), fatigue, and weight gain
Iron	Carries oxygen in the blood via hemoglobin and supports energy production	Red meat, beans, spinach, and fortified cereals	Fatigue, anemia, and weakened immunity

Mineral	Functions	Some Sources	Deficiency Symptoms
Magnesium	Supports muscle and nerve function, bone health, and energy production	Nuts, seeds, whole grains, spinach, and avocados	Muscle cramps, fatigue, and irregular heartbeat
Manganese	Helps with bone formation, metabolism, and antioxidant function	Nuts, whole grains, leafy greens, and in black, green, and some herbal teas	A deficiency is rare, but can include weak bones and poor metabolism
Phosphorus	Works with calcium for bone health and plays a role in energy production	Meat, fish, dairy, beans, and nuts	A deficiency is rare, but can include fatigue and muscle weakness
Potassium	Helps regulate fluid balance, muscle contractions, and nerve signals	Bananas, potatoes, oranges, and spinach	Weakness, fatigue, and muscle cramps
Selenium	Acts as an antioxidant and supports thyroid function	Brazil nuts, seafood, and whole grains	Weak immune function and fatigue
Sodium	Maintains fluid balance, aids in nerve transmission, and supports muscle function	Table salt, processed foods, and naturally in some vegetables and shellfish	A deficiency is rare, but can include dizziness and muscle weakness
Sulfur	Essential for protein synthesis and found in amino acids like methionine and cysteine	Meat, fish, eggs, onions, and garlic	A deficiency is rare, as it's abundant in protein-rich foods
Zinc	Supports immunity, wound healing, and cell growth	Meat, shellfish, legumes, and seeds	Slow wound healing, hair loss, and reduced immunity

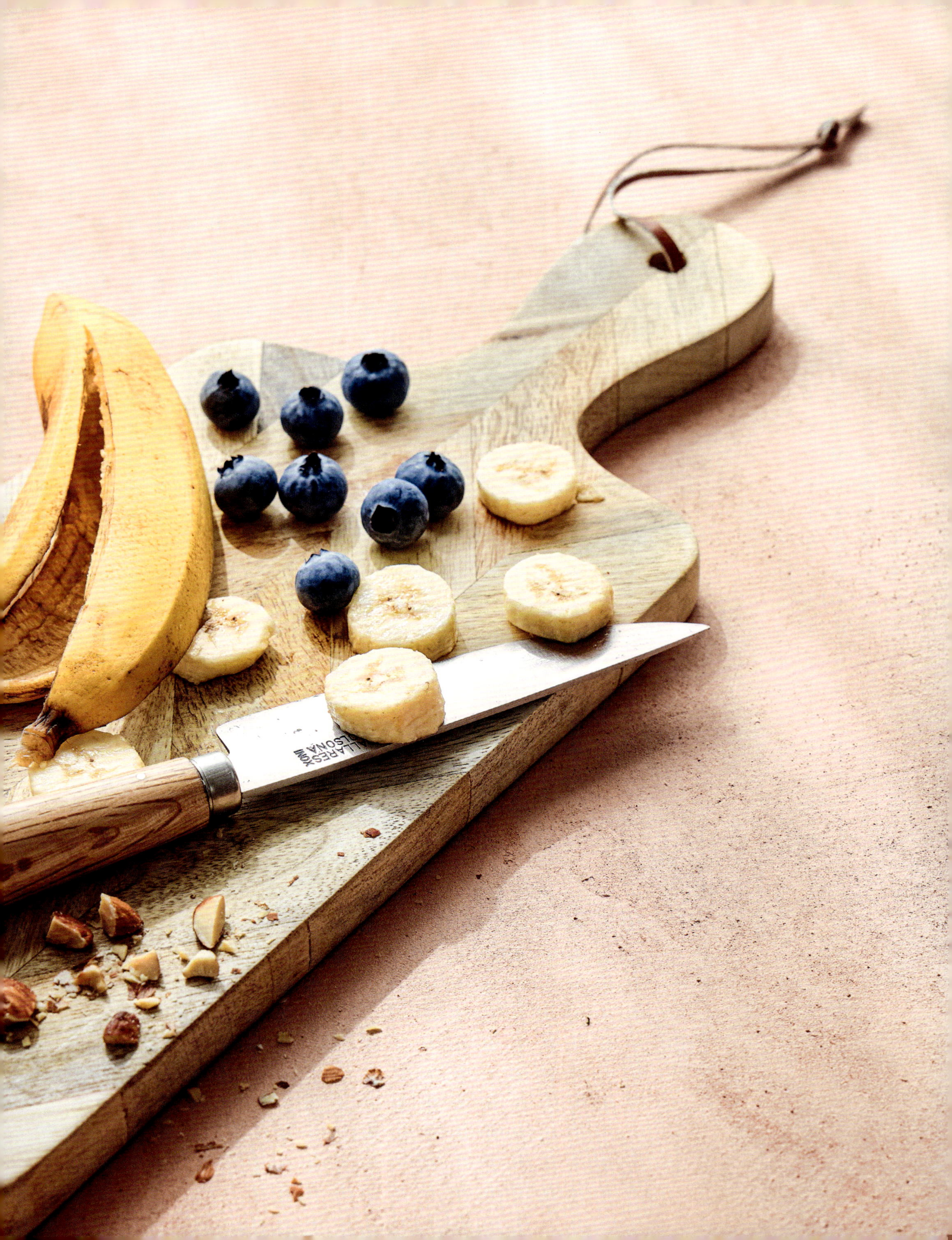

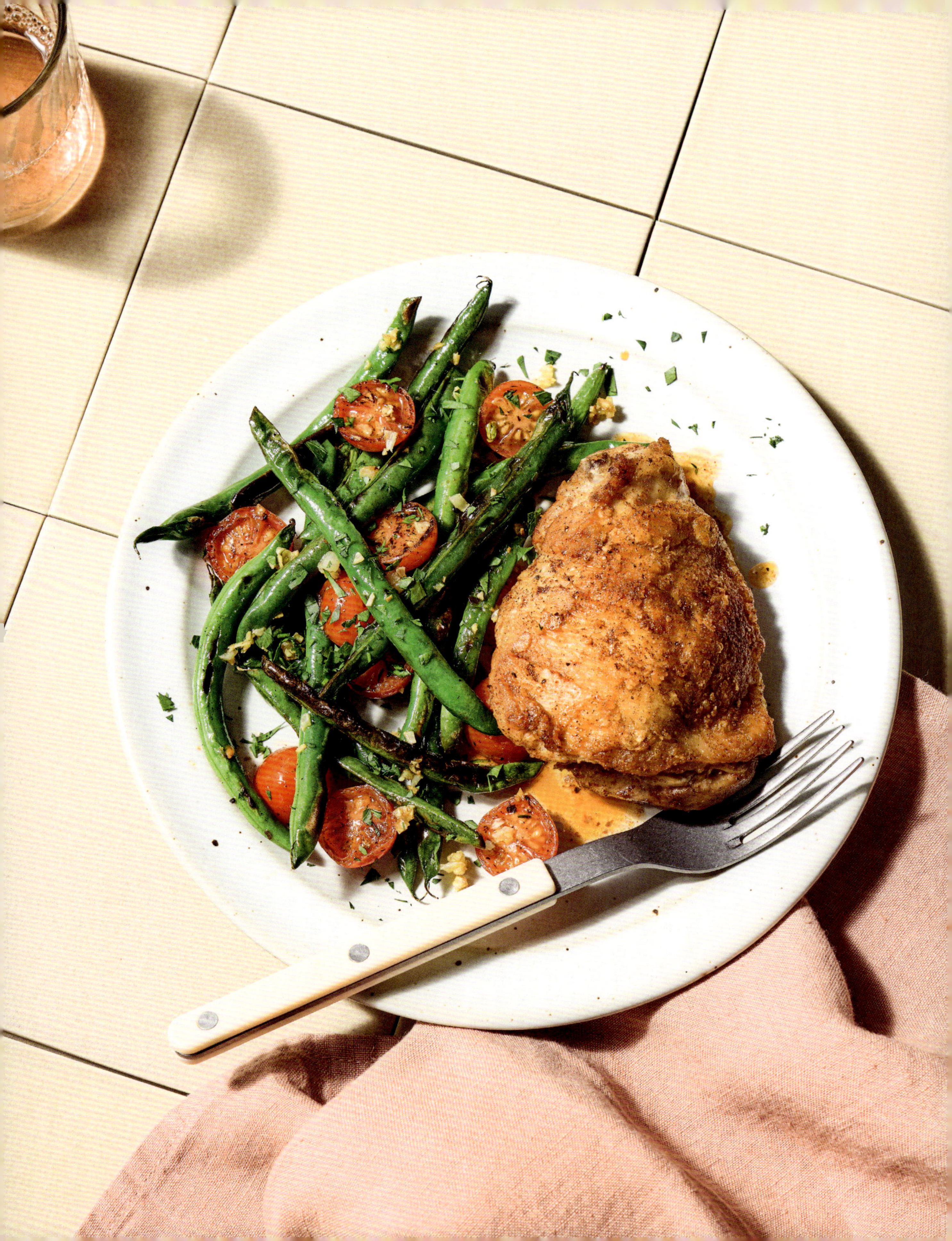

Mastering the Art of Balance

Now that you understand a bit better the building blocks of nutrition and how to properly fuel your body, it's time to put that knowledge into practice. Let me be clear, I don't count macros. (If you're not familiar, macro counting involves meticulously tracking the grams of carbohydrates, fats, and proteins that you consume each day. Personally, no thank you!) Instead, I aim for overall nutritional balance throughout the day.

I use my version of the plate method, a simple, sustainable, and flexible approach to balanced meals. Originally introduced by the USDA in 2011 as a replacement for the food pyramid, the plate method offers an intuitive way to make healthier choices without the hassle of counting calories or weighing portions. My version makes it even more practical and enjoyable. I've included some of my personal favorite tasty food examples here for each section of the plate. These lists are far from comprehensive.

Non-Starchy Veggies

Artichokes
Asparagus
Beets
Bell peppers
Bok choy
Broccoli
Brussels sprouts
Cabbage
Carrots
Cauliflower
Cucumbers
Eggplant
Green beans
Kale
Mushrooms
Parsnips
Romaine lettuce
Snap peas
Spinach
Tomatoes
Zucchini

Healthy Fats

Avocado
Cheese
Chia seeds
Eggs (also a protein)
Fatty fish (salmon—also a protein)
Flaxseeds
Hemp hearts
Nuts/nut butters
(peanut, almond, cashew)
Olives/olive oil
Pistachios
Pumpkin seeds

Fiber-Rich Carbs	
Apples	Oats
Barley	Popcorn
Berries (blackberries, raspberries, blueberries)	Quinoa
Brown rice	Sweet potatoes
Corn	White potatoes
Couscous	Whole-grain bread
Farro	Whole-wheat pasta
Green peas	Whole-wheat tortillas
	Winter squash

My Balanced Plate

Protein	
Beans (also fiber-rich carb)	Lentils (also fiber-rich carb)
Chicken breasts	Pork chops
Chicken thighs	Pork loin
Cottage cheese	Salmon
Eggs	Sirloin steak
Greek yogurt	Soy (edamame, tofu, tempeh)
Ground meat (chicken, beef, turkey)	Tofu
Kielbasa	Tuna

One-Half of the Plate: Non-Starchy Vegetables

These are your nutrient powerhouses. Non-starchy vegetables, such as leafy greens, broccoli, carrots, and bell peppers are packed with vitamins, minerals, and fiber. Plus, they make your plate colorful and inviting! They add bulk to your meals, support digestion, and help you feel full, without adding a lot of calories, aka energy. This is the largest section of the plate because vegetables should form the foundation of most meals. Eat your veggies!

One-Quarter of the Plate: Proteins

Protein is essential for muscle repair, immune function, and keeping you full and satisfied longer. Protein-packed foods also provide essential amino acids, making them key players in a balanced meal. This quarter of your plate should include lean proteins, such as chicken, lean red meat, fish, beans, tofu, or eggs. Plant-based protein options are just as good for you as animal-based.

One-Quarter of the Plate: Carbs (bonus points for fiber-rich carbs!)

Carbohydrates are your body's primary source of energy, and it's important to choose slow-digesting, nutrient-dense carbs that provide sustained energy and help stabilize blood sugar levels. This section of your plate should include whole grains, such as quinoa, brown rice, farro, or whole-wheat pasta; or starchy vegetables, such as sweet potatoes, winter squash, or corn. All of these deliver fiber and nutrients to keep your digestion on track and your energy full-steam and steady throughout the day. And don't worry if your carb isn't fiber-rich, you're still giving your body its preferred source of energy. The non-starchy veggies act as your fiber insurance policy!

Healthy Fats: Add in Moderation

While fats don't need a dedicated section of your plate, they're an essential (tiny but mighty!) part of a balanced diet. Healthy fats like olive oil, avocado, nuts, seeds, and fatty fish play a supporting role in nutrient absorption, heart health, brain health, and satiety. Adding a small amount to your meals, like a drizzle of olive oil or a handful of nuts, elevates both flavor and nutrition.

Hydration: Water & Low-Sugar Beverages

While also not a part of your plate, hydration is essential for a balanced meal. Drinking water, herbal tea, or a low-sugar beverage helps with digestion and ensures that your body absorbs nutrients efficiently. Proper hydration is key to overall health.

HERE'S AN EXAMPLE OF A BALANCED PLATE:

- **Roasted Brussels sprouts (non-starchy veggie):** Fill half the plate.
- **Grilled chicken (protein):** Add one to two pieces of light or dark meat.
- **Quinoa salad (fiber-rich carb):** Fill the remaining quarter of the plate.
- **Avocado slices (healthy fat):** Add this tasty topping for added flavor and nutrition.

Balanced Snacking

Snacks are an opportunity to nourish your body, and they can be balanced, too (see page 103)! Aim for snacks that include at least two food groups to keep your energy steady and your hunger at bay. I also recommend including at least one protein source in all of your snacks so that you balance protein intake throughout the day. For example:

Apple slices (fiber-rich carb) + almond butter (protein and fat).

Carrot sticks (veggie) + hummus (protein and fat).

These combinations provide a steady source of energy, support digestion, and keep you satisfied until your next meal. Think of snacks as mini-meals that help fill in any nutritional gaps throughout the day.

A Balanced Plate . . .

A balanced plate isn't just about portions—it's about fuel, focus, and full-body health. Once you incorporate the basics of it into your daily diet, you'll find that in addition to the delicious and nutritious aspect, it also . . .

- **Stabilizes Your Blood Sugar:** Prevents energy spikes and crashes, keeping you fueled and focused.
- **Supports Digestion:** Fiber from veggies and whole grains supports gut health and regularity.
- **Keeps You Satisfied:** Protein and healthy fats help you stay full and reduce the likelihood of overeating.
- **Boosts Overall Health:** You get a wide range of essential nutrients for daily functions and long-term health and well-being.

Pantry Power & Ingredients

When it comes to organizing your pantry, you know I have some tips for you. When I bought my house in late 2024, one of the first things that I did was set up my pantry. I am super into organization. I know, who the heck thinks nutrition *and* pantry organization are fun? I do!

Please make sure that whatever containers, organizers, or labels you use in your pantry are easy on the eyes. The more visually appealing they are, and your entire pantry is, the more likely you are to want to cook from it! Even if you are the only person who sees and uses your pantry? Yes! You matter.

Containers & Supplies

I highly recommend nice **clear, stackable containers** for your bulk and regularly consumed pantry items. They really help in terms of grab and go. You can quickly see what's inside—whether it's oats, rice, beans, pasta, etc.—so that you don't have to snoop around your own pantry, pulling up lids and cracking open boxes to determine what's what. Also, **labels**! Sometimes pantry items, such as various types of grains and beans, are pretty tricky to tell apart.

For canned items, I recommend using **one or two can racks, tiers, or organizers** so that they don't topple every which way. There are so many different styles for those. While you're at it, get **a few shelf bins or boxes**! Not everything neatly stacks, so you can place your odds and ends in these.

If you regularly feel like things are overfull in your pantry, consider an **over-the-door** organizer for bottles, cans, and jars. **Lazy Susans** and **pull-out organizers** can be very helpful, too.

Pantry Sections

If you are doing a big pantry organization or *reorganization,* start by **pulling out all pantry items,** so that you can consolidate and arrange everything on your kitchen counter or table. See what you have the most of and consider what you use most often.

Next up, organize your sections. **Group similar items together,** so that you're less likely to scratch your head wondering where you put that dang flaxseed meal. Place it with your seeds and nuts, or wherever it makes the most sense for it to be.

Now, figure out where each of these sections will live in your pantry. Place whatever you use most often in the prime eye-level, easiest-to-grab spot. Lesser used pantry items should be up tippity-top and down low. (I luckily don't have any out-of-reach pantry shelves. I'm grateful for that. I can grab from all my shelves without using a stepstool, or I can holler at my tall fiancé to come help me.)

You can get dialed in with all sorts of next-level pantry organization. Just make sure to always think about how often you use various ingredients. Do you really need an entire shelf devoted to dried fruits if you, well, don't really dig dried fruits? Nope! I favor practical organization rather than aspirational organization. Know thyself! Here's a sneak peek at the primary sections in my pantry:

Nutrition-Boosting Add-Ons

The top shelf section of my pantry is all about quick add-on macronutrients for dishes and snacks. It's where I store things like **flaxseeds, hemp hearts, all sorts of nuts, protein powders, and nutritional yeast.** I like my pistachios for protein, hemp hearts for healthy fats, and flax and chia seeds for fiber.

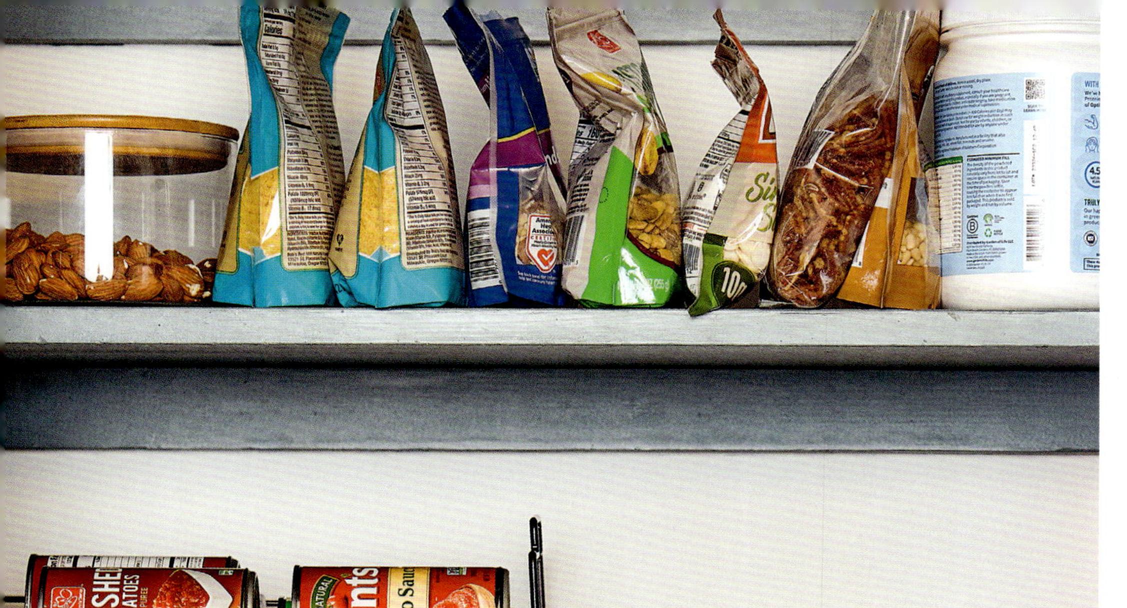

Nutrition-Boosting Add-Ons

Canned Goods + Lentils + Rice + Pasta

Nutrient-Dense Snacks + Grains + Breads

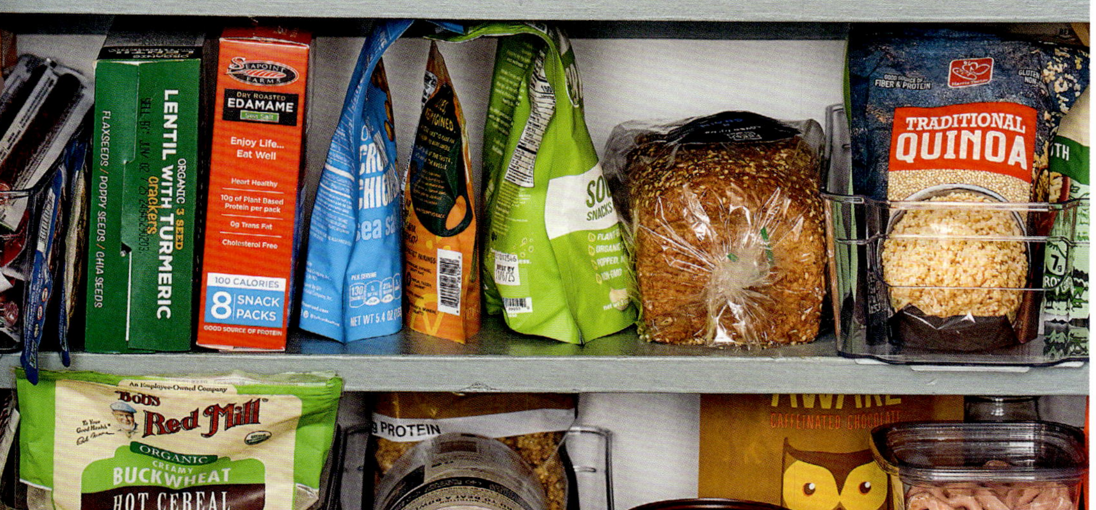

Breakfast Zone + Indulgent Snacks

Canned Goods + Lentils + Rice + Pasta

The second highest shelf in my pantry, just above eye-level for me, holds all my **canned items,** which is unsurprisingly a ton of beans. You know I love my beans (page 41)! I also keep a lot of **canned veggies, canned tuna, canned tomatoes, and tomato sauces** on hand in my pantry since all those items are in heavy rotation.

Next to that, on the same shelf, are my **lentils, rice, and pasta,** all of which I cook often. I almost always have a healthy supply of dried lentils in my pantry because I typically meal-prep them every or every other week. I try to stick with whole grains as much as possible except when it comes to pasta. I prefer regular semolina pasta over whole wheat thanks to my Italian heritage.

Nutrient-Dense Snacks & Grains & Breads

Moving down in my pantry, I store all my **nutrient-dense snacks** like pita chips and roasted nuts, as well as most of my **grains (not rice!) and breads**—sandwich bread, quinoa, couscous, farro, etc.

Breakfast Zone & Indulgent Snacks

Just below all of that is my **breakfast zone** with things like oats, buckwheat, boxed breakfast cereals, maple syrup, etc. Next to that are my **indulgent snacks**—everything from Oreos to chips.

Miscellaneous

And on the very bottom shelf of my pantry, well, that's **everything else**! It's generally quite a lot of bottled and jarred things that I don't use 24/7 but love, like nut butters, vinegars, oils, and hot sauces.

A to Z Ingredients

Everyone is different when it comes to how they stock their pantry and fridge. Some people rely primarily on canned goods and pasta that will last them for many months with fewer fresh ingredients. Survival-mode. Others, like me, prefer to have more variety and wide-ranging types of foods. And you know I consider the nutritional factors of each item! Here are a bunch of my favorite nutritious foods and ingredients that I like to have on hand.

Apple Cider Vinegar

I use raw, unfiltered apple cider vinegar with the "mother" in it (the cloudy, viscous fermentation substance) because it supports healthy blood sugar levels and aids digestion. I also like the way it tastes! I use it most often in salad dressings like my Honey Mustard Dressing (page 129).

Avocados

Avocados are creamy, spreadable, and full of flavor; a great substitute for mayonnaise and butter; and I eat a lot of them. They're rich in heart-healthy monounsaturated fats (for the low-down on healthy fats, see page 27) and loaded with fiber. One avocado contains roughly 13 to 14 grams of fiber. Storage tip: Keep halved or chopped avocado in an airtight container splashed with a bit of lemon juice to discourage browning.

Balsamic Vinegar & Glaze

Loaded with antioxidants and delicious, I drizzle balsamic glaze (see my homemade version on page 172)—a rich, syrupy balsamic reduction—over everything from roasted vegetables (Sheet-Pan Smashed Brussels Sprouts, page 212) and grilled meats to Caprese salads. It's sweet and tangy and elevates everything you add it to.

Bell Peppers

I almost always have bell peppers in my crisper. I appreciate how different they are when raw—sweet, crunchy, and juicy—versus when slow sautéed or roasted—soft and silky. I like all the different colors, too: red, orange, yellow, green. I once visited a bell pepper farm and learned that the difference between a red and green bell pepper is simply their ripeness.

Who knew? All types are loaded with vitamins A and C, potassium, folic acid, and fiber.

Breakfast Cereals

Almost all healthy breakfast cereals, whether hot or cold, are fortified with essential vitamins and minerals like iron, calcium, vitamin D, and B, so a morning bowl of cereal is like a tasty multivitamin! Please opt for high-fiber ones (whole grain is best) and avoid added sugar—many so-called healthy ones are loaded with it. Pair cereal with added protein and/or fiber—milk plus banana, for the win—and you're treating yourself right. My favorite cereal: whole-grain-oats-loaded Strawberry Cheerios Protein.

Broths

Bone broths have been very popular the past several years. If you are looking for higher protein content, go for stock or bone broth as opposed to a non-bone broth. They have high protein content due to the broken-down connective tissues. They're great, and I love them, too, but all broth is loaded with vitamins and minerals. I love how it enhances the flavor of grains—a lot of my recipes pair the two: Saucy Farro with Blistered Tomatoes (page 216) and Cheesy Zuke Rice (page 219). Meat broths contain collagen which is great for joint health. If you've never made homemade broth, it's super easy and a smart way to use leftover veggies, bones, and meat scraps destined for the trash or compost.

Canned Beans

I can't get enough of canned beans! I preach about them 24/7. They're affordable, tasty, easy to throw into and onto so many dishes, and loaded with plant-based protein, fiber, and nutrients. Please rinse and drain them. The canning liquid contains heaps of unnecessary sodium. By rinsing, you often reduce the overall sodium content by 40%!

Cannellini beans are one of my favorites. Mild and versatile, they're great in stews, hashes, salads, and spread over bread or toast with avocado. When I'm in a rush, I often crack open a can of cannellini beans for a snack. I sprinkle them with a little salt and pepper, and spoon them right out of the can. Yes, I know, I normally recommend rinsing, not when I'm in a rush, though, and eating them on their own!

Canned Soups

My pantry always has several canned soups stacked up in it. They're super convenient and filled with nutrients. I especially love lentil soups and vegetable soups. Both are high in fiber and you can always add a protein to make them into a complete and balanced meal. Amy's Kitchen Organic Soups—all of them—are my tried-and-true faves.

Canned Tomatoes & Tomato Paste

Canned tomatoes make me happy—diced, crushed, fire-roasted, tomato paste—all of them. They go into so many favorite dishes like my Cheesy Kielbasa Skillet (page 185) and Veggie-Loaded Chicken Tikka Masala (page 182). Fun canned tomato fact: Lycopene, a powerful antioxidant linked to heart health, becomes more bioavailable (easier for the body to absorb) when tomatoes are cooked. Since canned tomatoes are cooked during processing, they tend to contain more lycopene than fresh tomatoes.

Canned Tuna

One of my favorite quick go-to protein sources is canned tuna. It's a nutritional powerhouse with a 3-ounce serving clocking in with 20 to 25 grams of protein! Tuna is rich in omega-3 fatty acids, particularly EPA and DHA, which are known to reduce inflammation, lower blood pressure, reduce the risk of heart disease, and improve cardiovascular health. It's also high in vitamin D (most Americans are deficient), several B vitamins, including B_{12}, niacin (B_3), and B_6, which are amazing—see page 29. Eat your tuna!

Cheese

I'm absolutely in love with cheese, and lucky for me, it's full of protein and calcium. It pairs well with fruits, veggies, whole grains, and lean proteins. Try my Cheese & Crackers Remix with Apple Dippers (page 113)! I recommend hand-grating rather than buying pre-grated, because it's more affordable and it melts better. If you crave cheese but don't want so much fat, go for low-fat fresh mozzarella. It's delicious when hot, and lovely cold or at room temperature on things like Caprese salad.

Lactose-intolerant? Many cheeses contain little to no lactose since it's broken down during the cheesemaking process. In general, the longer a cheese is aged, the less lactose it contains. Cheese storage tip: Discard the original packaging if it's plastic and wrap it in waxed paper before storing it in a loosely sealed container.

Chia Seeds

These fun little seeds transform by plumping up and softening when hydrated and are rich in omega-3 fatty acids and loaded with fiber. Three tablespoons, slightly more than what goes into my Oats & Seeds Porridge (page 90), has a whopping 10 grams of fiber. I toss them into smoothies, and my Overnight Coconut Chia Seed Pudding with Mango (page 105) is so delicious.

Citrus Juice & Zest

I use a lot of citrus juice and zest in my food, and I especially love both in vinaigrettes. Some of my favorite citrus-loaded recipes: Lemony Salmon Orzo (page 175), Zesty Spinach & Broccoli (page 205), and Tunacado Toasties (page 130). Of course, citrus is loaded with vitamin C, which among other healthful things boosts iron absorption. When shopping for lemons and limes I opt for heavier ones with thinner unblemished skin that gives slightly when squeezed. They are often the ripest and juiciest.

If you're watching your salt intake, incorporate more citrus! Like salt, it's a flavor enhancer, natural tenderizer (breaks down collagen in meat and seafood), and preservation aid (extends shelf life and prevents browning).

Coconut Milk

Canned coconut milk is delicious and a great dairy substitute that I use mostly in curries, stews, and soups like my Curried Pumpkin-Lentil Soup (page 161) and my Creamy Chickpea Curry (page 166). I usually buy full-fat coconut milk because of how flavorful and creamy it is.

Cornstarch

Naturally gluten-free cornstarch is my kitchen go-to quick thickener for sauces, gravies, and soups. I use it a lot. I like it better than more gloopy flour. It makes sauces and dishes glossier. It's also high in carbs, so I sometimes add it to kick up the carbs in protein-rich meals.

Couscous

Couscous is a nice fiber-rich, plant-based-protein-loaded option for weeknight meals because it's tasty and cooks up (and fluffs up!) so quickly and easily. One of my favorite couscous dishes is my Chickpea, Couscous & Feta Bowl (page 140). In my pantry, I usually have what's called Moroccan couscous, the smallest and fluffiest variety. For a bit more bite and texture for a pilaf, a salad, or soups and stews, I'll use a larger pearl couscous.

Cottage Cheese

I eat *a lot* of cottage cheese. It's so tasty, plus it's high in protein. I blend it into all sorts of sweet and savory dips (see page 113). My preferred brand is thick and creamy live-culture Good Culture cottage cheese. It doesn't have any artificial additives and it's delicious.

Cucumbers

I prefer thin-skinned, skinny, minimal seeded, crunchy, and sweet English cucumbers to the softer, seedy salad cucumbers more readily available in grocery stores. (Persian cukes and many Asian varieties are similar to English cucumbers.) If you can get your hands on English cukes, I highly recommend them. Know though, that any cucumber is A-OK for the recipes in this book.

Dried Fruits

When it comes to snacking, dried fruits are your friends. They're yummy, convenient, portable, and shelf stable, and they're also great in prepared dishes. Dried fruit is also high in fiber (¼ cup of most has about 3.5 grams of fiber) and a natural sweetener. I particularly love and recommend . . .

- **Raisins:** High in iron and potassium
- **Dried apricots:** Contain vitamins A and C, potassium, and fiber
- **Prunes:** Great for digestion
- **Dates:** High in fiber and a good natural sweetener
- **Dried cranberries:** High in antioxidants and tasty in salads
- **Dried figs:** High in fiber

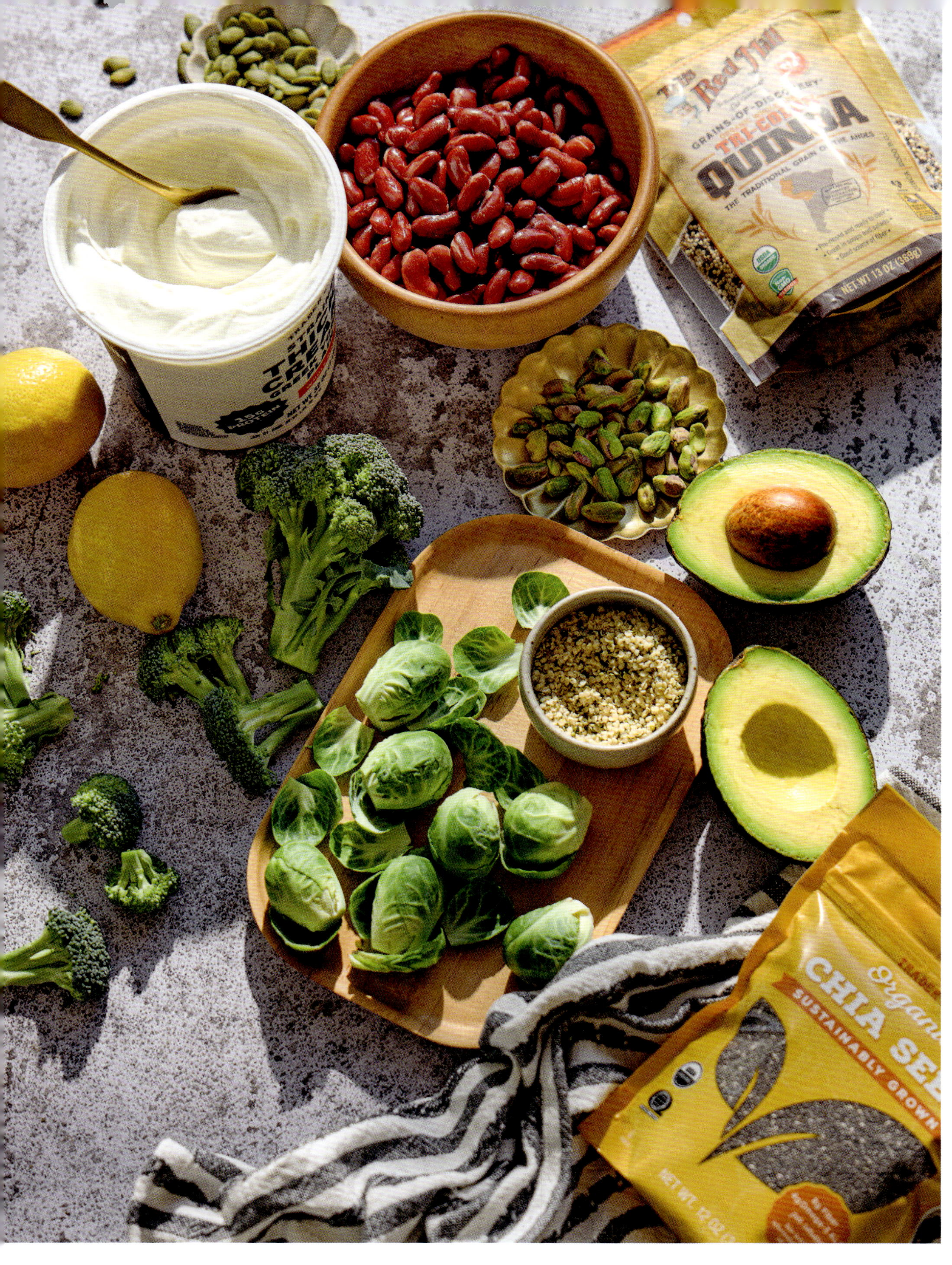
Bob's Red Mill
GRAINS-OF-DISCOVERY
THE TRADITIONAL GRAIN OF THE ANDES
NET WT 13 OZ (369g)
15g PROTEIN
SUSTAINABLY GROWN

Edamame

Edamame (young green soybeans) are in a bunch of my recipes—my Lizzo Salad (page 125), Doctored Instant Ramen (page 243), and Edamame Bowl (page 138) to name a few. I call for shelled (out of their pods) frozen edamame. Fresh are harder to source. Edamame are a complete source of protein—9 grams per ½ cup—and I love snacking on them. I simply steam them in the microwave, sprinkle with a pinch of salt, and YUM!

Eggs

Remember when everyone thought eggs were bad news for raising cholesterol? Well, now there is plenty of research that debunks that. Dietary cholesterol does not, in fact, increase blood cholesterol. The yolks of eggs are my favorite part, and they contain so much healthy fat and choline. Choline is super good for your brain and liver as well as for fetal development. So, if you're pregnant, eat your eggs!

Extra-Virgin Olive Oil

Hello, monounsaturated fats! I'm a big fan of the Mediterranean diet, and of course, olive oil is a main component. I use a lot of olive oil for everything from roasting veggies and making vinaigrettes, to cooking up skillets (pages 76 and 185). I *love* it.

Farro

Farro is higher in protein than most grains, with 5 to 7 grams of protein per ½ cup cooked, so it's a great choice for vegetarians, vegans, or anyone looking to increase protein intake. The protein in farro also contains several essential amino acids that are important for muscle repair and overall body function. One of my favorite farro dishes is my Saucy Farro with Blistered Tomatoes (page 216).

Flaxseeds & Flaxseed Meal

Both flaxseeds and flaxseed meal (ground flaxseeds) are rich in omega-3 fatty acids and high in dietary fiber. Whole flaxseeds are lovely as a crunchy topping for salads, yogurt, and oatmeal. I also like to add them to smoothies. Grinding flaxseeds breaks their hard outer shell and makes the nutrients (omega-3 fatty acids, fiber, lignans) more bioavailable and easier for the body to absorb. Flaxseed meal can be added to baked goods and hot cereals and used as a thickener for soups and sauces. It's also a pretty great vegan egg substitute for baking (1 tablespoon of flaxseed meal + 3 tablespoons of water = 1 egg).

Fresh Herbs

I use fresh herbs primarily to enhance flavor and aroma and to make my dishes look nice. It elevates a dish quickly and naturally without adding more salt, sugar, or unhealthy fats. My go-to herbs are . . .

- **Parsley:** Use it as a garnish; add it to salads, soups, and sauces, or mix it into dressings and marinades.
- **Cilantro:** Ideal for fresh salsas, guacamole, and salads, or as a garnish for curries, tacos, and soups.
- **Chives:** Great for garnishing soups, baked potatoes, eggs, and salads, or mixing into dips and spreads.
- **Thyme:** Pairs well with meats, poultry, vegetables, and sauces.
- **Basil:** Best used fresh and added at the end of cooking to preserve its flavor.

Frozen Fruits & Veggies

Frozen fruits and veggies are your friends. They're typically frozen at peak ripeness, when most nutrient-dense—locking in vitamins, minerals, and antioxidants. Not only are they often just as nutritious as their fresh counterparts, but they also tend to have higher nutrient levels than fresh produce that's been stored for extended periods. Frozen fruits and veggies are also convenient, cost effective, and obviously have a long shelf life (on your *freezer* shelf!). Less food waste for the win.

Garlic

Garlic is great for you! It contains heaps of vitamin C and antioxidants. Antioxidants protect your cells from the damage that free radicals (unstable reactive molecules) can cause. That makes me happy because the Italian in me absolutely craves garlic. I put it in just about everything! On average, I'd say I cook up and consume four to five cloves in various dishes a day. When a recipe in my book calls for two or three cloves of garlic, know that I'm probably using double that. My garlic motto: The more the merrier.

Greek Yogurt

Nonfat or low-fat plain Greek yogurt is almost always front and center in my fridge. I use it almost every day, and you'll find it in *so many* recipes in this book. I love its tang, texture, and versatility. I remember the first time I simply added ranch seasoning to it for a really quick ranch dressing (page 142) and was blown away. It's a great probiotic to have around for quick dressings, salads, sauces, a hot and cold cereal topper, and then some. Go, Greek yogurt! MVP.

Ground Meat

I love ground meat. It's affordable, accessible, and freezes well. I mostly use ground beef, chicken, and turkey. All are great for everything from meatloaves (page 193), burgers, and Stephwrap Supremes (page 153), to soups, stews, sauces, casseroles, and my Lazy Shepherd's Pie (page 187). I tend to favor leaner 90/10 (90% lean meat, 10% fat) for sauces and casseroles that don't rely heavily on fat for flavor, and a slightly higher fat content like an 85/15 for burgers, meatloaves, and other dishes where big flavor and juiciness is key.

Honey

I adore this natural tasty sweetener and use it often for dressings (Lizzo Salad, page 125), marinades and sauces, or glazes (Sheet-Pan Honey-Glazed Carrots & Parsnips, page 208), and as an a.m. hot or cold cereal topper (Overnight Oats, page 93). There are three types of honey I favor: Raw honey is minimally processed and retains the most antioxidants and enzymes; manuka honey is known for its antimicrobial properties; and local honey often has unique flavor profiles based on the flora where the bees have buzzed.

Hummus

Occasionally I make my own hummus, but mostly I use store-bought packs of this tasty Middle Eastern dip/spread. My favorite types of store-bought are roasted red pepper and garlic-heavy, but I'll take whatever you're serving. Hummus is filled with plant-based protein and fiber, and I think you'll like it in my Hummus & Pita Bento Box (page 116) as well as on my Hummus & Edamame Toast (page 73).

Kale

When I was doing my dietetic internship in grad school, I was on a very tight budget and I ate kale like popcorn, tearing off little hunks of it (I'm talking raw Tuscan kale from Trader Joe's) because I knew just how nutritious it was. Some people get triggered when foods are called "super foods"—I get it—*but* I am gonna say it just this once in my cookbook (and I have *a lot* of recipes for it in here), kale is a super food! Look at the daily value percentage of these nutrients in ONE cup of raw kale: 400% vitamin K, over 400% vitamin A, 60% vitamin C.

Kefir

If you haven't tried it before, I'll bet you've heard of or seen this protein-boost yummy fermented drink made from milk (dairy or nondairy) and kefir grains. Kefir grains aren't actual grains, they're an amalgam of the microscopic bacteria and yeast that ferments the beverage. As a result, kefir has a tangy, slightly sour taste similar to yogurt, but it's thinner and more drinkable. I often have a few bottles of it in my shopping cart. Its wide variety of probiotic strains helps you maintain a healthy balance of gut bacteria.

Kimchi

This traditional funky Korean fermented vegetable (often made from napa cabbage and radishes, along with chile pepper, garlic, ginger, and green onions) is also rich in beneficial bacteria (probiotics) including lactobacilli. I love it. Probiotics help you maintain a healthy balance of gut bacteria, which is essential for proper digestion, nutrient absorption, and prevention of digestive issues like constipation, diarrhea, and bloating.

Kosher Salt

I prefer kosher salt to table salt, because it has larger, coarser grains that are easier to pick up and sprinkle evenly over food. While developing the recipes for this book, I used Diamond Crystal. Just know that if you use a finer table salt (or Morton's kosher salt) in place of the kosher salt in any of my recipes, you'll want to use roughly half the volume since it is finer and denser. So, if a recipe calls for 1 teaspoon of kosher salt, use about ½ teaspoon of table salt (or Morton's kosher salt), then taste and adjust accordingly.

Lentils

I cook and prep lentils almost every week for various soups, salads, and bowls. They're an excellent source of plant-based protein, with about 18 grams of protein per 1 cup cooked, and they're also high in dietary fiber, with about 15 grams per cooked cup. Among my favorite lentil dishes are my Curried Pumpkin-Lentil Soup (page 161) and Warm Lentil Salad with Roasted Veggies (page 126).

Maple Syrup

Maple syrup is a uniquely delicious natural sweetener with beneficial minerals including manganese and zinc. I mean, it comes from TREES! Always go for pure maple syrup, rather than pancake syrups, which are typically made with corn syrup and artificial flavors.

Nut & Seed Butters

I use a lot of nut and seed butters—stirring them into everything from sauces and dressings, and hot breakfast cereals, to smoothies and yogurt. So tasty. Choose those that just contain the nuts or seeds and maybe a bit of salt. Even those touting "natural" on the label can contain added sugars and/or oils.

Nuts & Seeds

Need extra protein in a dish? Add nuts or seeds! They're crunchy, tasty, and fairly shelf stable. Peanuts have 7 grams of protein per ounce; almonds have 6 grams; pistachios have 6 grams; pumpkin seeds have 8 to 10 grams; and hemp hearts have 9 to 10 grams per 3 tablespoons.

Nutritional Yeast Flakes

I mostly use this savory deactivated yeast as a yummy popcorn, pasta, or pizza topper, but I also add it to soups, sauces, dips, and my Veggie "Tuna" Salad (page 146). It's an excellent source of B_{12} and it contains all nine essential amino acids, making it a complete protein. If you regularly use it as a topper like me, I recommend storing it in a countertop glass shaker, like ones used for red pepper flakes or grated Parmesan at pizza parlors.

Old-Fashioned Rolled Oats

Rolled oats are a great source of fiber, complex carbs, essential vitamins, and minerals, making them a breakfast staple in my house. I use them in my Overnight Oats (page 93).

Pastas—Traditional & Alternative

Considering my Italian heritage, you know I love pasta. My favorites are farfalle (bow tie), orzo (make my Lemony Salmon Orzo, page 175!), penne, spaghetti, and capellini (angel hair). I almost always pair pasta with protein and veggies for a balanced meal. When I'm in the mood for comfort food, I use alternative pastas made from chickpeas or lentils, which are more nutrient-dense and higher in protein. Craving satisfied—check!—dish balanced—check!

Pesto

And what goes better with pasta than pesto? It's delicious and high in healthy fats and antioxidants. Beyond pasta, I like to use pesto as a topper for chicken, fish, and veggies before roasting. I also spread it onto sandwiches and wraps like my Turkey Pesto Wrap (page 145). I often make my own pesto because it's more affordable and I get to control how garlicky, salty, and oily it is. It's really easy to make, if you never have. Mince up or food process about 1 cup of lightly packed fresh basil (or other leafy fresh herbs or greens), 2 garlic cloves, and 2 tablespoons of nuts (pine nuts are tasty but spendy, other nuts work great), grate ¼ cup of some hard Italian cheese and add it, drizzle in a heaping ¼ cup of extra-virgin olive oil and you're in business!

Popcorn

Fun fact: Popcorn is a whole grain, so it's naturally high in fiber. It's one of my favorite quick and affordable snacks. My go-to toppings and mix-ins are nutritional yeast, cashews, chocolate, cheese, and dried fruits. It's also great in trail mix—add it to mine (page 109)!

Quinoa

Quinoa is one of the few plant-based foods that's a complete source of protein (see page 26). I cook it a lot, and I think it's good at any temperature. I highly recommend my Eggy Quinoa Cups (page 61) for a quick-yummy breakfast on the go and my Stove Top Stuffing Remix (page 235) for nutritious, delicious comfort food. Remember to rinse your quinoa before cooking it—the grains are often covered in saponins (bitter and soapy tasting plant chemicals). No thank you!

Rice

I cook a lot of rice, most often using white and brown varieties. Brown rice is a whole-grain option with a nuttier flavor, chewier bite, and more fiber and nutrients. I prefer the taste of white rice, so I use it more often. When I need to up my fiber, I opt for brown rice.

Salmon

I like to cook salmon on Mondays when I'm at home—Sheet-Pan Salmon & Veggies (page 170) or Lemony Salmon Orzo (page 175). It's a great way to start my week and then I usually have yummy leftovers for Tuesday lunch. It's recommended that we all have fatty fish such as salmon twice a week. I toggle between farm-raised and wild-caught. Farm-raised is often fattier, but has different environmental implications. Wild-caught is leaner and generally higher in omega-3 fatty acids.

Soy Sauce

The umami (savory flavor) of soy sauce has no equal. Just a splash adds so much depth to dishes like Grilled Chicken Slaw Wrap (page 149) and Doctored Instant Ramen (page 243). It's made from fermented soybeans and wheat, although gluten-free tamari can be swapped in.

Spinach

Spinach is packed with vitamins A, C, and K plus iron and fiber. Storage tip: Wrap it in a paper towel and store it in a resealable bag or container in the fridge so that it doesn't wilt.

Sweet Potatoes vs. Yams

There is much confusion when it comes to these two tubers. I always call for the darker red-skinned, orange, and sweet on the inside sweet potatoes. However, sweet potatoes are often referred to as yams, depending on where you are in the country and what grocery store you're shopping at. A true yam has pale light-yellow flesh and the skin is typically dark brown. Yams often have "hairs" coming out of their skin, and they are starchier and denser than sweet potatoes.

In terms of nutritional value, sweet potatoes contain an incredible amount of beta-carotene. Beta-carotene is a precursor to vitamin A, meaning your body converts it into vitamin A (see the benefits on page 28). Orange-fleshed yams contain a good deal, too, just not as much. Sweet potatoes have a lower glycemic index than white or gold potatoes, which means they cause slower rise in blood sugars—great for folks who are diabetic or have insulin insensitivity.

Tofu

Tofu is another complete protein with all nine essential amino acids as well as a good deal of calcium and iron. I tend to use firm or extra-firm tofu in stir-fries, salads (my Warm Lentil Salad with Roasted Veggies *and tofu* is so good, page 126), and baked goods and use the silken or soft tofu when blending it into a dish or making an eggless scramble.

Tortillas

I almost always have one or two types of tortillas at home. I like flour tortillas since they're pliable and great for wraps (see pages 145 and 149), burritos, quesadillas, and my Stephwrap Supreme (page 153). I use corn tortillas for tacos and enchiladas and whole wheat tortillas when I need a meal with more fiber.

Turmeric

When consumed raw, fresh turmeric has significantly more antioxidants than its ground counterpart. It's strong tasting, though, so I tend to pair it with fresh ginger—I like the way they taste together—and add it to smoothies. While I was in grad school, I ate fresh turmeric raw because I loved what it was doing for my body and mind, particularly its anti-inflammatory benefits. These days, I'm more inclined to use dried and ground turmeric, which is also great for you.

Wine

I LOVE that my last item here is wine! While there certainly are negative effects from over-consumption, in moderation, wine is a delicious fermented beverage loaded with polyphenols (antioxidant plus anti-inflammatory) *and* it makes me feel good and happy. Crave, cook, and nourish! On nights in, I love to pour myself a glass of red wine, put on some Brazilian bossa nova, and set into some easy breezy cooking.

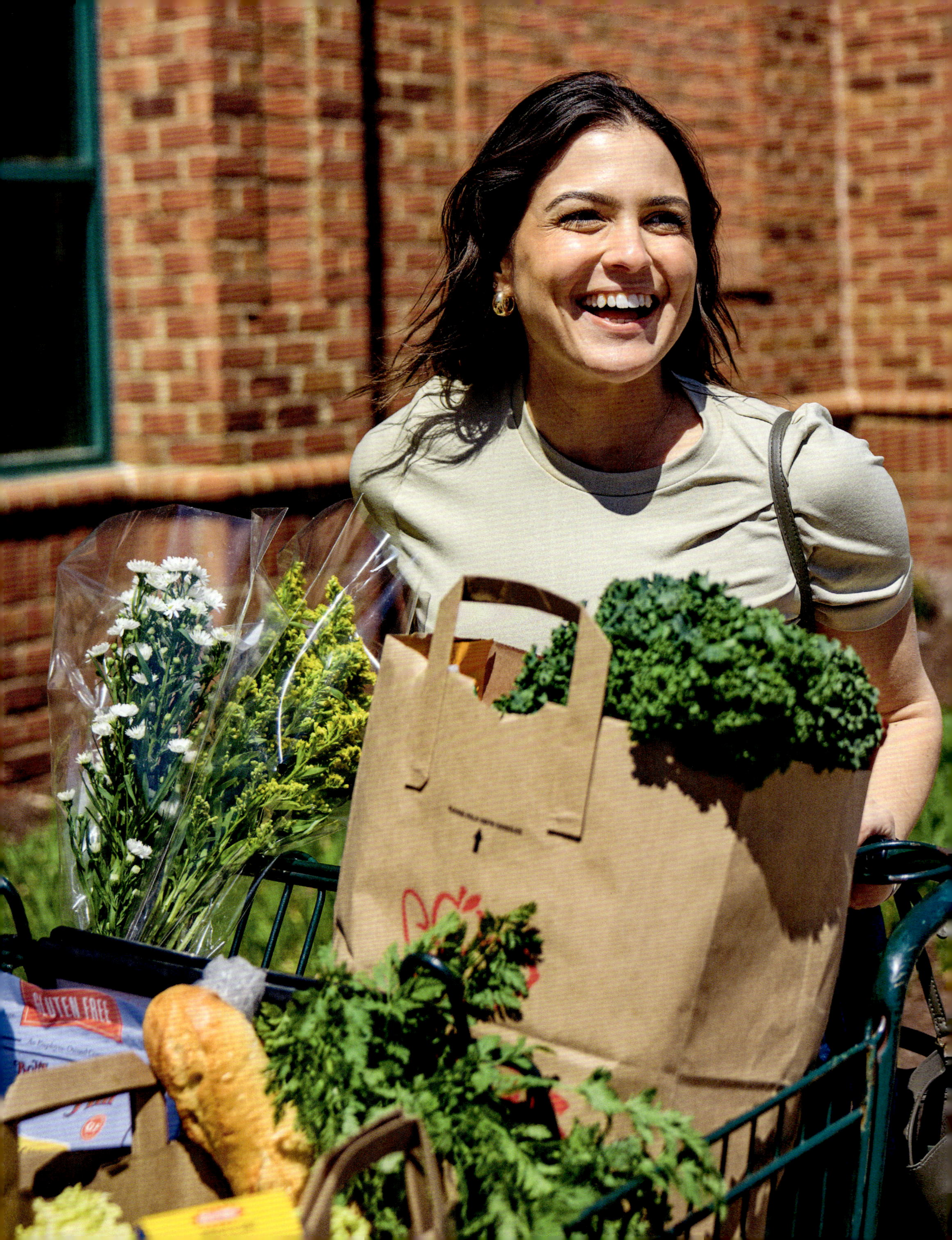
GLUTEN FREE

Grocery Shopping & Meal-Prep Tips & Hacks

I love grocery shopping, and I take my time doing it. I know that I'm the odd woman out on this, and that it's generally more stressful than enjoyable for most people, but I seriously adore it. It's one of my many forms of therapy.

On the weekend, I look forward to waking up, making coffee, pouring it into a to-go mug, and heading to my local grocery store for a long leisurely shop. Sometimes it feels a little like window shopping, only it's aisle shopping. I'm not in a rush, so please go ahead and pass me in the fast lane if you are!

Of course, I'm gathering things in my cart that I'll be purchasing all along the way, but I'm also checking out sections of the store that I don't plan to buy a thing from. I like to take my time and roll with it—see what's out there, what's stocked and available, what's new and heavily marketed, even if it's not ultimately going to feed me that week. It feeds my curiosity! I get all sorts of meal inspo and cooking ideas from slowly cruising the store.

I don't have a favorite grocery store. Most of them make me happy, since I love food and shopping so much. That said, I particularly appreciate a well-stocked and vibrant produce section, with plenty of local, farm-fresh options. I also love an inviting little grocery store café area. Added bonuses: a well-appointed salad bar and a stand-alone olive bar. The truth is, my favorite grocery store is whichever one I'm currently shopping in.

I'm sure I'll get some eyerolls here, but one fun way to make a grocery shopping trip more enjoyable is to dress like you're going on a first date. I often do this. For real! I'm talking leave your sweats and hoodie at home, and put on something that makes you feel good. And to be clear, I'm not talking about doing this in order to meet someone, I'm talking about doing this for *you*!

There are other ways to make the grocery shopping experience more enjoyable. Pop in your earbuds and listen to a fun playlist or podcast while you shop. Lizzo is my jam, and maybe you listen to her while shopping for all the goodies in my Lizzo Salad (page 125) and cruising the aisles? I also highly recommend getting and using cute reusable bags for your haul. Save the planet one bag at a time!

Also, every once in a while, friendly engagement with a stranger at the grocery store is really good for you, good for them, and good for community. We're all on our phones and devices so much these days, and real-time human face-to-face interactions are opportunities! A friendly face can turn a not-so-great day into a beautiful day ultrafast. The love you have, is the love you give.

Divide & Conquer

My biggest piece of advice, when it comes to meal planning, grocery shopping, and meal-prepping for the week, is to divide and conquer. Please, please don't try to do everything all at once! That can be quite overwhelming, and we do not want that. That is not enjoyable; not even for me, Ms. Grocery Shopping Is My Jam. Whenever and however it fits best in your schedule, I recommend taking three days for the whole endeavor.

Day 1: Meal plan

Day 2: Grocery shop

Day 3: Meal prep

Day 1: MEAL PLAN

I encourage you to start your meal planning on whatever day is the last day of your work week. For me, that's Friday. I'm usually still in work mode and on my computer, but the weekend is just around the corner. Before the good times roll, I take care of this important personal task by powering through and planning out some upcoming weekday meals, and some snacks, depending on how much energy I still have.

Crave

I get meal inspo from all sorts of places including TikTok, Pinterest, cookbooks, my own tried-and-true recipes, and my food-focused imagination. Start looking for dishes that sound the most delicious to you for the week.

Choose some recipes that you are craving. Don't worry about balancing anything at this point, just focus on what sounds good. Do you want something creamy and cheesy? Are you more in the mood for crunchy and fresh? What exactly are you craving?

Breakfast: **2**
Lunch: **1**
Dinner: **3–5**
Snacks: **2**

Step 1: Choose Your Recipes

Breakfast 1	Pumpkin Protein Pancakes with Cinnamony Yogurt	(page 100)
Breakfast 2	Overnight Oats	(page 93)
Lunch 1	Turkey Pesto Wrap	(page 145)
Dinner 1	Cheesy Kielbasa Skillet	(page 185)
Dinner 2	Lemony Salmon Orzo	(page 175)
Dinner 3	Gardened-Up Frozen Pizza	(page 239)
Dinner 4	Curried Pumpkin-Lentil Soup	(page 161)
Snack 1	Cheese & Crackers Remix with Apple Dippers	(page 113)
Snack 2	Quick Sweet Potato Snack	(page 121)

Step 2: Schedule Your Recipes

	Monday	Tuesday	Wednesday	Thursday	Friday
Breakfast	Breakfast 1	Breakfast 2	Breakfast 1	Breakfast 2	Breakfast 1
Lunch	Lunch 1	Dinner 1 leftovers	Dinner 2 leftovers	Lunch 1	Dinner 4 leftovers
Dinner	Dinner 1	Dinner 2	Dinner 3	Dinner 4	All leftovers
Snacks	Snack 1	Snack 2	Snack 1	Snack 2	Snack 1

Nourish

Now's the time to start thinking about balance. There are all sorts of cool and diverse micronutrients in our food. I go through all of them in detail on pages 25 to 31 if you want to get into it. If not, I hear you, simply make sure you are getting a good balance of protein, fiber, fats, and carbs in all your meals for the week. If any of the recipes are lacking one or more, simply add and adjust the recipe as needed.

Step 3: Balance Your Recipes

Lunch & Dinner Recipes	Protein	Carb	Non-starchy Veggie	Bonus: Healthy Fats
Turkey Pesto Wrap (page 145)	Greek yogurt Mozzarella Turkey	Flour tortilla	Green leaf lettuce Tomato	Avocado
Cheesy Kielbasa Skillet (page 185)	Kielbasa	Farfalle pasta	Mushrooms Spinach Yellow squash	
Lemony Salmon Orzo (page 175)	Salmon	Frozen green peas Orzo	Spinach	(salmon)
Gardened-Up Frozen Pizza (page 239)	Kielbasa	Crust	Mushrooms Spinach	Olive oil
Curried Pumpkin-Lentil Soup (page 161)	Cannellini beans Greek yogurt Lentils	Cannellini beans Lentils Pumpkin	Red bell pepper	

Balance Your Recipes

Breakfast & Snack Recipes	Protein	Fiber-Rich Carb	Bonus: Healthy Fats
Pumpkin Protein Pancakes with Cinnamony Yogurt (page 100)	Cottage cheese Eggs Greek yogurt Milk	Oats Pumpkin puree	Eggs
Cinnamon Nut Crunch Overnight Oats (page 94)	Milk	Banana Oats	Almonds Flaxseed meal Nut butter
Cheese & Crackers Remix with Apple Dippers (page 113)	Cheddar cheese Cottage cheese Greek yogurt	Apple Whole-grain crackers	Olive oil
Quick Sweet Potato Snack (page 121)	Greek yogurt	Sweet potato	Chopped nuts

Write Your Shopping List & Swap Ingredients

Compile a list of the ingredients you'll need for each dish that you are planning to cook for the week. Look over all of the ingredients required for your recipes and see which ones you can combine and/or swap. Let's say one dish that you're craving calls for quinoa, and one calls for rice. In that case, think: Is it okay to make both with rice or both with quinoa? If so, which would taste better and feel better? Basically, streamline your shopping list so that it's not too long and unwieldy.

Finalize Your Shopping List

It's almost time for you to head to your local grocery store! Give your shopping list a final look-through and make sure that you don't already have any of the items on it.

That's what Friday typically looks like for me. All of that usually takes me 20 to 30 minutes max. Once you're in the habit of doing all of this, it will feel like clockwork. Less like a chore and more like a treat. Remember, you're taking good care of yourself!

I highly recommend checking out Paprika Recipe Manager if you haven't used it already. It's a meal planning app that takes all your recipes and categorizes the ingredients within them that you'll need. One of the coolest features is that it organizes your shopping list by grocery store aisle or section.

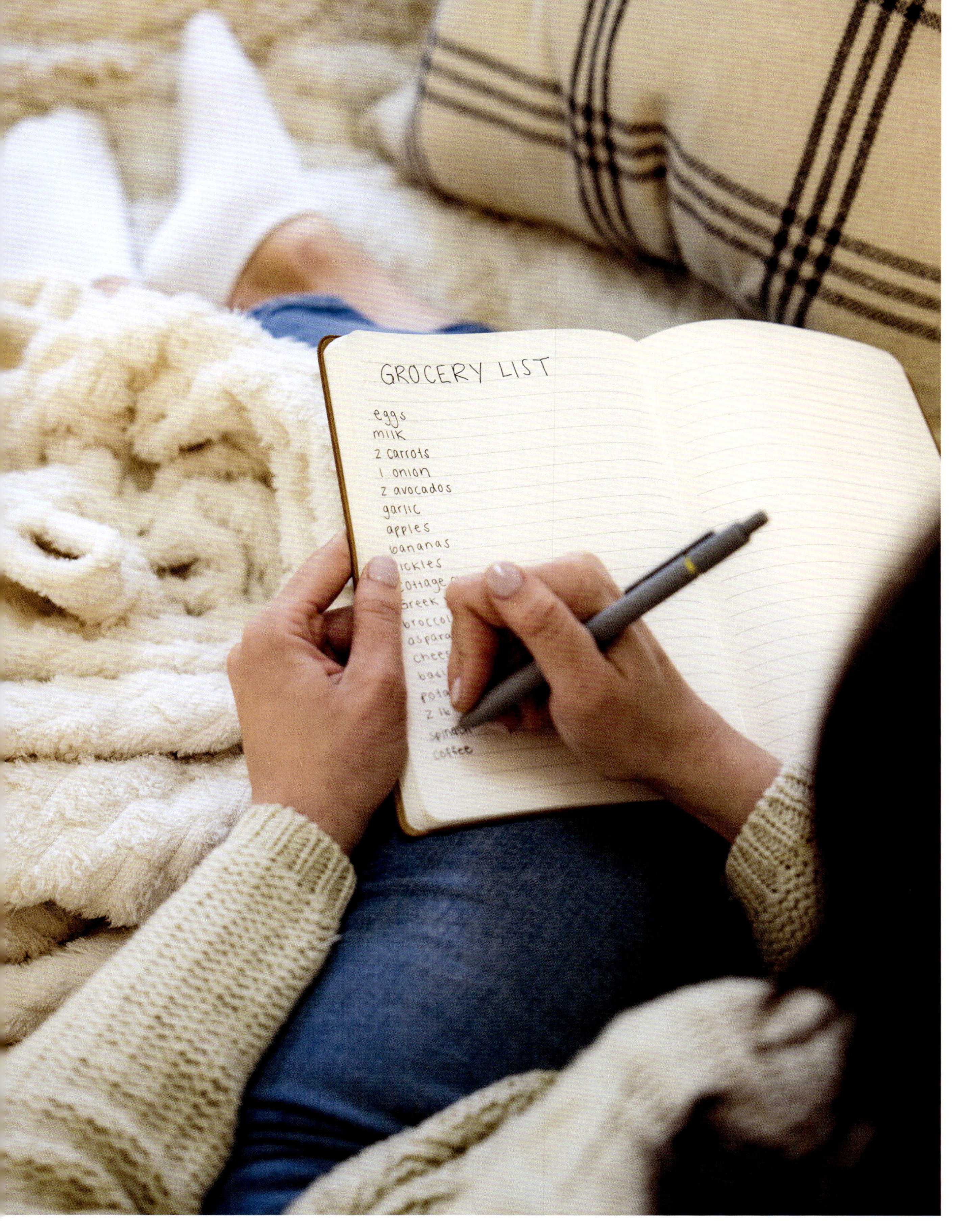
GROCERY LIST
eggs
milk
2 carrots
1 onion
2 avocados
garlic
apples
bananas
coffee

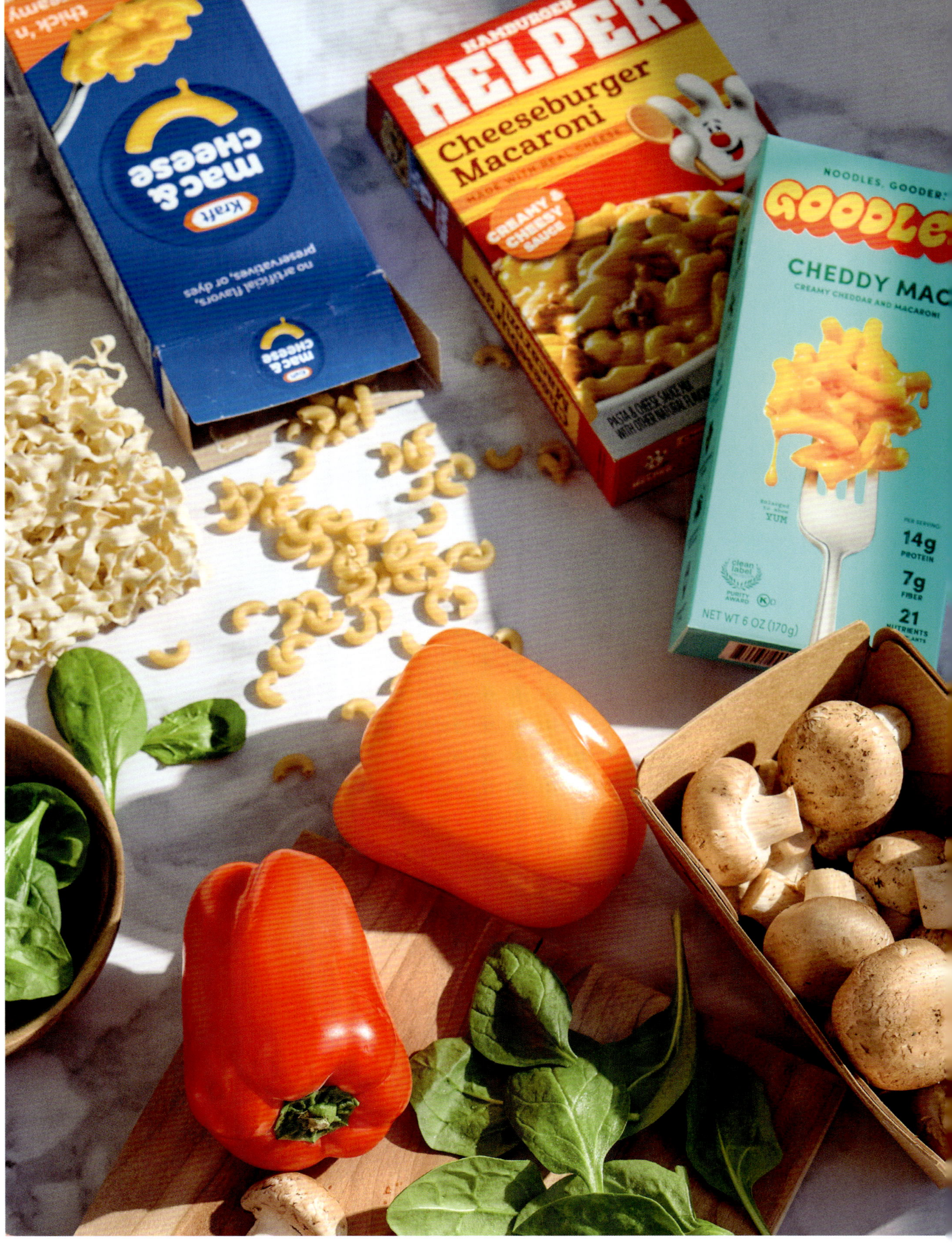
Kraft
mac & cheese
no artificial flavors, preservatives, or dyes
HAMBURGER
HELPER
Cheeseburger Macaroni
MADE WITH REAL CHEESE
CREAMY & CHEESY SAUCE
NOODLES, GOODER.
CHEDDY MAC
CREAMY CHEDDAR AND MACARONI
YUM
14g PROTEIN
7g FIBER
NET WT 6 OZ (170g)

Day 2: GROCERY SHOP

The next day (Saturday, for me!) is grocery shopping day! Hot tip: Grocery stores are often kind of slow on Saturday a.m. My fiancé has let me know that I sort of shop like a shark. I grocery shop by slowly circling the various sections and aisles: produce, then meat and seafood, then dairy, then into the aisles.

First up is produce. I think it's always great to start your grocery shop trip in produce. Here's to plant power! And it's especially beneficial when you're shopping while you're hungry; impulse fruit and veggie buys are pretty good for you. Whatever fruits and veggies I don't find in produce, I grab later in the frozen or the canned aisles.

Next up, I head to the meat and seafood counter and pick out whatever fresh protein I plan to cook during the week. After that, it's dairy. Once that's done, I stop my Jaws-theme-music-playing shark circling and head into the aisles. I start with the frozen aisle for all the frozen fruits and veggies needed.

After that, I cruise all of the other store aisles, and I grab everything from canned goods, popcorn, nuts, and seeds to bread, pasta, and then some.

Yes, navigating grocery stores can certainly be frustrating. Even though I love it, I do feel the pain from time to time, especially when a store is enormous, and there are numerous special sections or aisles like "health foods" or "gluten-free." In that scenario, you might be looking *everywhere* for chia seeds—in cereals, in grains, in health foods—and find them only after you've zigged and zagged the entire store more than once, in the GF aisle. That's why I tend to favor and shop at the same grocery stores regularly. Once you know the general layout, you won't have to retrace your footsteps as often.

Shopping on a Budget

BUY IN BULK: Stock up on oats, rice, beans, and frozen foods when they're on sale.

CHECK YOUR PANTRY BEFORE SHOPPING: Use what you already have before shopping for more of the same.

CHOOSE STORE BRANDS: House brands often cost less and are of the same quality.

COMPARE UNIT PRICES: Check the price per ounce or pound to get the best deal.

COOK MORE AT HOME: Homemade meals are cheaper and healthier than takeout.

OPT FOR AFFORDABLE PROTEINS: Eggs, beans, tofu, canned tuna, and Greek yogurt are all typically budget friendly.

PLAN AHEAD: Make a weekly meal plan and grocery list to avoid impulse buys.

REDUCE FOOD WASTE: Freeze leftovers, repurpose extra ingredients, and store food properly.

SHOP SEASONALLY: Choose in-season fruits and veggies for better prices and quality.

SKIP OVERPRICED CONVENIENCE FOODS: Buy whole produce and prep at home.

USE FROZEN & CANNED FOODS: Frozen veggies and canned beans are cost-effective and last longer.

Reading a Nutrition Label

In order to make informed and healthy diet choices, it's important to know how to read a nutrition label. They aren't the most user-friendly part of food packaging, that's for sure. Here's the gist . . .

Nutrition Facts

8 servings per container

Serving Size	**2/3 cup (55g)**
Amount per serving	
Calories	**230**
	% Daily Value*
Total Fat 8g	**10%**
Saturated Fat 1g	**5%**
Trans Fat 0g	
Cholesterol 0mg	**0%**
Sodium 160mg	**7%**
Total Carbohydrate 37g	**13%**
Dietary Fiber 4g	**14%**
Total Sugars 12g	
Includes 10g Added Sugars	**20%**
Protein 3g	
Vitamin D 2mcg	**10%**
Calcium 260mg	**20%**
Iron 8mg	**45%**
Potassium 235mg	**6%**

*The % Daily Value (DV) tells you how much a nutrient in a serving of food contributes to a daily diet. 2,000 calories a day is used for general nutrition advice.

Serving Size & Portions

Always check the serving size and servings per container. Many labels list values for a single serving, which may be smaller than what you typically eat.

Calories & Energy Balance

Calories indicate energy intake. Use this to compare foods based on your personal needs. Consider calories in context of nutrient density (e.g., 200 calories of nuts vs. 200 calories of soda).

Pay attention to the energy per serving.

% Daily Value (% DV)

- 5% DV or less = Low in that nutrient.
- 20% DV or more = High in that nutrient.
- Use % DV to compare similar products (picking lower sodium or higher fiber options).

Macronutrients (Carbs, Protein, Fats)

- **Carbohydrates:** Look at total carbs, fiber, and sugars (including added sugars).

  Higher fiber (>3g per serving) is ideal for sustained energy and digestion.

  Limit added sugars (aim for less than 10% of daily calories from added sugars).
- **Protein:** Helps with muscle maintenance and satiety.

  High protein: >10g per serving.

  Good source of protein: 5 to 9g per serving.

  Moderate protein: 2 to 4g per serving.
- **Fats:** Healthy fats (unsaturated fats like olive oil, nuts, avocado) are beneficial.

  Limit saturated fats (aim for less than 10% of daily calories).

  Avoid trans fats (look for "partially hydrogenated oils" in the ingredients list).

Micronutrients (Vitamins & Minerals)

- Aim for higher % Daily Value (DV) in key nutrients: Fiber, vitamin D, calcium, iron, and potassium are often under-consumed.
- High sodium (over 20% DV per serving) can contribute to high blood pressure.

Ingredient List

Ingredients are listed in descending order by weight—the first few items make up the bulk of the product.

THE 3-3-2-2-1 Hack When You Don't Have Time to Meal-Prep

So, what happens if you forgot, or simply didn't have time to meal plan and draw up an organized grocery list for the week? You don't want to cruise the grocery store in a haphazard way and end up with a bunch of impractical impulse purchases. This is my hack for those times so you can still shop and eat nutritiously. It's as simple as this:

Move through the store and shop for . . .

3 VEGGIES—ONE veggie to pair with a meal, ONE leafy green, and ONE veggie for snacking.

3 PROTEINS—ONE meatless protein (BEANS!), ONE seafood protein (tuna, salmon, etc.), and ONE meaty dinner entrée like chicken or beef.

2 GRAINS—ONE grain for dinner, such as quinoa or rice, and ONE grain for breakfast like whole-grain toast or oatmeal.

2 FRUITS—ONE for snacking (an apple, grapes) and ONE for a meal (fruit topping for salad or oatmeal).

1 DIP OR SPREAD—ONE hummus pack, yogurt dip, etc.

That's it! Easy.

Day 3: MEAL PREP

Sunday, my Day #3, is usually when I do my weekly meal prep. And I'm not talking about lining up a bunch of same size and shape containers on my kitchen counter and putting the same chicken, broccoli, rice, etc. into them. That would mean that you're basically eating the same thing every day of the week. No thank you very much! I like to diversify my meals and am way more flexible and fun when it comes to my meal prep.

First, I prep grains and lentils for the week. Grains that I often cook a big batch of for the week include farro, barley, quinoa, rice, oats, etc. And I love all lentils—red, brown, green, black, gimme! All of these can be in the fridge for several days and ready to go for any meal of the day.

Then, I'll prep a good deal of my fruits and vegetables, especially if they're doubling as the week's snacks. That means different things for different fruits and veggies, but I basically peel, slice, and chop them up (or rinse and spin them if they're greens), so that they're ready to eat. If I'm hungry during the day on a weekday, and I see a big watermelon that's uncut, there's little to no way I'm going to get out my knife then and there and chop and slice that up. Instead, I'm more than likely to reach for that bag of chips, or something junkier and easier.

As far as prepped produce storage goes, I tend to put all my fruit in one tightly lidded container, all of my rinsed and spinned/dried leafy greens in another, and all of my prepped veggies in another.

That's the gist. Sometimes I'll cook a big pot of something on the weekend for the week—a curry, soup, or stew—or I'll roast a bunch of veggies and protein—but usually I just cook a grain or lentil and prep some produce, and that gets me in good enough shape for easy to whip up a.m. to p.m. meals and snacks.

That's my advice and flexible how-to for meal planning + shopping + prepping. I hope it helps you. There are obviously weeks when none of this happens. Sometimes, life is just too chaotic to make it work. I try to stick to this as much as possible, though, because it feels good, tastes good, and it makes my week brighter and better.

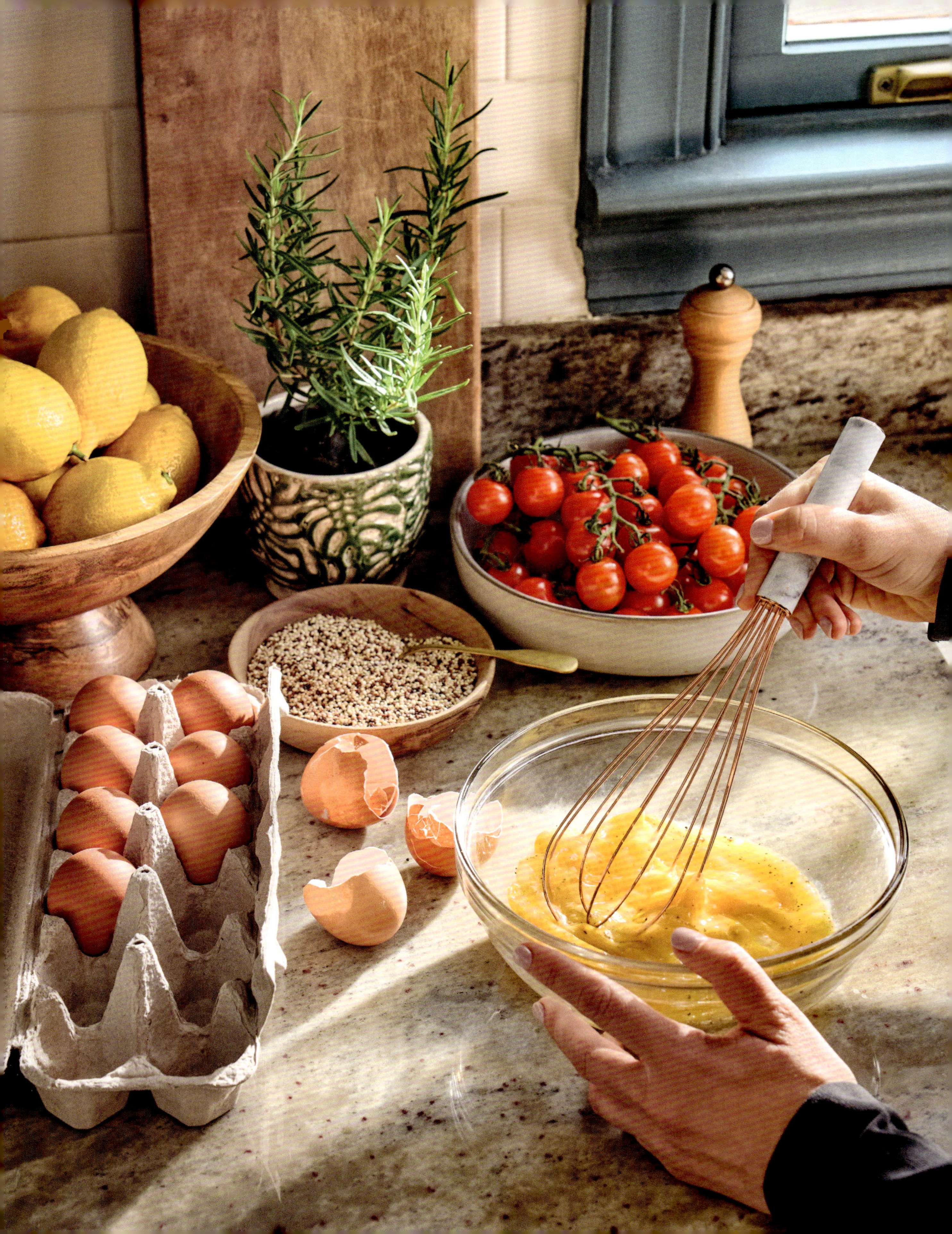

Savory Start to the Day

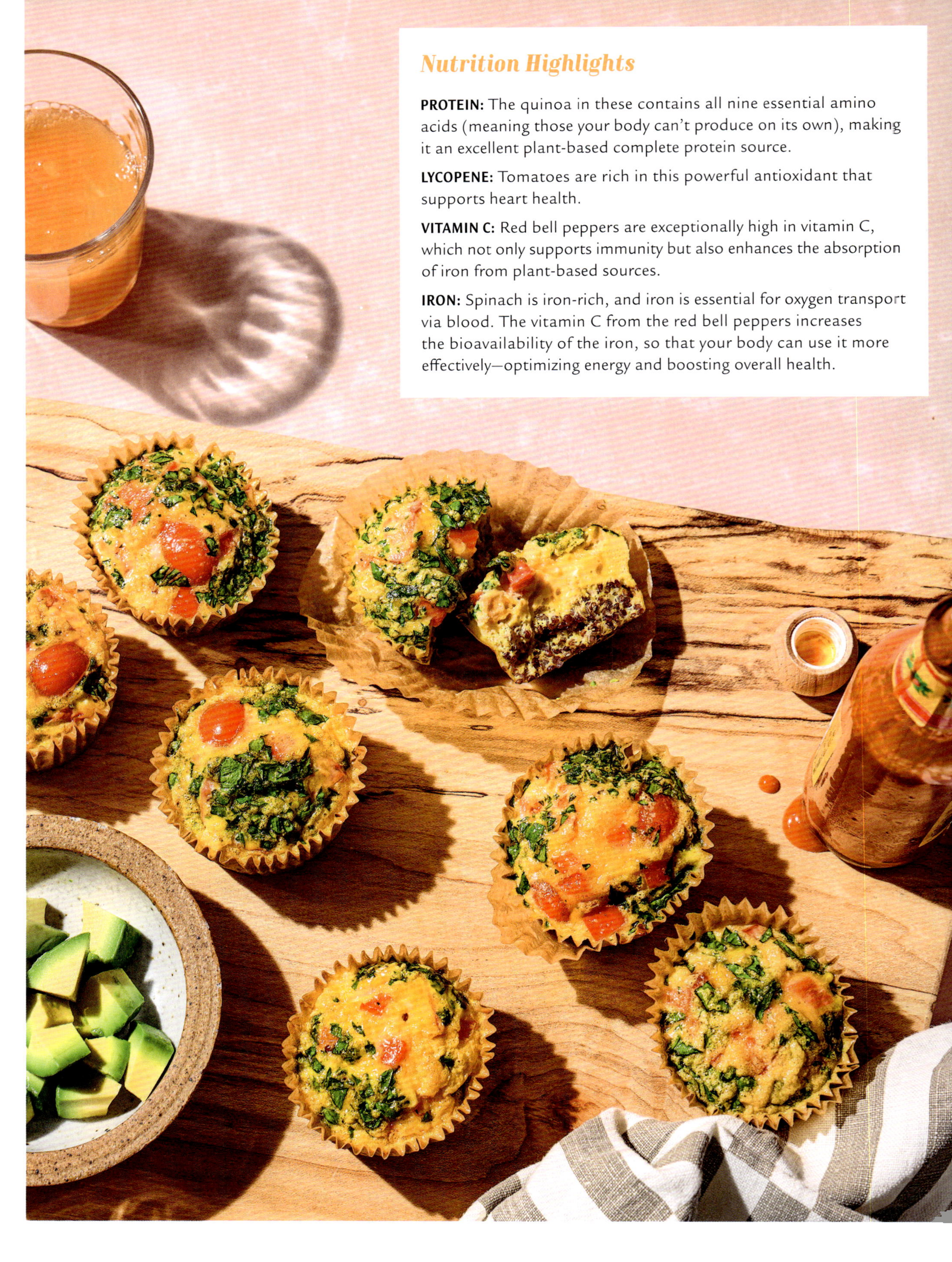

Nutrition Highlights

PROTEIN: The quinoa in these contains all nine essential amino acids (meaning those your body can't produce on its own), making it an excellent plant-based complete protein source.

LYCOPENE: Tomatoes are rich in this powerful antioxidant that supports heart health.

VITAMIN C: Red bell peppers are exceptionally high in vitamin C, which not only supports immunity but also enhances the absorption of iron from plant-based sources.

IRON: Spinach is iron-rich, and iron is essential for oxygen transport via blood. The vitamin C from the red bell peppers increases the bioavailability of the iron, so that your body can use it more effectively—optimizing energy and boosting overall health.

Eggy Quinoa Cups

MAKES 12 | SERVES 4 TO 6
PREP TIME: 10 minutes
COOK TIME: 40 minutes

PER SERVING:	CALORIES 315 kcal	PROTEIN 18g	FAT 20g	CARBOHYDRATE 14g	FIBER 5g

Cooking spray or neutral oil, for the muffin tin

2 cups chicken broth (or preferred broth)

1 cup quinoa, rinsed

1 cup grated sharp Cheddar cheese

8 large eggs

1 teaspoon onion powder

½ teaspoon kosher salt

¼ teaspoon freshly ground black pepper

½ cup quartered cherry tomatoes

¾ cup diced red bell pepper

1 cup lightly packed baby spinach, chopped

1 avocado (optional), sliced or diced

Hot sauce (optional), for serving

I really love frittatas, but I only make them for special occasions since they take so long to prepare. These cute little egg cups, essentially mini frittatas, come together quickly and are easily portioned for serving.

I like them at any temperature, which is why I often eat them straight out of the fridge on busy mornings. The recipe calls for sharp Cheddar but any cheese will work—Parmesan, pepper Jack for a little heat, creamy goat cheese. And feel free to use different veggies!

Preheat the oven to 350°F. Lightly grease 12 cups of a standard muffin tin with cooking spray or oil or line with muffin liners.

In a medium pot, combine the broth and quinoa and bring to a boil over high heat. Once boiling, give it a quick stir and decrease the heat to low. Cover and simmer until the quinoa is tender and the broth is completely absorbed, 12 to 15 minutes. Residual broth in the quinoa will make the cups too moist and they will fall apart.

Transfer the cooked quinoa to a medium bowl and stir in the Cheddar until it's combined and melty. In another medium bowl, whisk the eggs with the onion powder, salt, and pepper.

Fill each muffin cup with a scant ¼ cup of the cheesy quinoa, pressing down lightly to form them. Top each cup evenly with the tomatoes, bell peppers, and spinach. Pour the egg mixture evenly over each cup ( ), about 2 heaping tablespoons per cup. The cups will be quite full.

Transfer the muffin tin to the oven and bake until the cups are set in the middle and cooked through, 20 to 25 minutes. Insert a knife into the middle of one or more to check. The veggies at the top of the cups will be juicy, but the quinoa and egg should be fairly firm and set.

Set aside to cool for about 10 minutes before removing the quinoa cups from the muffin tin. If you are not using muffin liners, use a small rubber spatula or table knife, along with a small spoon to carefully scoop them out.

If desired, serve garnished with avocado or hot sauce.

STORAGE + REHEAT

Once cooled, store airtight in the refrigerator for up to 4 days. To reheat, warm in a pan over medium heat or microwave. Add the avocado or hot sauce right before serving.

STEPH'S TIP

To avoid a mess, transfer the whisked eggs to a liquid measuring cup. Pour them from it into a tablespoon over each muffin cup.

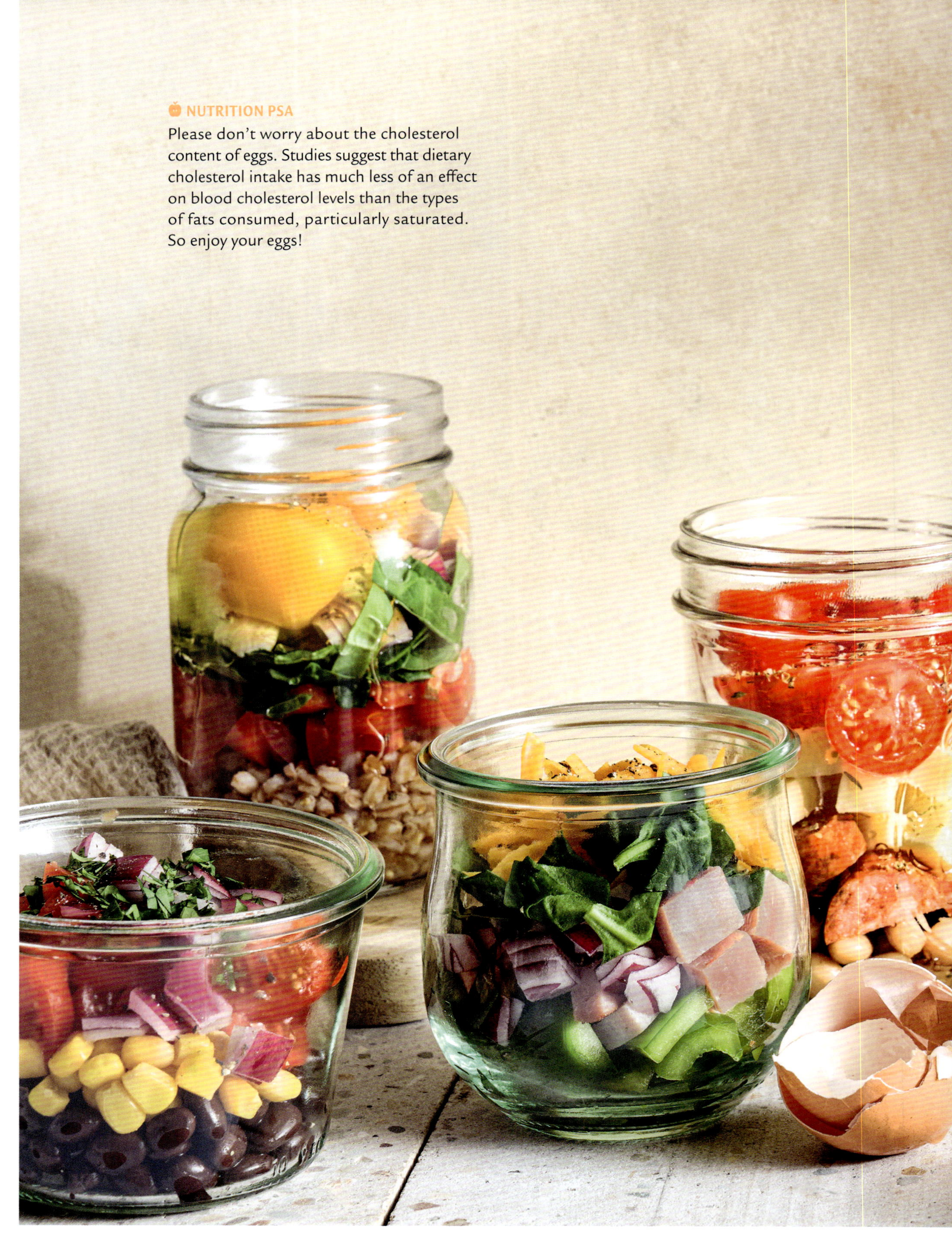

NUTRITION PSA

Please don't worry about the cholesterol content of eggs. Studies suggest that dietary cholesterol intake has much less of an effect on blood cholesterol levels than the types of fats consumed, particularly saturated. So enjoy your eggs!

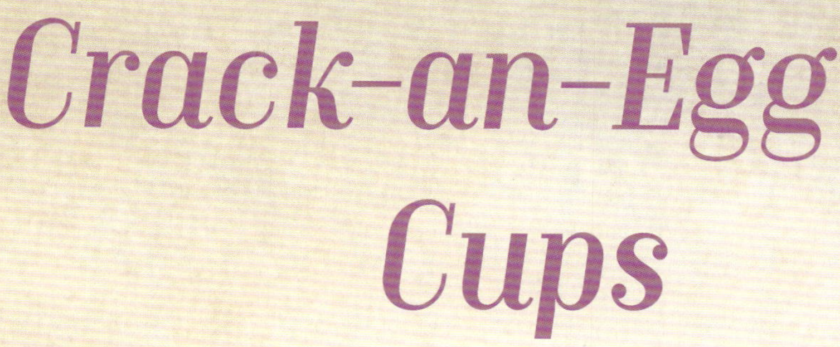

Crack-an-Egg Cups

My Crack-an-Egg Cups are all about boosting protein intake and sneaking in some a.m. veggies. Meal prep made easy.

For the following recipes, you simply chop up the veggies, prep additional ingredients, and layer everything in your jar. In the morning, crack in a couple eggs, season, stir, and pop it in the microwave. In just a few minutes, you've got breakfast! I love how the eggs expand and fluff up in the jar as they cook.

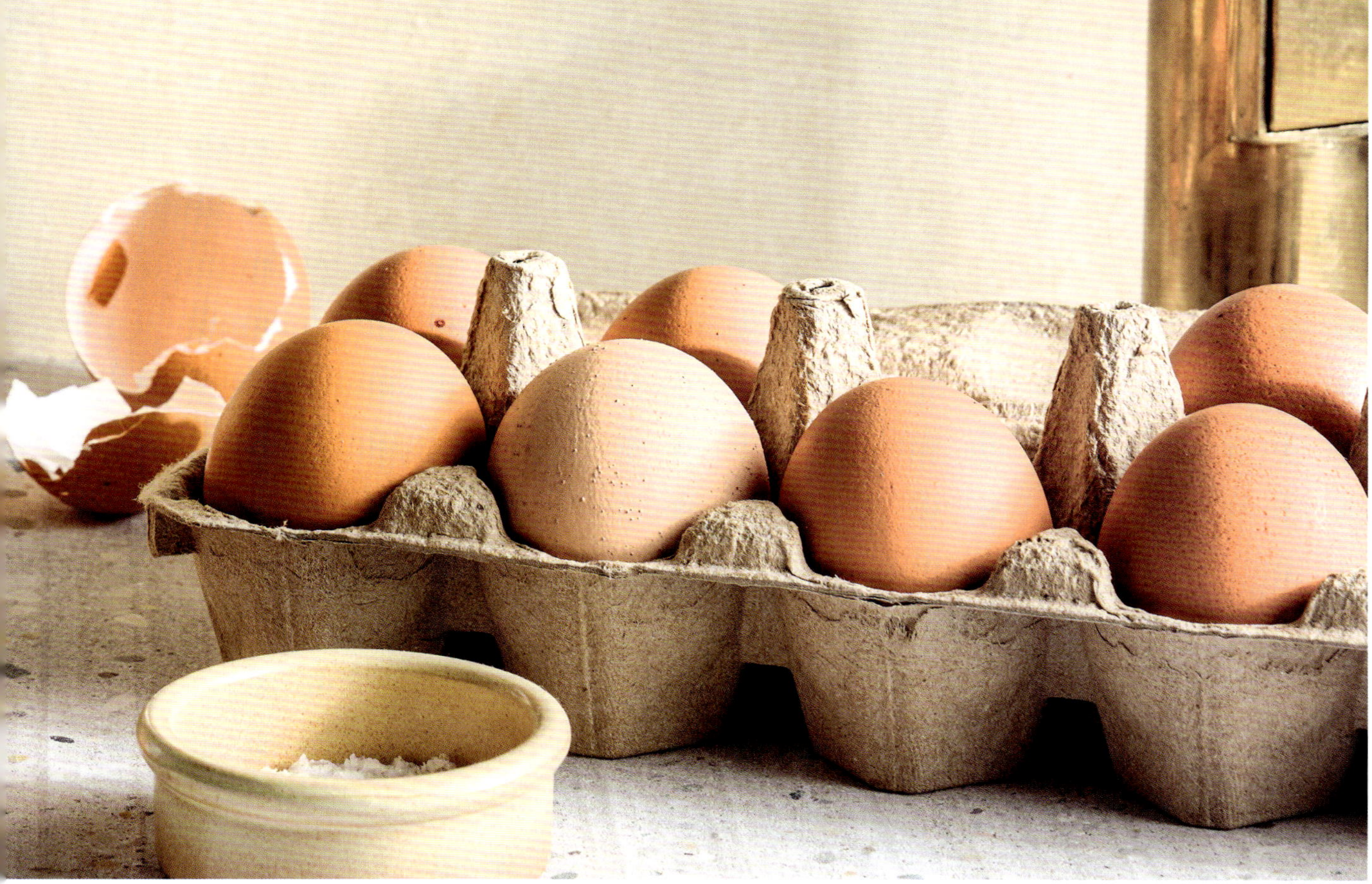

Farro, Feta & Tomato Egg Cup

SERVES 1
PREP TIME: 5 minutes
COOK TIME: 3 minutes

PER SERVING:	CALORIES 253 kcal	PROTEIN 17g	FAT 12g	CARBOHYDRATE 18g	FIBER 3g

- ⅓ cup cooked farro
- ¼ cup chopped tomatoes
- ⅓ cup lightly packed spinach, chopped
- 1 tablespoon finely chopped red onion
- 1 tablespoon crumbled feta cheese
- 2 large eggs
- ⅛ to ¼ teaspoon kosher salt
- A pinch to ⅛ teaspoon freshly ground black pepper

Farro is an ancient grain chock-full of fiber, protein, and magnesium. And, as a whole, rather than refined, grain it delivers long-lasting energy, focus, and satiety. Coupling it with the feta, spinach, red onion, and tomatoes, as I do here, makes for a colorful, flavorful start to your day.

In a 1-pint canning jar, add the cooked farro ( ), tomatoes, spinach, onion, and feta. Secure with a lid and refrigerate for up to 5 days.

When ready to cook, crack the eggs into the jar, season with the salt and pepper to taste, and stir well with a fork, breaking up the yolks as you stir.

Microwave for 1 minute, then carefully stir again. The eggs should be a little frothy with parts starting to set. Microwave for an additional 1½ to 2½ minutes, checking the egg cup every 30 seconds or so, until the eggs are fully set and cooked through. Carefully remove the jar from the microwave and enjoy right away! It's best enjoyed day of.

YOU DO YOU

Instead of farro, use the same amount of cooked or canned chickpeas or any leftover cooked grain. Or try goat cheese instead of the feta.

STEPH'S TIP

To cook the farro, start with 1 cup of farro. (It will yield 2 cups and having leftover cooked farro is never a bad thing. Toss it into salads, soups, wraps, etc.) In a small pot, combine 3½ cups of lightly salted water and the farro and bring to a boil. Cover, lower the heat, and simmer until the farro is tender, has a slight bite, and has absorbed most of the water, 25 to 45 minutes (cook times vary widely). Drain off any remaining water, and enjoy. Store in an airtight container and refrigerate for up to 5 days.

Cannellini Bean, Sausage & Mozzarella Egg Cup

SERVES 1
PREP TIME: 5 minutes
COOK TIME: 3 minutes

PER SERVING:	CALORIES 353 kcal	PROTEIN 30g	FAT 24g	CARBOHYDRATE 15g	FIBER 3g

¼ cup canned cannellini beans, drained and rinsed

⅓ cup diced precooked Italian sausage or another preferred meat or veggie sausage

¼ cup halved or quartered cherry tomatoes

2 tablespoons cubed mozzarella cheese

2 large eggs

⅛ to ¼ teaspoon kosher salt

¼ teaspoon Italian seasoning

This is my a.m., eggy, get-you-going version of a slice of pizza or baked pasta. And it's healthy! You get protein from the eggs and Italian sausage, healthy carbs from the beans, and essential vitamins from the cherry tomatoes.

In a 1-pint canning jar, add the beans, sausage, tomatoes, and mozzarella. Secure with a lid and refrigerate for up to 5 days.

When ready to cook, crack the eggs into the jar, season with the salt to taste and Italian seasoning, and stir well with a fork, breaking up the yolks as you stir.

Microwave, uncovered, for 1 minute, then carefully stir again. The eggs should be a little frothy with parts starting to set. Microwave for an additional 1½ to 2½ minutes, checking the egg cup every 30 seconds or so, until the eggs are fully set and cooked through. Carefully remove the jar from the microwave and enjoy right away! It's best enjoyed day of.

Black Bean, Corn & Tomato Egg Cup

SERVES 1
PREP TIME: 5 minutes
COOK TIME: 3 minutes

PER SERVING:	**CALORIES** 241 kcal	**PROTEIN** 18g	**FAT** 9g	**CARBOHYDRATE** 23g	**FIBER** 7g

⅓ cup canned black beans, drained and rinsed

¼ cup corn kernels, canned, fresh, or thawed frozen

¼ cup chopped tomatoes

1 tablespoon finely chopped red onion

2 large eggs

⅛ to ¼ teaspoon kosher salt

A pinch to ⅛ teaspoon freshly ground black pepper

Chopped fresh cilantro (optional), for garnish

This is my simplified spin on huevos rancheros—in a cup! The corn adds a touch of natural sweetness and gives you energy thanks to the carbs. Along with the protein-rich eggs and beans, and all the fiber-full veggies, you'll be ready to tackle the day.

In a 1-pint canning jar, add the black beans, corn, tomatoes, and onion. Secure with a lid and refrigerate for up to 5 days.

When ready to cook, crack the eggs into the jar, season with the salt and pepper to taste, and stir well with a fork, breaking up the yolks as you stir.

Microwave, uncovered, for 1 minute, then carefully stir again. The eggs should be a little frothy with parts starting to set. Microwave for an additional 1½ to 2½ minutes, checking the egg cup every 30 seconds or so, until the eggs are fully set and cooked through. Carefully remove the jar from the microwave, top it with the cilantro (if using), and enjoy right away! It's best enjoyed day of.

Ham, Spinach & Cheddar Egg Cup

SERVES 1
PREP TIME: 5 minutes
COOK TIME: 3 minutes

PER SERVING:	**CALORIES** 283 kcal	**PROTEIN** 26g	**FAT** 17g	**CARBOHYDRATE** 6g	**FIBER** 1g

⅓ cup diced ham

¼ cup chopped green bell pepper

¼ cup finely chopped red onion

⅓ cup lightly packed spinach, chopped

2 tablespoons grated Cheddar cheese

⅛ to ¼ teaspoon kosher salt

A pinch to ⅛ teaspoon freshly ground black pepper

2 large eggs

I always feel like I'm eating a little diner omelet in a cup—ham, Cheddar, green bell pepper, spinach—when I make this one. It's very satisfying. Feel free to use a different protein if you like. I just recommend using a precooked protein, such as ham or a precooked sausage, because then you don't have an additional step.

In a 1-pint canning jar, add the ham, bell pepper, onion, spinach, and Cheddar. Secure with a lid and refrigerate for up to 5 days.

When ready to cook, crack the eggs into the jar, season with the salt and pepper to taste, and stir well with a fork, breaking up the yolks as you stir.

Microwave, uncovered, for 1 minute, then carefully stir again. The eggs should be a little frothy with parts starting to set. Microwave for an additional 1½ to 2½ minutes, checking the egg cup every 30 seconds or so, until the eggs are fully set and cooked through. Carefully remove the jar from the microwave and enjoy right away! It's best enjoyed day of.

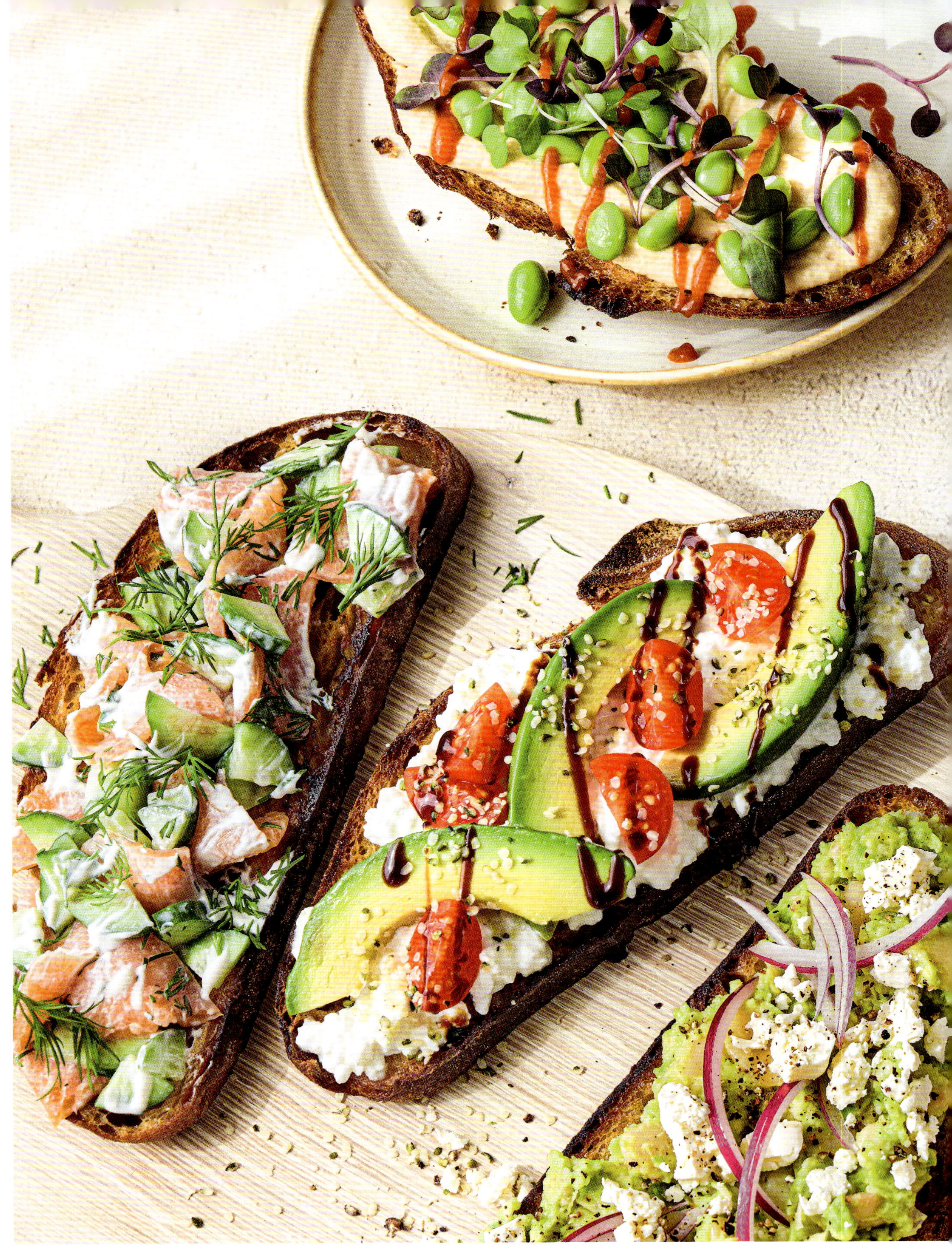

Savory Toasts

I'm Team Savory 100 percent. These four nutrition-loaded savory toasts are my kind of breakfast. I highly recommend a multi-seed, hefty, wide sandwich bread for them. You want plenty of room for all the toppings and a substantial bread (nothing thin or mushy) that can hold up. Also, feel free to butter or drizzle any of these toasts with olive oil before topping them. I often do.

White Bean, Feta & Avocado Toast

SERVES 1
PREP TIME: 5 minutes
COOK TIME: 2 to 3 minutes

PER SERVING:	**CALORIES** 370 kcal	**PROTEIN** 14g	**FAT** 21g	**CARBOHYDRATE** 42g	**FIBER** 16g

½ avocado

½ cup canned or cooked Great Northern, butter, navy, or cannellini beans, drained and rinsed if canned

1 teaspoon fresh lime juice

Kosher salt and freshly ground black pepper

1 large slice sandwich bread

4 to 6 thin slices red onion, to taste

2 tablespoons crumbled feta cheese

The avocado toast trend has been going strong for a while, which is great since avocado is rich in healthy fats that are both good for your heart and for lowering cholesterol. I *love* avocado toast, but sadly most renditions don't include protein. Hello, white beans! I've got you.

In a small bowl, combine the avocado and beans. Using a potato masher or the bottom of a canning jar or sturdy cup, mash together until they are fairly smooth. Add the lime juice and salt and pepper to taste and stir to combine.

Toast the bread until golden brown and nicely crisped. Spread the avocado/bean mixture evenly over the toast. Top with the red onion and feta. Finish it with salt and pepper to taste. Slice the toast in half, if you like, and enjoy right away!

NUTRITION PSA
Draining and rinsing canned beans can reduce their sodium content by up to 40%!

Cottage Cheese, Tomato & Avocado Toast

SERVES 1
PREP TIME: 5 minutes
COOK TIME: 2 to 3 minutes

PER SERVING:	**CALORIES** 340 kcal	**PROTEIN** 16g	**FAT** 18g	**CARBOHYDRATE** 29g	**FIBER** 10g

1 large slice sandwich bread

⅓ cup 2% cottage cheese or whatever fat content you prefer

¼ cup halved or quartered cherry tomatoes

½ avocado, sliced

1½ teaspoons hemp hearts (hulled hemp seeds)

Kosher salt and freshly ground black pepper

Drizzle of Balsamic Glaze, homemade (page 172) or store-bought

I've been a fan of cottage cheese forever, well before it was trending. This is one of my favorite savory toasts, and it keeps you going for hours after eating it. Don't skimp on the hemp hearts! They're delicious and nutritious with a lovely bite—they're also in my Lizzo Salad (page 125), Hearty Kidney Beans & Sweet Potato Bowl (page 139), and Veggie Crafted Beef Mac & Cheese (page 232).

Toast the bread until golden brown and nicely crisped. Spread the cottage cheese evenly over the toast. Arrange the tomatoes and avocado on top. Sprinkle with the hemp hearts and salt and pepper to taste, and drizzle with the balsamic glaze. Slice the toast in half, if you like, and enjoy right away!

Smoked Salmon & Cucumber Toast

SERVES 1
PREP TIME: 5 minutes
COOK TIME: 2 to 3 minutes

PER SERVING:	**CALORIES** 199 kcal	**PROTEIN** 18g	**FAT** 4g	**CARBOHYDRATE** 21g	**FIBER** 3g

2 ounces smoked salmon, chopped (heaping ⅓ cup)

¼ cup thinly sliced quartered English or salad cucumber

2 tablespoons nonfat or low-fat Greek yogurt

1½ teaspoons chopped fresh dill, plus more for garnish

1 teaspoon fresh lemon juice

Kosher salt and freshly ground black pepper

1 large slice sandwich bread

I've always been a lox plate enthusiast. This toast basically turns all those components into a creamy, crunchy, citrusy toast topper. Yum! Lucky you, salmon is quite high in omega-3 fatty acids, which are crucial for heart health and brain function.

In a small bowl, stir together the salmon, cucumber, yogurt, dill, lemon juice, and salt and pepper to taste.

Toast the bread until golden brown and nicely crisped. Spread the salmon mixture evenly over the toast. Garnish with more fresh dill, slice the toast in half, if you like, and enjoy right away!

Hummus & Edamame Toast

SERVES 1
PREP TIME: 5 minutes
COOK TIME: 2 to 3 minutes

PER SERVING:	**CALORIES** 231 kcal	**PROTEIN** 13g	**FAT** 9g	**CARBOHYDRATE** 29g	**FIBER** 7g

1 large slice sandwich bread

¼ cup hummus (whatever homemade or store-bought type you prefer)

⅓ cup lightly packed microgreens

¼ cup shelled edamame, cooked (I use frozen and follow package cooking directions)

1 teaspoon fresh lemon juice

Kosher salt and freshly ground black pepper

Sriracha sauce (optional), for serving

Edamame do not get the attention they deserve. They're a complete source of protein (one of only a handful of plant proteins that are!) loaded up with all nine essential amino acids. They're also high in fiber, really easy to source (in the freezer aisle!) and to prepare (I usually boil or cook them in the microwave), and super tasty. The hummus is basically savory glue for the edamame and microgreens.

Toast the bread until golden brown and nicely crisped. Spread the hummus evenly over the toast and top it with the microgreens and edamame. Drizzle with the lemon juice and season with salt and pepper to taste. Drizzle with the Sriracha (if using) and slice the toast in half if you like. Enjoy right away!

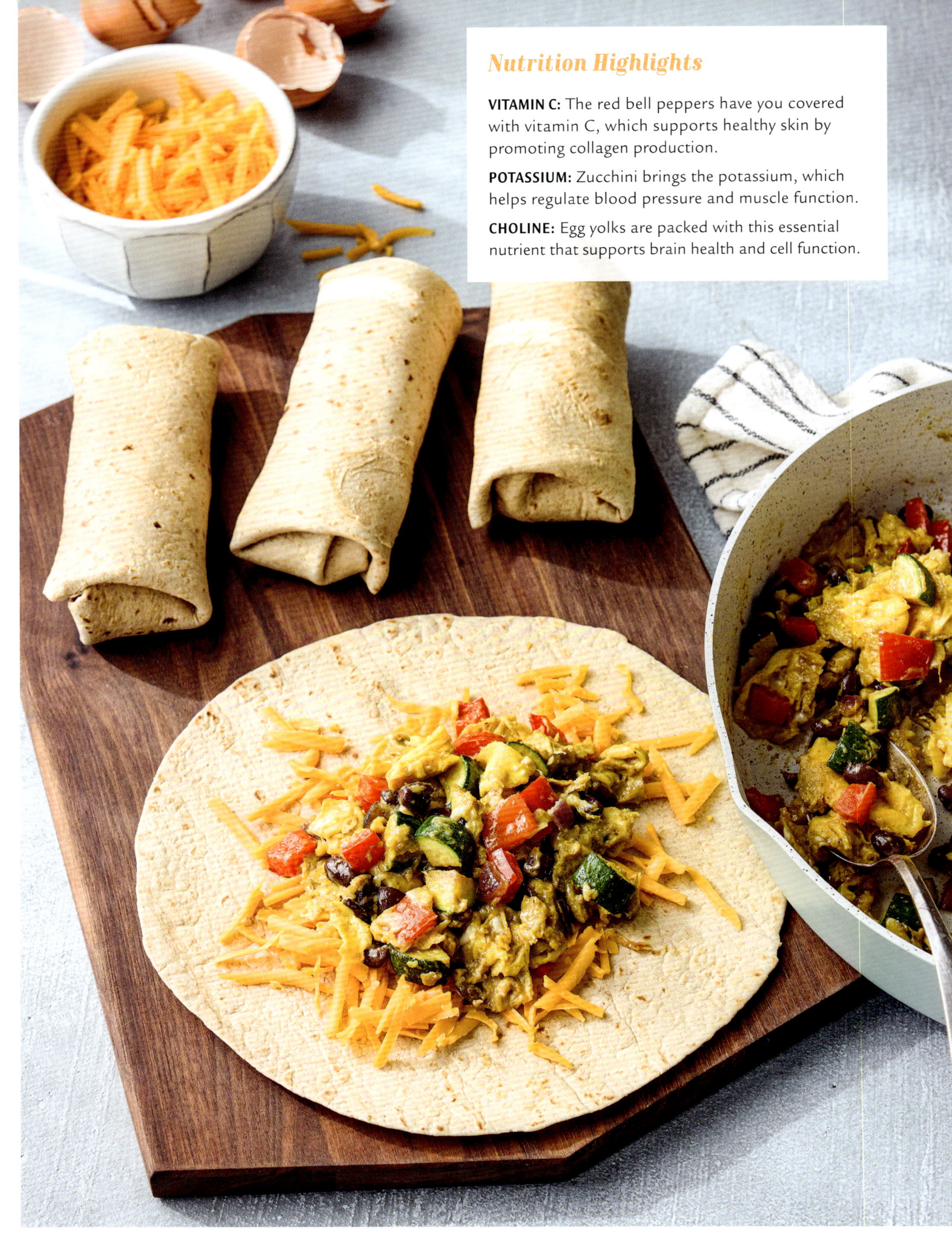

Nutrition Highlights

VITAMIN C: The red bell peppers have you covered with vitamin C, which supports healthy skin by promoting collagen production.

POTASSIUM: Zucchini brings the potassium, which helps regulate blood pressure and muscle function.

CHOLINE: Egg yolks are packed with this essential nutrient that supports brain health and cell function.

Freezer-Friendly Breakfast Burritos

SERVES 6
PREP TIME: 15 minutes
COOK TIME: 15 minutes

PER SERVING:	CALORIES 391 kcal	PROTEIN 22g	FAT 21g	CARBOHYDRATE 31g	FIBER 7g

- 1 tablespoon extra-virgin olive oil
- 2 red bell peppers, diced
- 1 zucchini, diced
- 1 small red onion, diced
- 1 teaspoon chili powder
- 1 teaspoon ground cumin
- 1 teaspoon garlic powder
- 1 teaspoon kosher salt, divided
- ½ teaspoon sweet paprika
- ¼ teaspoon freshly ground black pepper
- 8 large eggs
- 1 cup canned or cooked black beans, drained and rinsed if canned
- 6 large burrito-size whole-wheat or flour tortillas
- 1½ cups grated Cheddar cheese, divided

These are perfect for busy mornings. They're satisfying, easy to prepare in advance, and great with whatever veggies you have on hand. The combo of protein, fiber, and healthy fats equals a well-rounded, energy-sustaining, tasty start to the day.

In a large pan, heat the olive oil over medium heat until hot. Add the bell peppers, zucchini, and onion. Cook, stirring occasionally, until the vegetables have softened, about 5 minutes. Stir in the chili powder, cumin, garlic powder, ½ teaspoon of the salt, the paprika, and pepper. Cook until the spices are fragrant, 2 to 3 minutes.

In a medium bowl, whisk the eggs. Pour them over the vegetable mixture and cook, lightly stirring, nudging, and folding everything with a heatproof spatula or wooden spoon, until the eggs are fully cooked, about 2 minutes. Add the black beans, and the remaining ½ teaspoon salt and cook for about 1 minute, until the beans are warmed through. Remove from the heat and set aside.

Lay out the tortillas on a clean flat surface. Place 2 to 3 tablespoons of the Cheddar in the middle of each tortilla. Top with 1 heaping cup of the egg and veggie mixture, leaving about a 1-inch border all around. Evenly top each with the remaining cheese, about 1 heaping tablespoon per burrito.

Carefully fold the tortilla up from the bottom over the filling, then fold in the sides, and roll the burrito until it is snug and sealed. For easier handling, and to prevent any filling from falling out, tightly wrap each burrito that you are going to eat right away in parchment or waxed paper, tucking in the ends as you roll the same way that you rolled up the burrito. Enjoy right away.

STORAGE + REHEAT

If making for later, cool to room temperature and then refrigerate for up to 3 days.

To freeze: Once cooled to room temperature, wrap each tightly with plastic wrap and freeze them individually overnight (8 hours or more). Once frozen, place them all in a large resealable freezer bag or airtight container for up to 3 months.

To reheat: Transfer the frozen burrito to the refrigerator the night before. Once fully thawed, microwave on high for 1 to 4 minutes, flipping the burrito about halfway through, or heat in a pan over medium-low heat for about 5 minutes on each side, until heated through.

Eggy Bean Hash Skillet *with* Turkey Sausage

SERVES 4 TO 6
PREP TIME: 10 minutes
COOK TIME: 25 minutes

PER SERVING:	CALORIES 475 kcal	PROTEIN 28g	FAT 26g	CARBOHYDRATE 30g	FIBER 8g

3 tablespoons extra-virgin olive oil, divided

4 uncooked sweet Italian turkey sausages (about 1 pound total), Italian chicken sausage, or 1 pound seasoned bulk turkey or chicken sausage, coarsely sliced

½ red onion, diced

1 red bell pepper, diced

1 zucchini, diced

One 15-ounce can pinto beans (or 1½ cups cooked beans), drained and rinsed

One 15-ounce can cannellini beans (or 1½ cups cooked beans), drained and rinsed

1 teaspoon smoked paprika

1 teaspoon kosher salt, plus more to taste

½ teaspoon garlic powder

¼ teaspoon red pepper flakes

4 large eggs

Freshly ground black pepper

½ avocado, sliced

Hot sauce (optional)

This is my go-to breakfast on a slow and cozy Sunday after a late night out or a few glasses of wine at home. It satisfies my comfort food craving and also replenishes my body with nutrients. It's also an excellent way to clear the week's left behind veg from the fridge before they pass the point of no return. Dice them up and throw them in. Here's to food waste prevention! I often make this on the weekend for future me. I enjoy a bit then, and the leftover hash is easy to reheat and eat during the week.

In a large pan, heat 1 tablespoon of the olive oil over medium heat. When hot, add the sausage and cook, breaking it apart with a heatproof spatula or wooden spoon as it cooks, until it is nicely browned, 7 to 9 minutes. Transfer the cooked turkey sausage to a plate. Set aside.

Add the remaining 2 tablespoons olive oil and the onion to the same pan (no need to wipe it out or wash it) and cook, stirring occasionally, until the onion begins to soften, about 3 minutes. Add the bell pepper and zucchini and cook, stirring occasionally, until they are tender, about 5 minutes. Add the pinto beans, cannellini beans, sausage, smoked paprika, salt, garlic powder, and pepper flakes. Cook for 3 to 4 minutes, stirring occasionally, to heat through.

Use a spoon or spatula to create four small wells or pockets in the hash. Gently crack an egg into each well. Decrease the heat to medium-low, cover the pan, and cook until the egg whites are set but the yolks are still runny, 4 to 5 minutes ( ). For firmer yolks, cook a bit longer.

Remove the pan from the heat. Season with salt and pepper to taste, divide among serving plates, and add the avocado and hot sauce (if using).

STORAGE + REHEAT

Once cooled, store airtight in the refrigerator for up to 3 days. To reheat, warm in a pan over medium heat until heated through, or microwave. For best results, add the avocado and hot sauce (if using) right before serving.

STEPH'S TIP

If you prefer sunny-side up eggs with golden yolks, don't cover the pan, and continue to cook the hash and eggs for about the same amount of time, carefully nudging the whites down and into the hash, and breaking them up gently, so as not to pierce the yolks, as the eggs set.

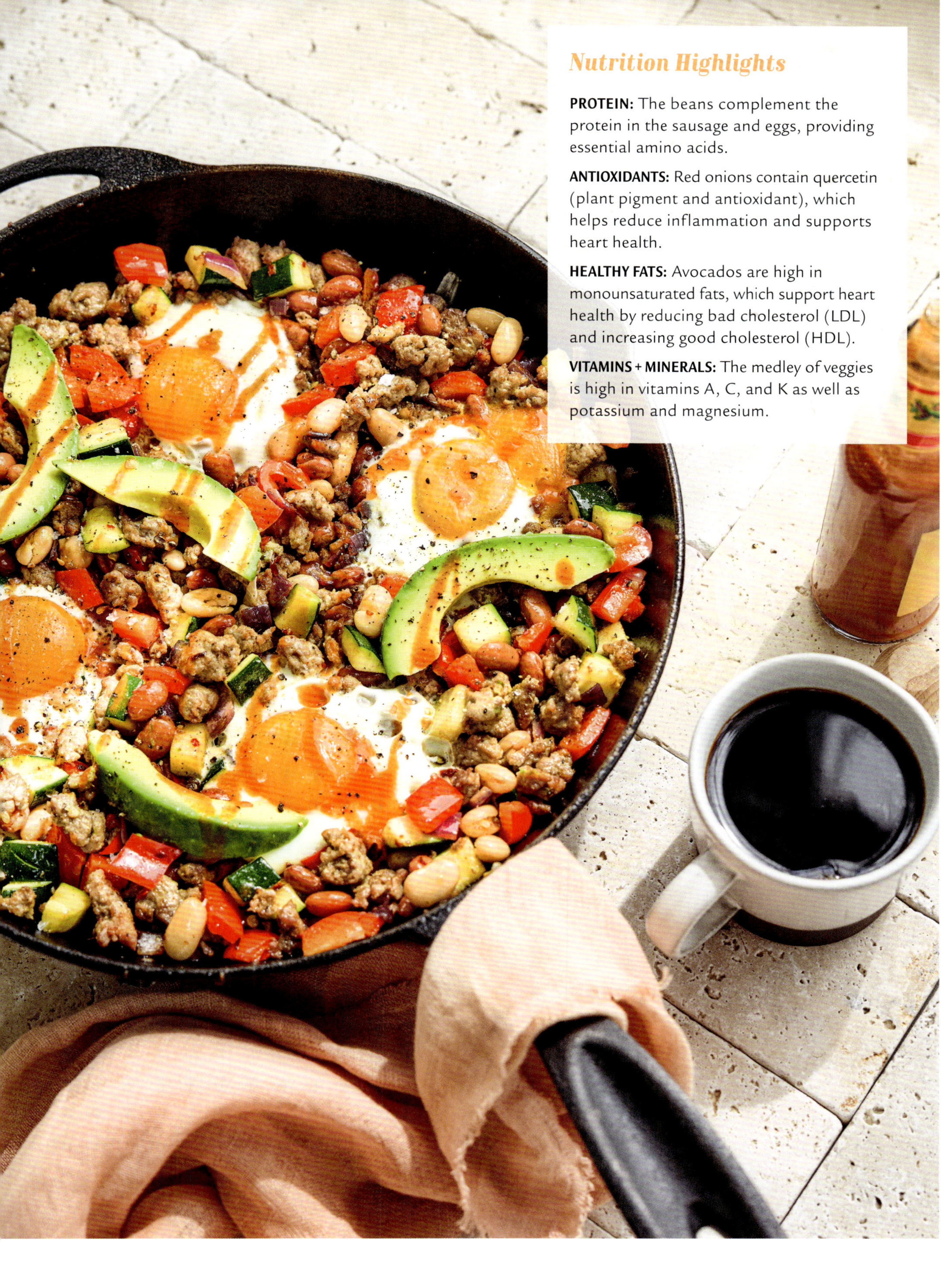

Nutrition Highlights

PROTEIN: The beans complement the protein in the sausage and eggs, providing essential amino acids.

ANTIOXIDANTS: Red onions contain quercetin (plant pigment and antioxidant), which helps reduce inflammation and supports heart health.

HEALTHY FATS: Avocados are high in monounsaturated fats, which support heart health by reducing bad cholesterol (LDL) and increasing good cholesterol (HDL).

VITAMINS + MINERALS: The medley of veggies is high in vitamins A, C, and K as well as potassium and magnesium.

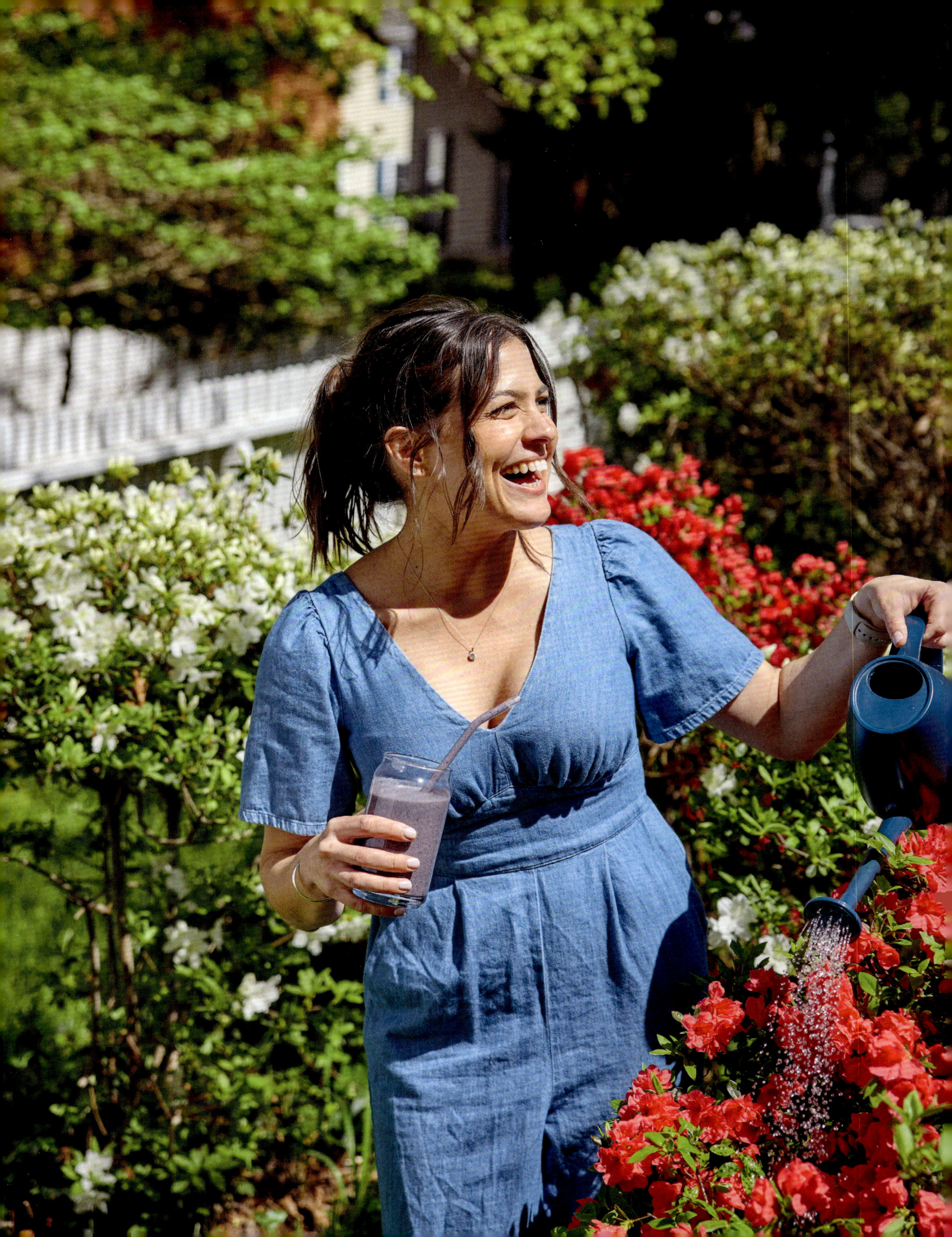

Morning

Sweet Tooth

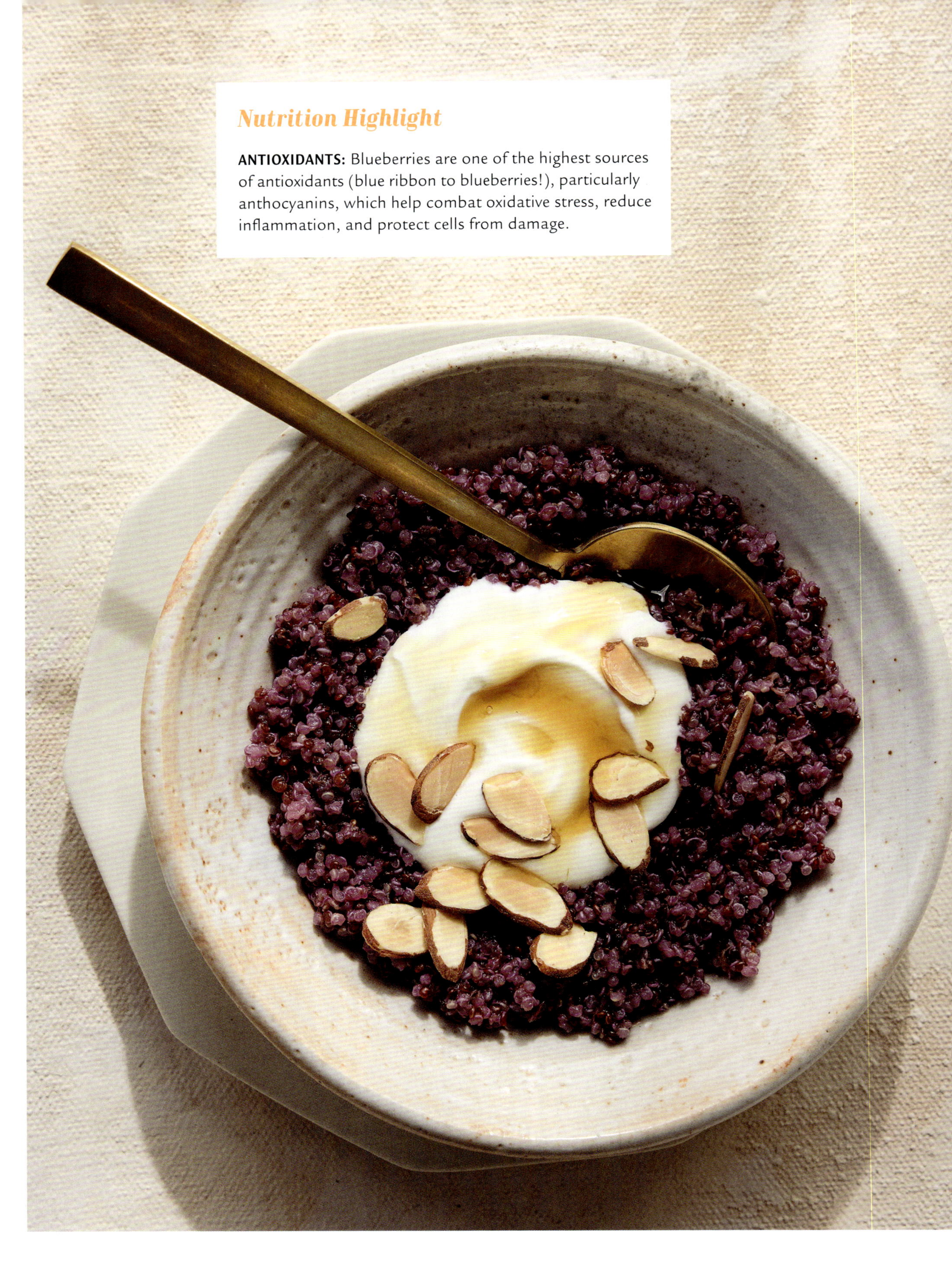

Nutrition Highlight

ANTIOXIDANTS: Blueberries are one of the highest sources of antioxidants (blue ribbon to blueberries!), particularly anthocyanins, which help combat oxidative stress, reduce inflammation, and protect cells from damage.

Blueberry Quinoa Breakfast Bowl

SERVES 1
PREP TIME: 5 minutes
COOK TIME: 15 minutes

PER SERVING:	CALORIES 533 kcal	PROTEIN 20g	FAT 15g	CARBOHYDRATE 84g	FIBER 9g

1 cup water

⅓ cup quinoa, rinsed

½ cup blueberries, fresh or frozen

2 tablespoons maple syrup, divided

2 teaspoons fresh lemon juice

⅓ cup nonfat or low-fat Greek yogurt

¼ cup sliced almonds

This bowl is a fun and tasty way to sneak protein into breakfast without cracking any eggs. Egg prices can put a dent in your wallet. This is in no small part why I get *tons* of requests online for egg-free breakfast ideas.

You get much-needed protein here from the quinoa. Consuming protein for breakfast always keeps you more satiated with stable energy levels throughout the a.m. Quinoa is loaded with other essential nutrients, and it contains all nine essential amino acids, making it a rare complete protein source among plant-based foods. Amino acids play a crucial role in building and repairing tissues, supporting immune function, producing enzymes and hormones, and maintaining overall health.

In a small pot, combine the water, quinoa, blueberries, and 1 tablespoon of the maple syrup. Stir well to incorporate and bring the mixture to a boil over medium heat. Once boiling, decrease the heat to low, cover, and simmer, stirring occasionally, until the quinoa is tender and most of the liquid has been absorbed, 12 to 15 minutes.

Remove from the heat and let the quinoa sit, covered, for 2 to 3 minutes to absorb any remaining liquid. Drizzle the quinoa with the lemon juice and fluff it with a fork.

Transfer the quinoa to a serving bowl and top it with the yogurt, almonds, and the remaining 1 tablespoon maple syrup. This dish is best enjoyed day of.

NUTRITION PSA

Reduce the carbs by 27 grams by leaving out the maple syrup.

STORAGE + REHEAT

Store airtight in the refrigerator for up to 2 days. To reheat, warm in a pan over medium-low heat until heated through, or microwave. Add a splash of water if needed to restore moisture.

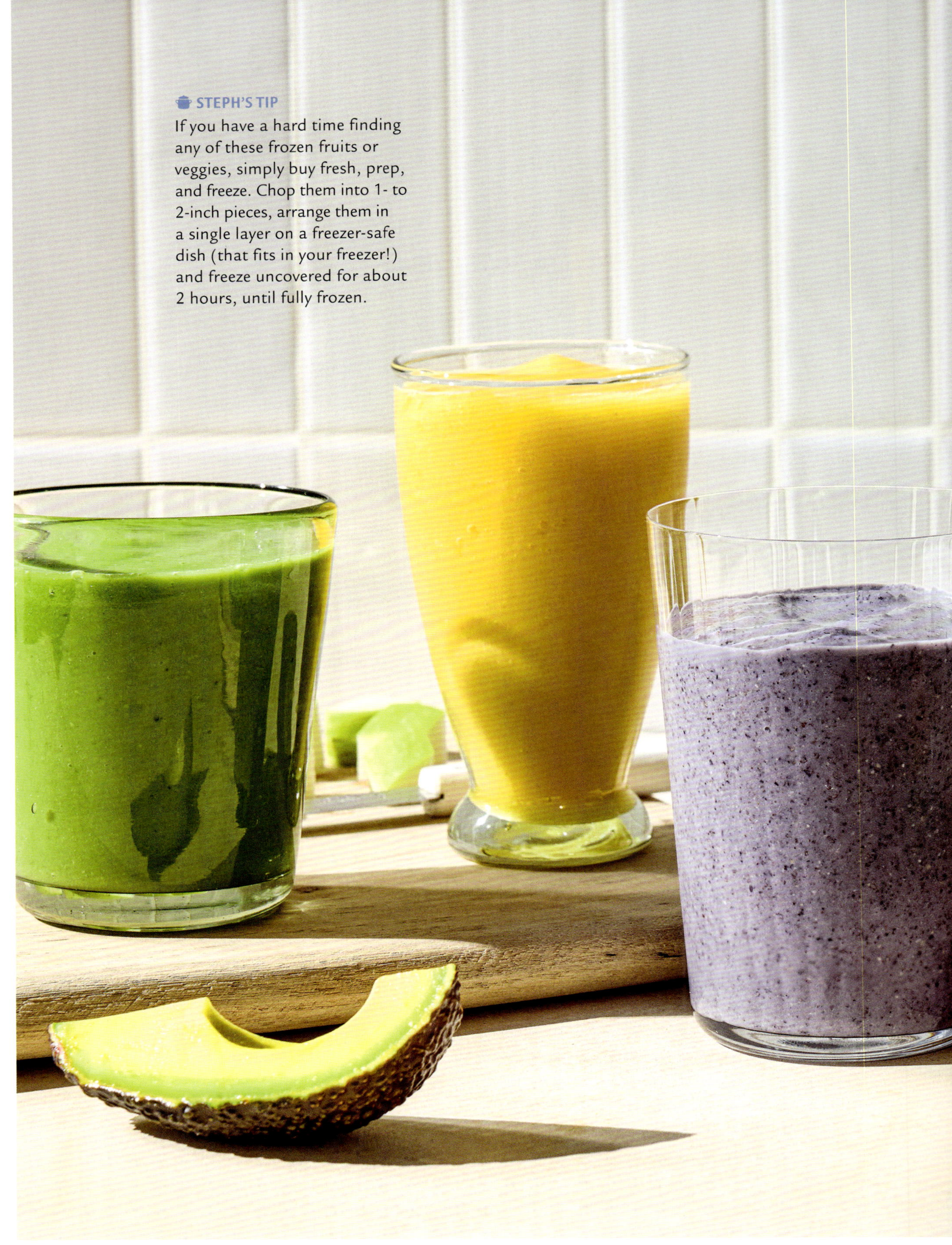

STEPH'S TIP

If you have a hard time finding any of these frozen fruits or veggies, simply buy fresh, prep, and freeze. Chop them into 1- to 2-inch pieces, arrange them in a single layer on a freezer-safe dish (that fits in your freezer!) and freeze uncovered for about 2 hours, until fully frozen.

Hidden Veggie Smoothies

Being a dietitian doesn't mean I don't know how to have a good time. I enjoy going out for drinks with friends, too, but afterward I sometimes wake up feeling a bit ugh. You too? That's when I put my professional dietitian knowledge to work and get straight to restoring my hydration and nutrient levels. Smoothies to the rescue!

Smoothies take diverse ingredients that often don't seem like they'd meld and, with the wave of a wand—or more accurately the push of a blender button—turn them into a.m. or snacky good-for-you deliciousness. Post-workout smoothies are also my jam.

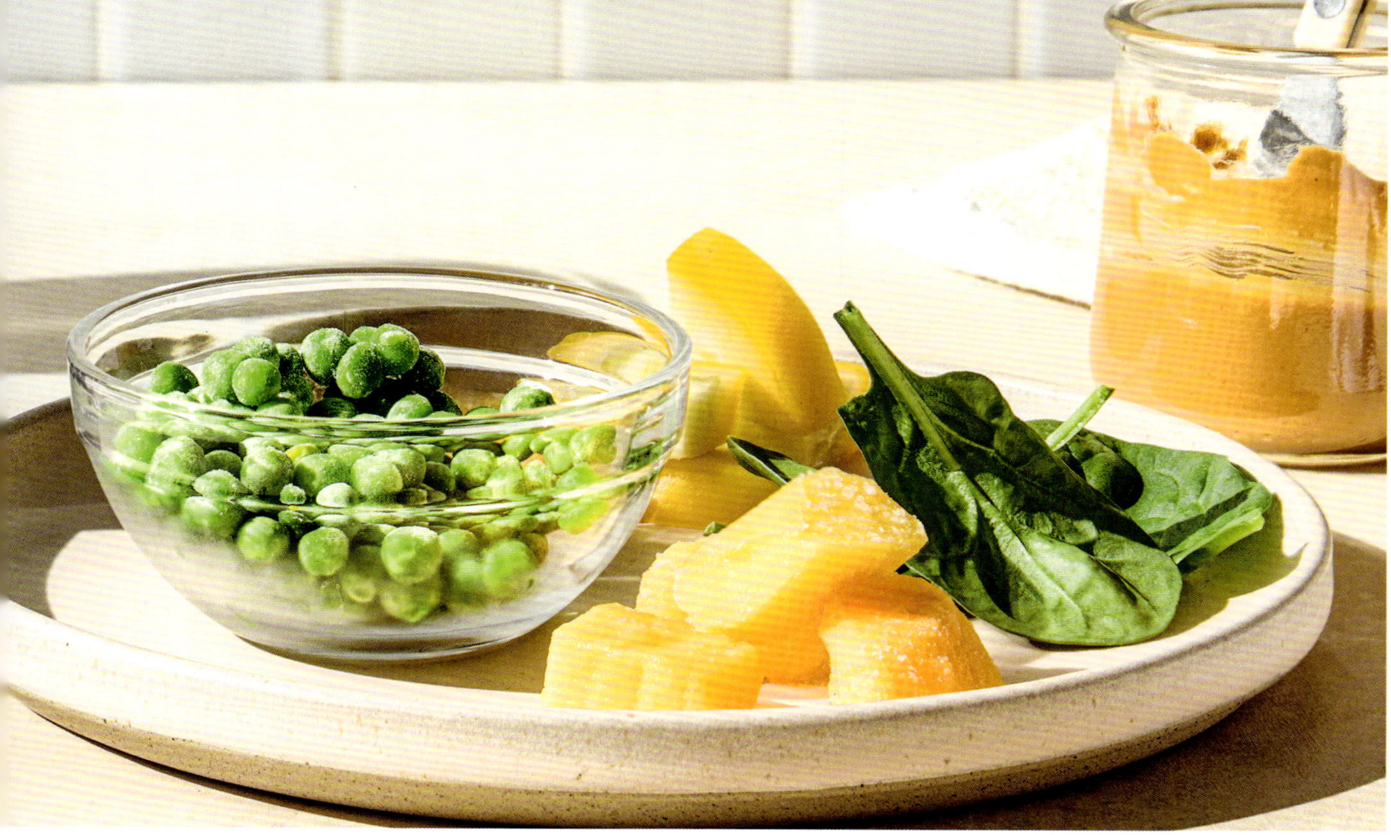

Sunshine Squash

MAKES ONE 16-OUNCE SMOOTHIE
PREP TIME: 5 minutes

PER SERVING:	CALORIES 148 kcal	PROTEIN 2g	FAT 1g	CARBOHYDRATE 28g	FIBER 3g

1 cup coconut water

1½ teaspoons apple cider vinegar

½ cup frozen yellow squash

½ cup frozen pineapple

½ cup frozen mango

¼ teaspoon ground turmeric

When we first started dating, my fiancé Miles mentioned that he froze squash and popped it into his smoothies. Genius. Now I add frozen veg to most of my smoothies. This smoothie is an excellent source of electrolytes, so it's the perfect go-to for mornings after a late night out. The coconut water, yellow squash, mango, and pineapple are rich in potassium and magnesium, essential for hydration and muscle recovery. To keep your blood sugar levels balanced, I recommend pairing it with a protein source such as yogurt, eggs, or cottage cheese.

Pour the coconut water and vinegar into a blender. Add the squash, pineapple, mango, and turmeric. Blend, starting at low and slowly increasing to high, for 1 to 3 minutes until smooth. Drink right away and enjoy!

Violet Cauliflower

MAKES ONE 16-OUNCE SMOOTHIE
PREP TIME: 5 minutes

PER SERVING:	**CALORIES** 408 kcal	**PROTEIN** 16g	**FAT** 16g	**CARBOHYDRATE** 53g	**FIBER** 11g

1 cup milk (dairy or nondairy)

¾ cup frozen riced cauliflower

¾ cup frozen blueberries

½ banana, chopped

1 tablespoon chia seeds

1 tablespoon unsalted peanut butter

This tasty smoothie—one of my faves—is loaded with nutrients that support your immune system, fight inflammation, and keep you energized. Cauliflower is high in vitamin C and glucosinolates (allies in chronic disease protection), and blueberries deliver anthocyanins (antioxidant plant pigments that lower blood pressure and improve brain function).

Pour the milk into a blender. Add the cauliflower, blueberries, banana, chia seeds, and peanut butter. Blend, starting at low and slowly increasing to high, for 1 to 3 minutes until smooth. Drink right away and enjoy!

Whirled Peas

MAKES ONE 16-OUNCE SMOOTHIE
PREP TIME: 5 minutes

PER SERVING:	**CALORIES** 302 kcal	**PROTEIN** 10g	**FAT** 7g	**CARBOHYDRATE** 58g	**FIBER** 12g

1 cup orange juice

1½ teaspoons apple cider vinegar

1 cup frozen peas

½ green apple, chopped

¼ avocado

½ cup lightly packed spinach

A common smoothie nutrition pitfall is too much fruit. Fruit is so tasty, but without balance, you'll peak and crash. Hello, veggie protein! This bright green, tart and lovely smoothie is super high in protein thanks to the peas. It contains 8 grams of frozen pea protein per cup! For even more of an electrolyte boost, I add magnesium-rich spinach. Like Popeye, I love my greens!

Pour the orange juice and vinegar into a blender. Add the peas, apple, avocado, and spinach. Blend, starting at low and slowly increasing to high, for 1 to 3 minutes until smooth. Drink right away and enjoy!

Cereal Glow-Up *with* Banana, Blueberries & Almonds

SERVES 1
PREP TIME: 5 minutes
COOK TIME: 5 minutes

PER SERVING:	**CALORIES** 522 kcal	**PROTEIN** 23g	**FAT** 13g	**CARBOHYDRATE** 89g	**FIBER** 11g

½ cup nonfat or low-fat Greek yogurt

½ cup milk (dairy or nondairy)

2 tablespoons maple syrup

1 cup multi-bran flakes cereal

½ banana, sliced

½ cup blueberries, fresh or thawed frozen

2 tablespoons chopped almonds

As a dietitian who loves cereal, I often hear judgy things like, "What kind of dietitian eats cereal?!" I'm here to say, without a shadow of a doubt, that cereal, when done right, is a nutritious—and delicious, quick, and easy!—a.m. option loaded with vitamins and minerals.

When I was little, I *loved* drinking the milk left in the bowl after my breakfast cereal. It usually had this amazing subtle maple flavor, so I've added maple syrup for you here. It's my favorite part! I also love this cereal hack: a 1:1 ratio of milk and Greek yogurt. The yogurt blends right in (you barely notice it) and you get its big protein and resulting steady blood sugar levels. The other tasty treats in the mix—banana, blueberries, and almonds—significantly boost your nutrient intake. I make this cereal a lot on busy weekdays, when I need to hustle hard until lunch. It's a breeze to whip up, it's comforting and yummy, and it really keeps me going.

In your serving bowl, stir together the yogurt, milk, and maple syrup until fully incorporated. Add the cereal and stir to combine. Top with the banana, blueberries, and almonds and enjoy! This bowl is best enjoyed day of.

CEREAL FIBER & SUGAR CHECK

Do a quick fiber check before you purchase boxed cereals. I recommend aiming for at least 3 to 5 grams per serving. Fiber slows down the absorption of sugar in your bloodstream, which means steady blood sugar levels. Also, be mindful of added sugars. Many breakfast cereals contain high amounts, which cause blood sugar spikes and crashes. I look for no more than 5 to 6 grams of added sugar per serving.

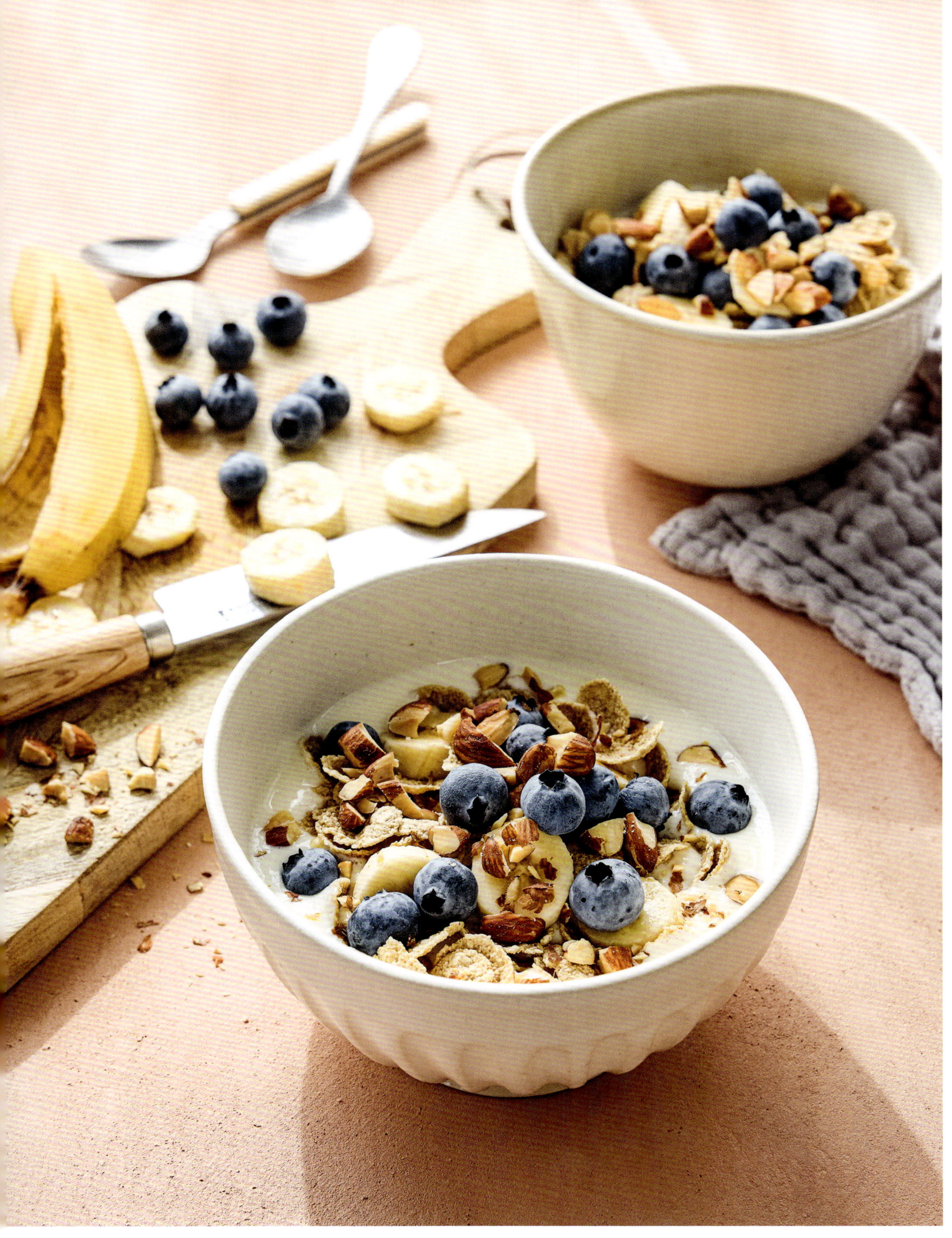

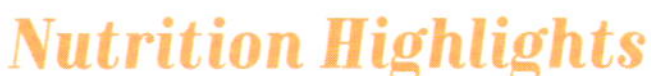

Nutrition Highlights

FIBER + ANTIOXIDANTS: Berries not only add their sweet and tart flavor, they're also rich in both of these essentials for immune and gut health.

HEALTHY FATS: Almonds and walnuts are loaded with healthy fats that support everything from brain function and energy storage to cell structure and function. For even more texture and healthy fats, top the parfait with granola or chia seeds.

PROTEIN: Hello, Greek yogurt! Protein provides long-lasting energy, and it also builds and repairs tissue, muscles, skin, hair, etc. If you prefer nondairy yogurt, go for it. It also delivers protein.

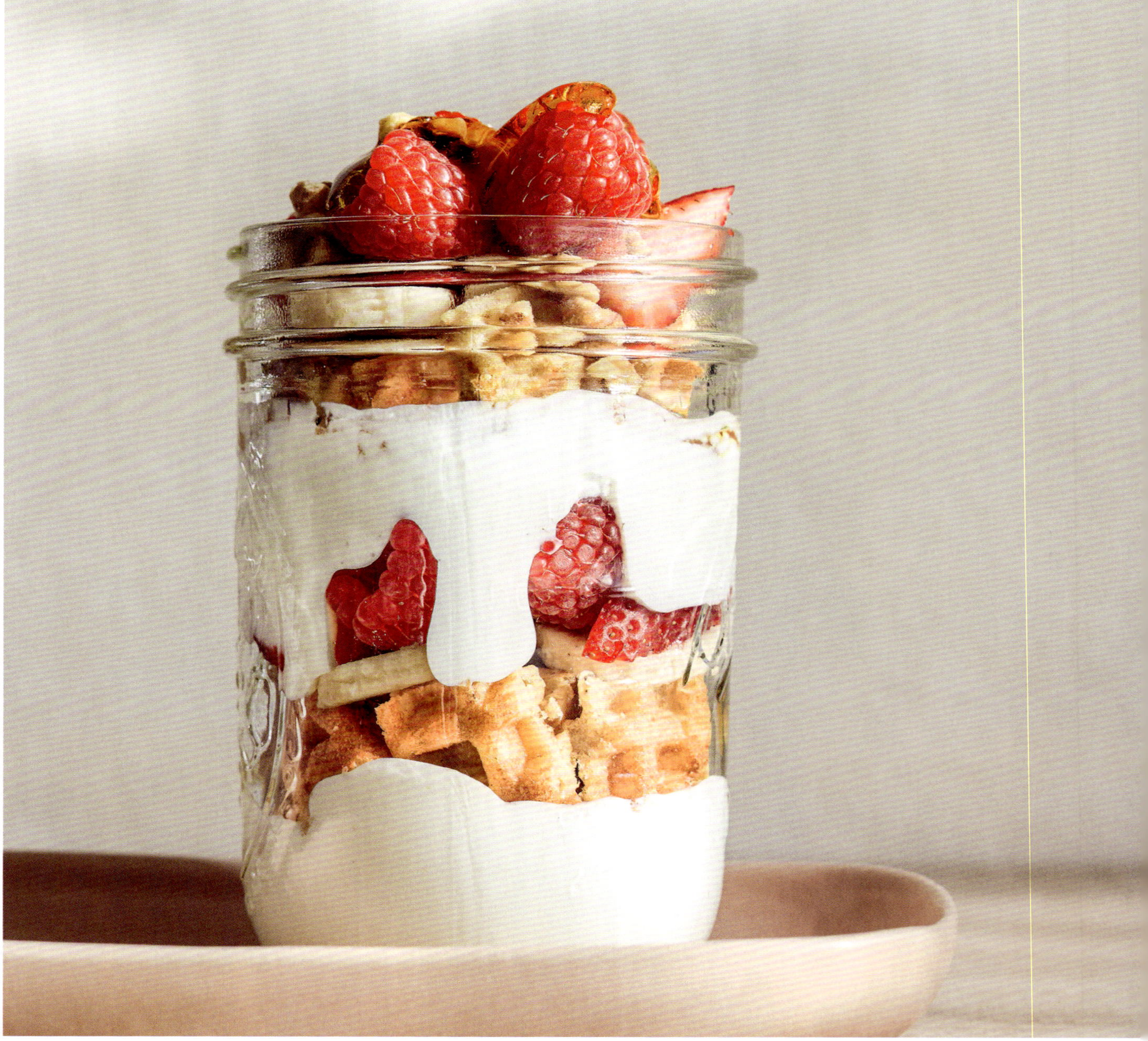

Crispy Banana-Berry Waffle Parfait

SERVES 1
PREP TIME: 5 minutes
COOK TIME: 3 minutes

PER SERVING:	**CALORIES** 415 kcal	**PROTEIN** 16g	**FAT** 7g	**CARBOHYDRATE** 70g	**FIBER** 8g

2 frozen waffles (any type and flavor works, even GF!), divided

½ cup nonfat or low-fat Greek yogurt, divided

3 teaspoons maple syrup, divided

½ banana, sliced, divided

⅔ cup mixed fresh berries (I like a mix of blueberries, raspberries, and strawberries), divided

1½ teaspoons sliced almonds or chopped walnuts

In high school, I used to eat a few frozen waffles every morning. Looking back, it's no surprise I'd crash by mid-morning—all carbs and no balance! As a dietitian, I've found that the perfect way to level things out and make frozen waffles not just delicious but also nutritious is to add protein and fiber. This parfait will keep you energized and satisfied until lunch. And, feel free to get creative with the layers. Add a drizzle of peanut butter, scoop in flavored yogurt, or add some chocolate chips. Have fun with it.

Toast the waffles until golden brown and nicely crisped. Once cool enough to handle, slice them into bite-size pieces.

In a pint-sized glass or serving bowl (I prefer something glass or see-through for this, so that you can see the parfait layers), spoon ¼ cup of the Greek yogurt onto the bottom. Top it with half of the toasted waffle pieces. Drizzle the waffle pieces with 1 teaspoon of the maple syrup. Place half of the banana slices and half of the mixed berries over the waffle pieces. Repeat the layers with the remaining ¼ cup yogurt, waffle pieces, 1 teaspoon of the maple syrup, banana slices, and berries.

Top the parfait with the almonds or walnuts, drizzle with the remaining 1 teaspoon of maple syrup, and enjoy! This parfait is best enjoyed day of.

Oats & Seeds Porridge

SERVES 1
PREP TIME: 5 minutes
COOK TIME: 5 minutes

PER SERVING:	**CALORIES** 572 kcal	**PROTEIN** 22g	**FAT** 21g	**CARBOHYDRATE** 80g	**FIBER** 18g

½ cup old-fashioned rolled oats

2 tablespoons chia seeds

2 tablespoons flaxseed meal

1 cup milk (dairy or nondairy)

1 tablespoon maple syrup, plus more (optional) for serving

Pinch of kosher salt

½ banana, sliced

Ground cinnamon (optional), for garnish

This porridge is warm, wholesome, and feels like a hug in a bowl—perfect for chilly mornings or whenever you need something quick, comforting, and super nourishing. It will keep you full for hours thanks to the fiber-packed rolled oats, chia seeds, and flaxseed meal, which deliver fiber, omega-3s, *and* protein. Top it with whatever you're craving, including any fresh fruit, a handful of chopped nuts, a sprinkle of spice, a drizzle of syrup, or all of the above. I love that it's ready in just FIVE minutes in the microwave! So, you can have your warm, creamy, and satisfying breakfast in no time.

In a microwave-safe medium bowl, combine the oats, chia seeds, flaxseed meal, milk, maple syrup, and salt. Stir until everything is well incorporated. Microwave on high for 2 to 3 minutes, stirring about halfway through, until the porridge has thickened and the oats are tender.

Carefully remove the bowl from the microwave (it will be hot!) and give it a quick stir. Set it aside for 1 to 2 minutes, so that the chia seeds plump up and thicken the porridge. Stir the porridge again. Drizzle it with additional maple syrup if using, top it with the banana, sprinkle it with the cinnamon (if using), and enjoy! This bowl is best enjoyed day of.

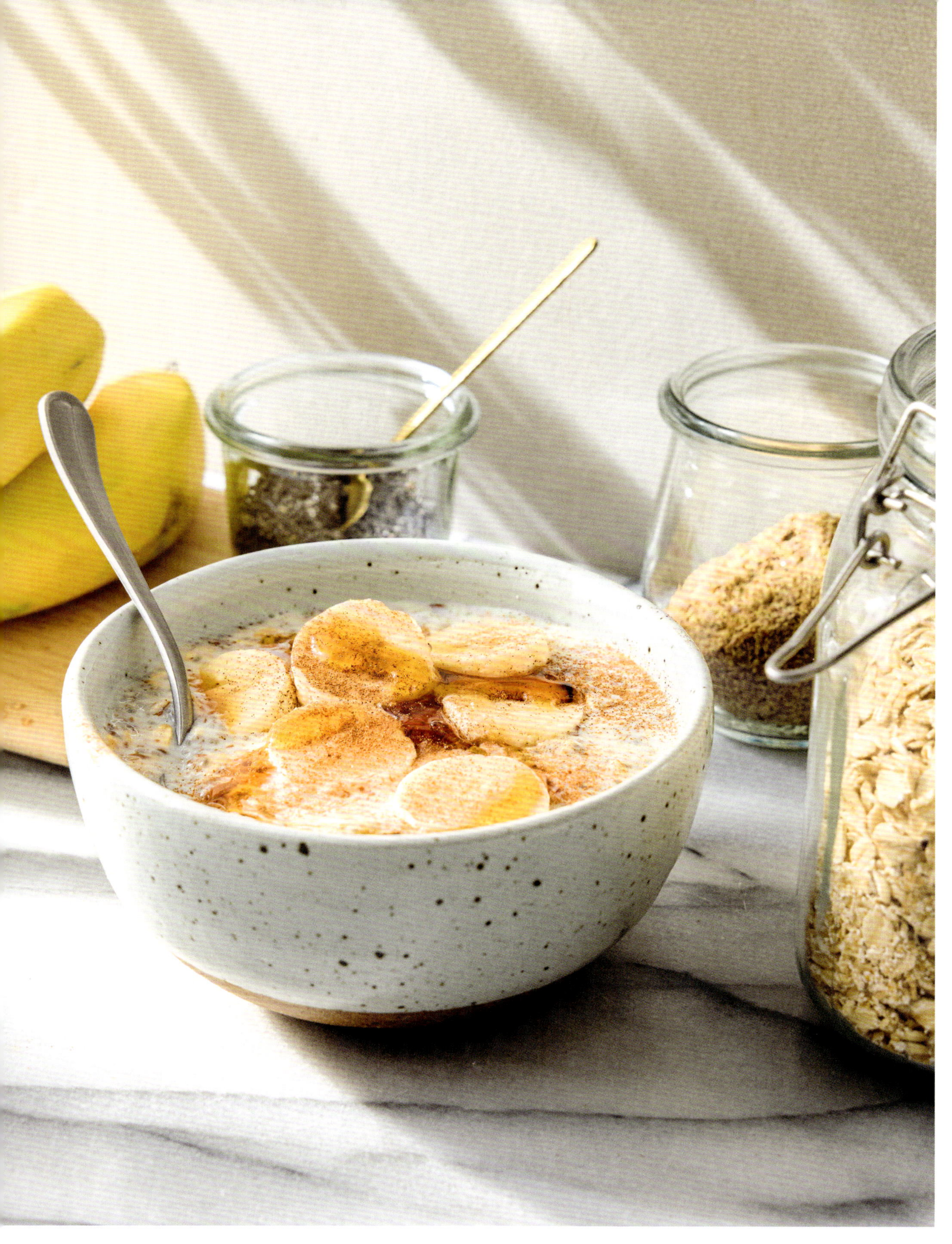

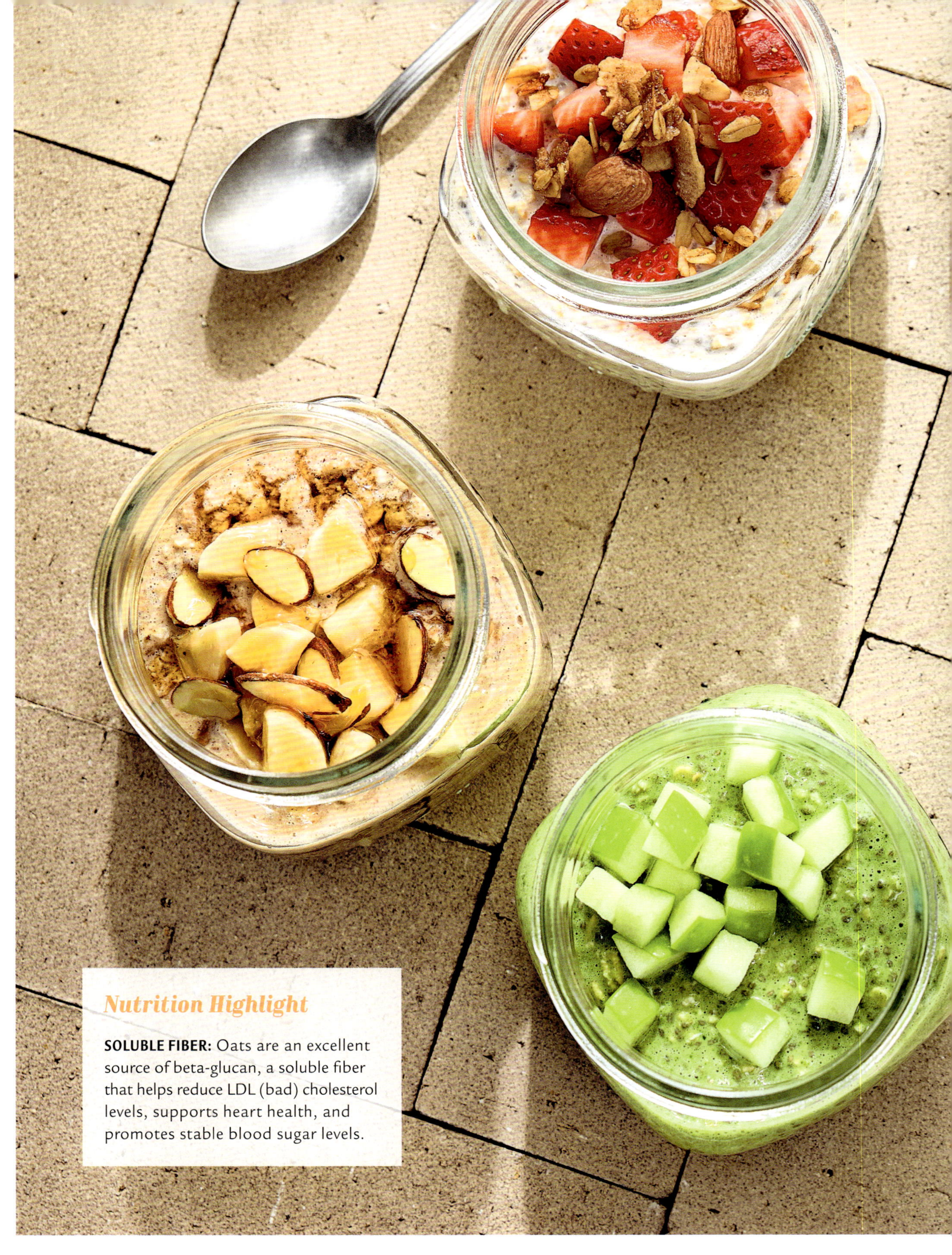

Nutrition Highlight

SOLUBLE FIBER: Oats are an excellent source of beta-glucan, a soluble fiber that helps reduce LDL (bad) cholesterol levels, supports heart health, and promotes stable blood sugar levels.

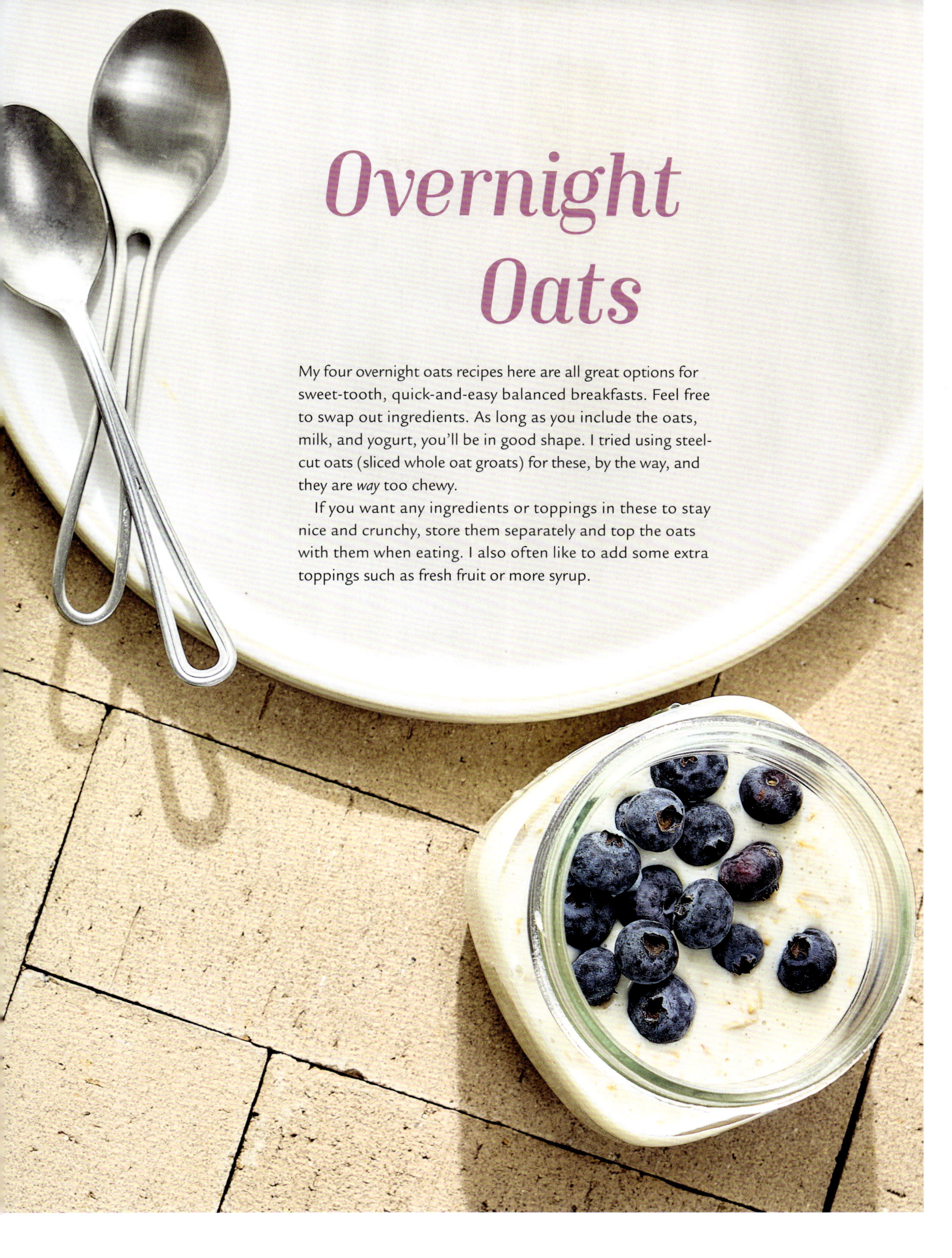

Overnight Oats

My four overnight oats recipes here are all great options for sweet-tooth, quick-and-easy balanced breakfasts. Feel free to swap out ingredients. As long as you include the oats, milk, and yogurt, you'll be in good shape. I tried using steel-cut oats (sliced whole oat groats) for these, by the way, and they are *way* too chewy.

If you want any ingredients or toppings in these to stay nice and crunchy, store them separately and top the oats with them when eating. I also often like to add some extra toppings such as fresh fruit or more syrup.

Cinnamon Nut Crunch Overnight Oats

SERVES 1
PREP TIME: 5 minutes
REFRIGERATION TIME: 6 hours or overnight

PER SERVING:	CALORIES 528 kcal	PROTEIN 19g	FAT 25g	CARBOHYDRATE 65g	FIBER 11g

½ cup old-fashioned rolled oats
¾ cup milk (dairy or nondairy)
1 tablespoon flaxseed meal
1 tablespoon nut butter
½ teaspoon ground cinnamon
½ teaspoon vanilla extract
½ banana, sliced
2 tablespoons sliced almonds
1½ teaspoons maple syrup

This is the first overnight oats combo that I ever made—so tasty and satisfying. I've been enjoying this a.m. cup of nut butter plus banana yum for years. Now you get to!

In a wide-mouth 1-pint canning jar or another lidded roughly 2-cup container, stir together the oats, milk, flaxseed meal, nut butter, cinnamon, and vanilla until everything is well mixed and the nut butter is fully blended. Top with the banana and almonds and drizzle with the maple syrup.

Cover and refrigerate for at least 6 hours or overnight and then enjoy! These keep for up to 3 days refrigerated, but after day one, the oats get mushy and the other ingredients lose their brightness and bite.

Strawberry Shortcake Overnight Oats

SERVES 1
PREP TIME: 5 minutes
REFRIGERATION TIME: 6 hours or overnight

PER SERVING:	**CALORIES** 536 kcal	**PROTEIN** 20g	**FAT** 18g	**CARBOHYDRATE** 76g	**FIBER** 13g

½ cup old-fashioned rolled oats

½ cup milk (dairy or nondairy)

½ cup strawberry yogurt (regular or Greek)

1 tablespoon chia seeds

½ teaspoon vanilla extract

⅔ cup diced strawberries

⅓ cup granola

Strawberry shortcake is my all-time favorite dessert and go-to birthday sweet treat. That love has been channeled into these overnight oats. You're going to really like the strawberry yogurt, fresh strawberries, granola, and everything else in this one. It's too good not to share.

In a wide-mouth 1-pint canning jar or another lidded roughly 2-cup container, stir together the oats, milk, yogurt, chia seeds, and vanilla until everything is well mixed. Top with the strawberries and granola.

Cover and refrigerate for at least 6 hours or overnight then enjoy! These keep for up to 3 days refrigerated, but after day one, the oats get mushy and the other ingredients lose their brightness and bite.

Lemon Blueberry Cheesecake Overnight Oats

SERVES 1
PREP TIME: 5 minutes
REFRIGERATION TIME: 6 hours or overnight

PER SERVING:	**CALORIES** 352 kcal	**PROTEIN** 15g	**FAT** 7g	**CARBOHYDRATE** 57g	**FIBER** 7g

½ cup old-fashioned rolled oats

½ cup vanilla yogurt (regular or Greek)

½ cup milk (dairy or nondairy)

1½ teaspoons fresh lemon juice

1 teaspoon maple syrup

½ cup blueberries

It's certainly not advisable nutritionally speaking to eat cheesecake in the a.m., *but* even without the cream cheese, these overnight oats hit all the same notes and are a breakfast of champions. Creamy vanilla yogurt, bright lemon, plus sweet burst-in-your-mouth blueberries. It's a healthy twist on dessert without all the saturated fat.

In a wide-mouth 1-pint canning jar or another lidded roughly 2-cup container, stir together the oats, yogurt, milk, lemon juice, and maple syrup until everything is well mixed. Top with the blueberries.

Cover and refrigerate for at least 6 hours or overnight then enjoy! These keep for up to 3 days refrigerated, but after day one, the oats get mushy and the other ingredients lose their brightness and bite.

Super Green Overnight Oats

SERVES 1
PREP TIME: 5 minutes
REFRIGERATION TIME: 6 hours or overnight

PER SERVING:	**CALORIES** 510 kcal	**PROTEIN** 19g	**FAT** 15g	**CARBOHYDRATE** 88g	**FIBER** 18g

1 cup lightly packed spinach

½ cup milk (dairy or nondairy)

½ banana, broken into a few pieces

2 tablespoons nonfat or low-fat Greek yogurt

½ cup old-fashioned rolled oats

2 tablespoons chia seeds

2 teaspoons honey

½ teaspoon vanilla extract

½ green apple, diced

If you want to trick yourself or a loved one into eating more veggies, make these yummy overnight oats, because I promise that you cannot taste the spinach. At all.

In a blender, combine the spinach, milk, banana, and yogurt. Blend, staring at low and slowly increasing to high, for 1 to 2 minutes until smooth.

In a wide-mouth 1-pint canning jar or another lidded roughly 2-cup container, stir together the oats, blended spinach/banana milk, chia seeds, honey, and vanilla until everything is well mixed. Top with the apple.

Cover and refrigerate for at least 6 hours or overnight then enjoy! These keep for up to 3 days refrigerated, but after day one, the oats get mushy and the other ingredients lose their brightness and bite.

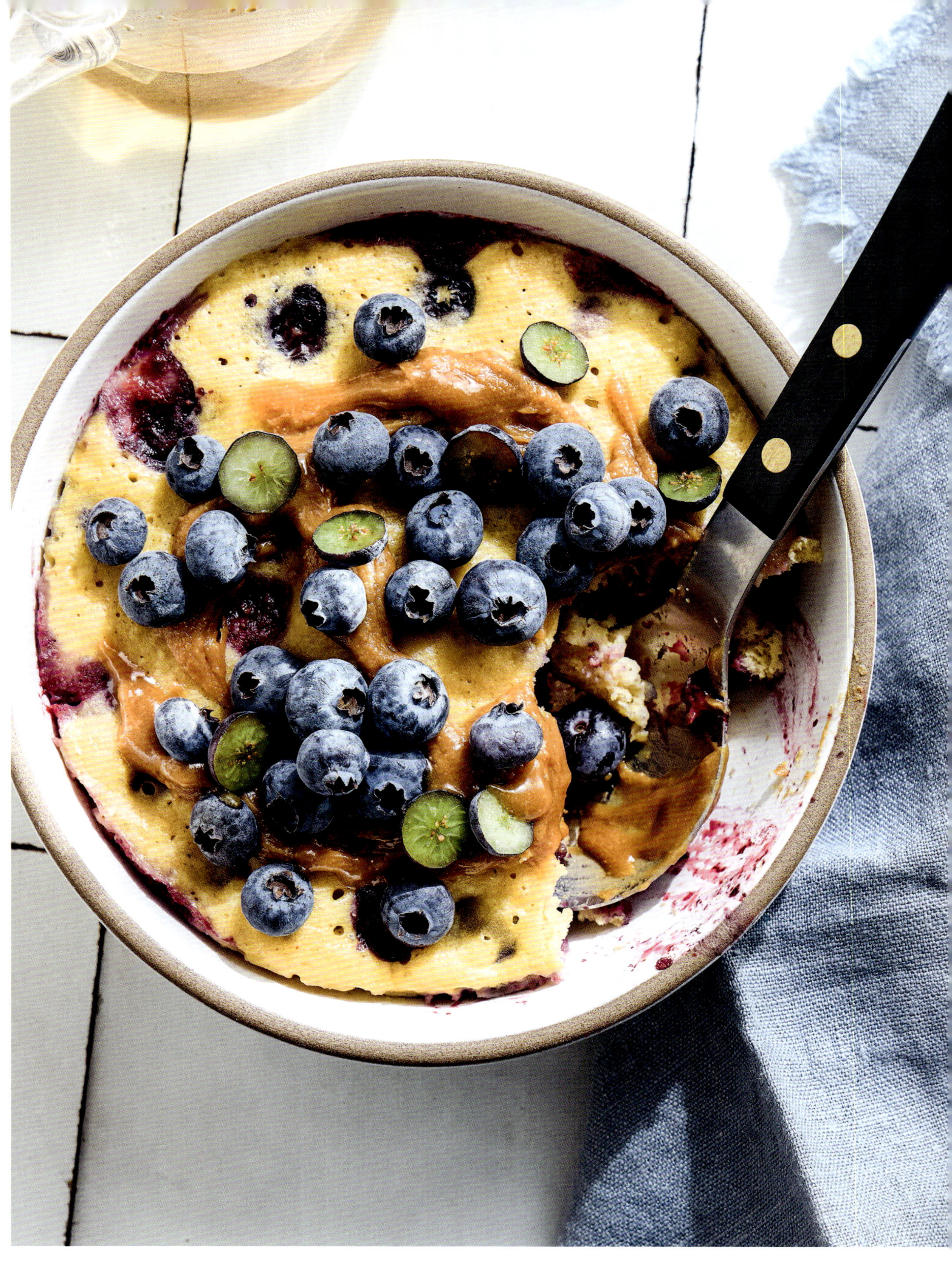

PB&J Microwave Pancake Bowl

SERVES 1
PREP TIME: 5 minutes
COOK TIME: 5 minutes

PER SERVING:	**CALORIES** 536 kcal	**PROTEIN** 22g	**FAT** 23g	**CARBOHYDRATE** 70g	**FIBER** 8g

½ banana

¼ cup pancake mix (any type and flavor works, even GF!)

1 large egg

1 tablespoon nonfat or low-fat Greek yogurt

½ teaspoon vanilla extract

⅛ teaspoon kosher salt

2 tablespoons unsalted peanut butter, divided

½ cup blueberries, fresh or thawed frozen, plus more for garnish

1 to 2 tablespoons maple syrup

I adore pancakes, but I don't make them at home all that often for a few reasons. They're time-consuming, they're messy, and I usually end up with way too much batter and extra pancakes. This microwaveable pancake bowl is a game changer. It's super tidy—everything goes right into the microwave-safe bowl—and it's ready in just a few minutes. Plus, it's perfectly portioned for one.

Blueberries are the nutrition star here. They contain anthocyanins, which give them their blue color and all sorts of healthful properties including lowering inflammation. They also contain flavonoids that support cognitive function by promoting blood flow to the brain and reducing neuroinflammation.

I *love* that as the blueberries cook in the peanut buttery batter, they burst and get all nice and jammy. That said, feel free to use whatever fruits and syrupy toppings that sound yummy to you. Come fall, pumpkin puree and cinnamon with a straight-up maple syrup sounds just as delightful. Now you and I can enjoy quick-and-easy homemade pancakes any day of the week!

In a wide, roughly 1-quart microwave-safe bowl or dish ( ), mash the banana with a fork until it is fairly smooth. Add the pancake mix, egg, yogurt, vanilla, and salt. Mix with the fork or a small whisk until everything is incorporated and the batter is fairly smooth. Some small chunks of banana are okay. Add 1 tablespoon of the peanut butter and stir to combine. Gently fold in the blueberries.

Microwave on high for 2 to 5 minutes, opening the microwave and checking the batter every minute or so, until the pancake is fully set (pay special attention to the middle of the batter) and cooked through. The batter will puff up and bubble, much like pancakes do in the pan. Microwave power varies widely, so make sure to keep an eye on the batter!

In a small bowl, combine the remaining 1 tablespoon peanut butter with the maple syrup and stir until smooth. If you want it to be thinner and sweeter, use more syrup!

Drizzle the maple/peanut butter syrup over the pancake bowl, garnish with blueberries, and enjoy!

NUTRITION PSA

Add a scoop of protein powder to the batter if you want or use a high-protein pancake mix like Kodiak.

STEPH'S TIP

As the pancake bowl cooks in the microwave, the pancake will rise to two to three times the initial batter height. Make sure your microwavable bowl or dish is large and deep enough for that.

Pumpkin Protein Pancakes *with* Cinnamony Yogurt

MAKES 3 PANCAKES | SERVES 1
PREP TIME: 5 minutes
COOK TIME: 15 minutes

PER PANCAKE:	**CALORIES** 156 kcal	**PROTEIN** 9g	**FAT** 5g	**CARBOHYDRATE** 20g	**FIBER** 3g
YOGURT SAUCE:	**CALORIES** 173 kcal	**PROTEIN** 10g	**FAT** 0g	**CARBOHYDRATE** 34g	**FIBER** <1g

1 cup old-fashioned rolled oats

⅓ cup canned pumpkin puree

⅓ cup 2% cottage cheese (or whatever fat content you prefer)

¼ cup milk (dairy or nondairy)

2 large eggs

1 tablespoon maple syrup, plus more for serving

1 teaspoon pumpkin pie spice

Cinnamony Yogurt

½ cup nonfat or low-fat Greek yogurt

2 tablespoons maple syrup

½ teaspoon ground cinnamon

½ teaspoon vanilla extract

Cooking spray or neutral oil, for greasing

I usually whip these pumpkiny pancakes up when the days are getting shorter and that first crisp breeze hits. They pack a serious punch of protein plus fiber, making them a great get-up-and-go breakfast or post-workout bite. Each serving has 40 grams of protein for muscle repair and satiety. Cottage cheese and Greek yogurt are protein rock stars, while oats bring plant-based protein and fiber to the mix. Greek yogurt is a fantastic pancake topper—creamy, tangy, and full of probiotics to keep your gut happy.

In a blender, combine the oats, pumpkin puree, cottage cheese, milk, eggs, maple syrup, and pumpkin pie spice. Blend on low speed, gradually increasing the speed to high, for about 2 minutes until fully blended. This is thicker than average pancake batter, so you'll need a rubber spatula to get it all out of the blender.

Make the cinnamony yogurt: In a small bowl, stir together the yogurt, maple syrup, cinnamon, and vanilla until well combined. Set aside.

Lightly grease a large nonstick pan or griddle with cooking spray or oil and set over medium heat. When the pan or griddle is hot, pour a heaping ½ cup of the batter onto it ( ). You will likely be able to cook 2 to 3 medium pancakes at once.

Cook the pancakes for about 3 minutes on each side, adjusting the heat as necessary, until they are golden brown on both sides and cooked through. Repeat with any remaining batter and add more oil to the pan as needed. Serve the hot pancakes with generous dollops of the cinnamony yogurt on top. Drizzle with additional maple syrup if desired.

STEPH'S TIP

Pumpkin puree is not just for pies! Add it to your breakfast repertoire to sneak in a.m. veggies. Plus, pumpkin is loaded with beta-carotene, which your body turns into vitamin A to support vision, immune health, and glowing skin.

STORAGE + REHEAT

Once cooled, store the pancakes airtight in the refrigerator for up to 3 days. Store the cinnamony yogurt separately in an airtight container in the refrigerator for up to 3 days. To reheat, warm pancakes in a pan over medium heat until heated through, or microwave.

YOU DO YOU

You can make your pancakes any size you like, of course. I like ½ cup per pancake to end up with 3 medium pancakes.

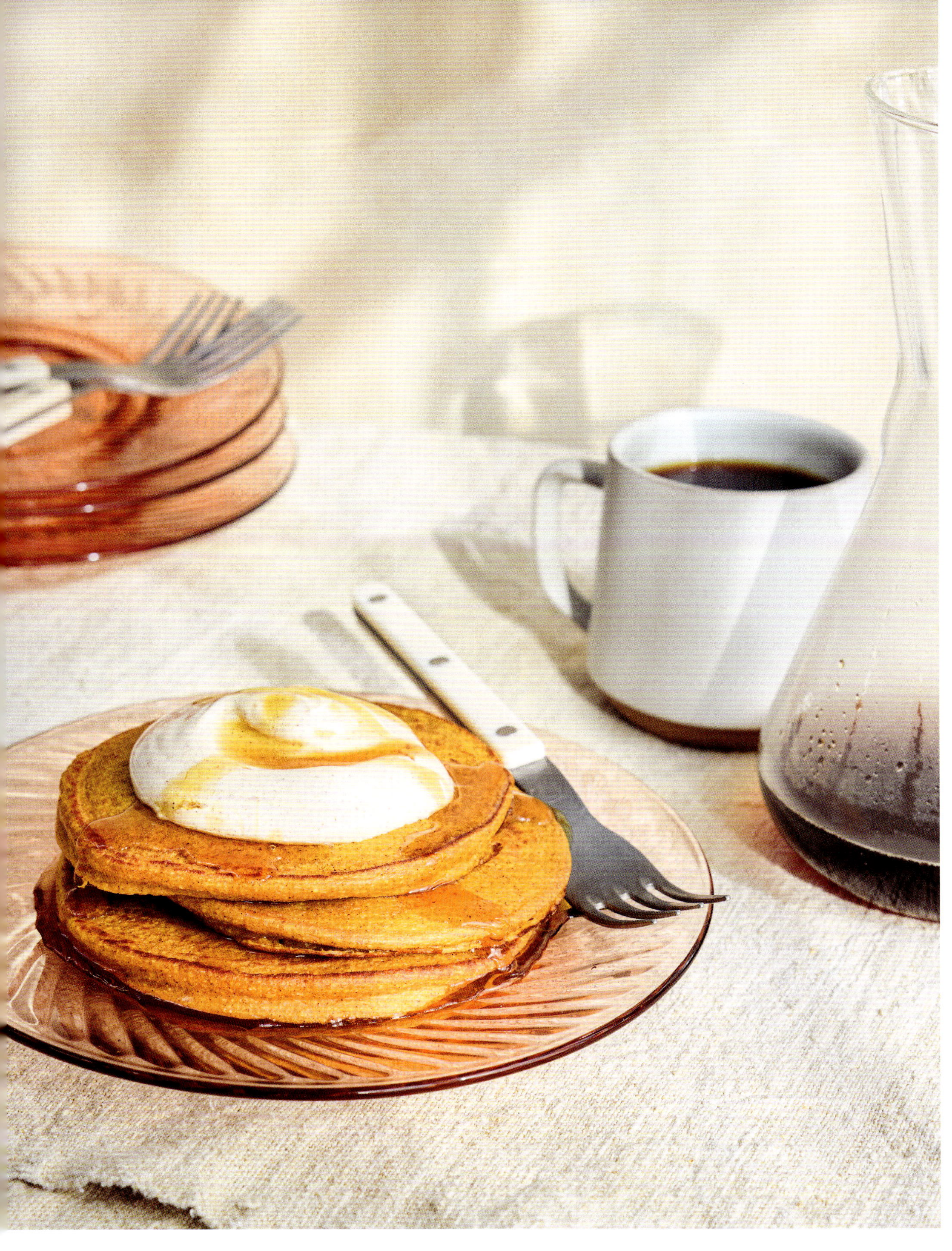

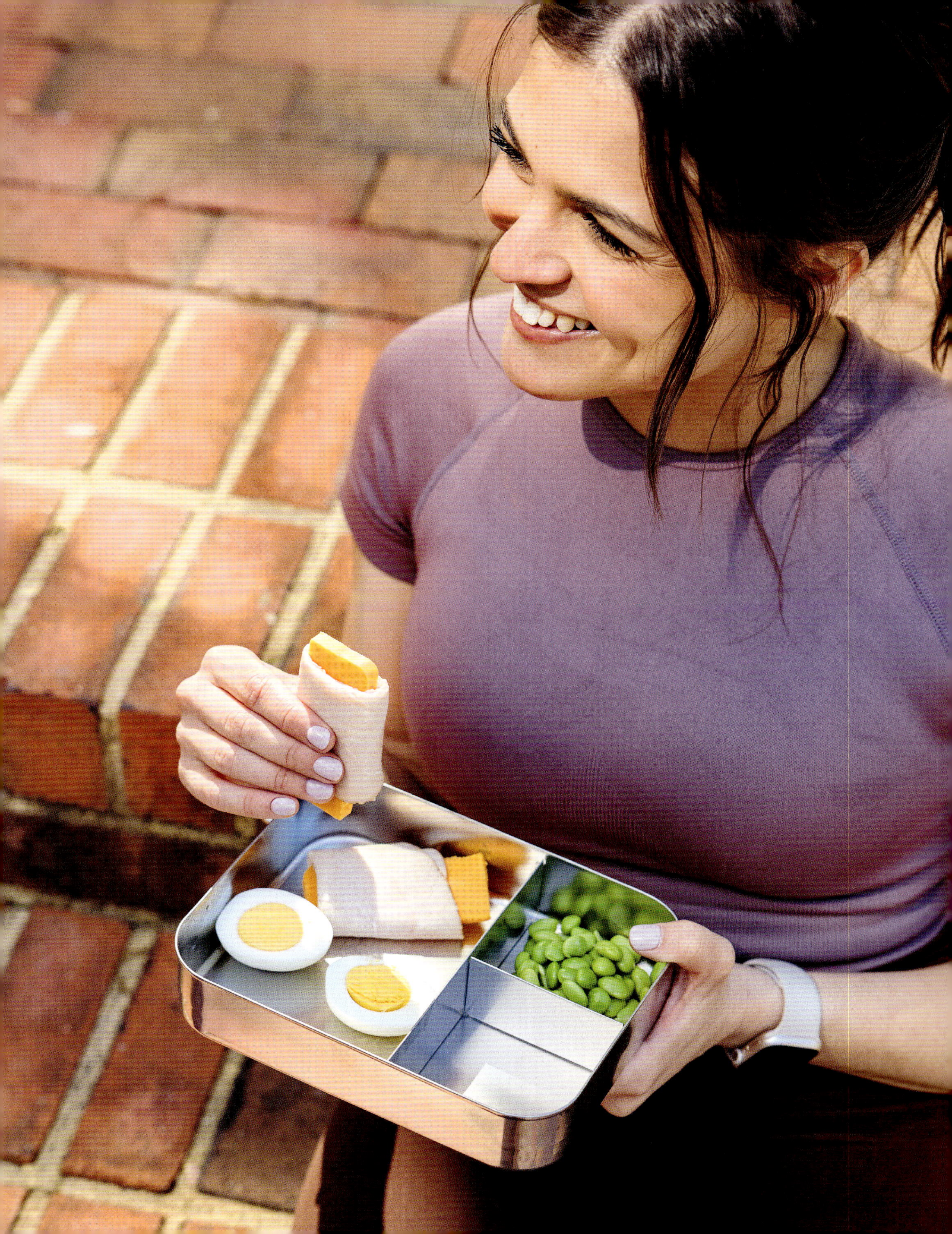

Balanced Snacking

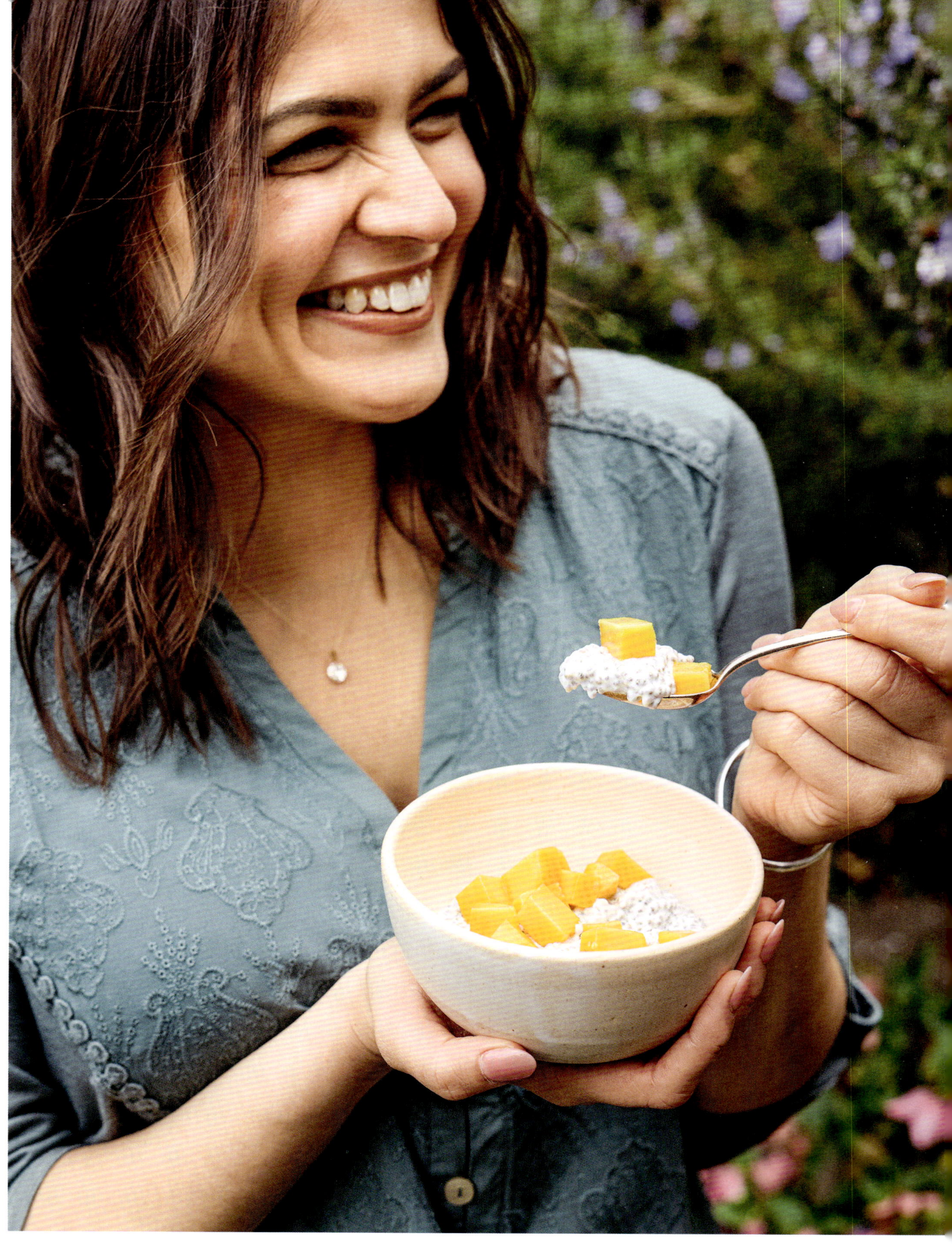

Overnight Coconut Chia Seed Pudding *with* Mango

SERVES 4
PREP TIME: 10 minutes
REFRIGERATION TIME: 8 hours or overnight

PER SERVING:	**CALORIES** 375 kcal	**PROTEIN** 10g	**FAT** 24g	**CARBOHYDRATE** 32g	**FIBER** 10g

One 13.5-ounce can full-fat coconut milk

1 cup nonfat or low-fat Greek yogurt

2 tablespoons maple syrup

1 teaspoon vanilla extract

½ cup chia seeds

2 cups diced mango (about 1 large)

This chilled snack is as nutritious as it is beautiful. I love the yellowy-orange color of the diced mangoes on top of the bright white coconut milk and yogurt plus the pops of black from the chia seeds. Gorgeous.

Nutritionally speaking, this snacker is a fiber powerhouse with 10 grams per serving. The recommended daily fiber intake is around 25 grams for women, and 38 grams for men, depending on age and other factors. Mangoes are fantastic for us, too—high in vitamins A plus C. They also are filled with polyphenols like mangiferin, quercetin, and catechins, all of which protect against oxidative stress (which leads to cell and tissue damage) and inflammation. Eyes glossing over? The gist: Mangoes are the bomb.

In a blender or food processor, combine the coconut milk, yogurt, maple syrup, and vanilla. Blend on medium speed until smooth, 15 to 20 seconds.

In each of four 1½- to 2-cup serving dishes or containers, add 2 tablespoons of the chia seeds. Evenly pour a heaping ½ cup of the blended pudding mixture over the seeds in each dish. Stir well and cover. Refrigerate the pudding overnight (for 8 or more hours) to allow the chia seeds to swell and the pudding to set.

Top each pudding with ½ cup diced mango before serving.

STORAGE

Store airtight in the refrigerator for up to 5 days. For best results, add the fresh mango right before serving.

'Nana Milk

MAKES ABOUT 2 CUPS | SERVES 1
PREP TIME: 2 minutes

PER SERVING:	CALORIES 227 kcal	PROTEIN 9g	FAT 5g	CARBOHYDRATE 39g	FIBER 3g

1 overripe banana, broken into a few pieces

1 cup milk (dairy or nondairy)

This recipe is dedicated to my four-year-old nephew, Ruben. There was a point when my sister, her husband, my nephew, and I lived with my parents. We were all going through house moving transitions, and it just made sense. During those few months, my sister would often blend an overripe banana with whatever milk was in the fridge and pass it to little Ruben. He loved it.

Bananas are a wonderful source of potassium, which is important for growing bodies. It supports heart health, proper muscle function, and nerve signals. The calcium and protein in milk (if you're using cow or goat milk) supports strong bones and teeth, as well as growth and development. 'Nana milk is also a nice natural sugars alternative to all the added-sugar drinks out there. And it's not just for kids! I drink it all the time—as a snack, breakfast addition, or post-workout refuel. Added bonus: It's a great way to use up overripe bananas before they go south, and it's way faster than baking banana bread.

In a blender, combine the banana and milk and blend on low speed, gradually increasing the speed to high, for 1 to 2 minutes until fully blended and lightly frothy. Serve right away over ice. 'Nana milk is best enjoyed day of.

NUTRITION PSA

For extra nutrition, and a more smoothie-consistency, blend in a handful of spinach, a tablespoon of nut butter, a scoop of protein powder, or all three!

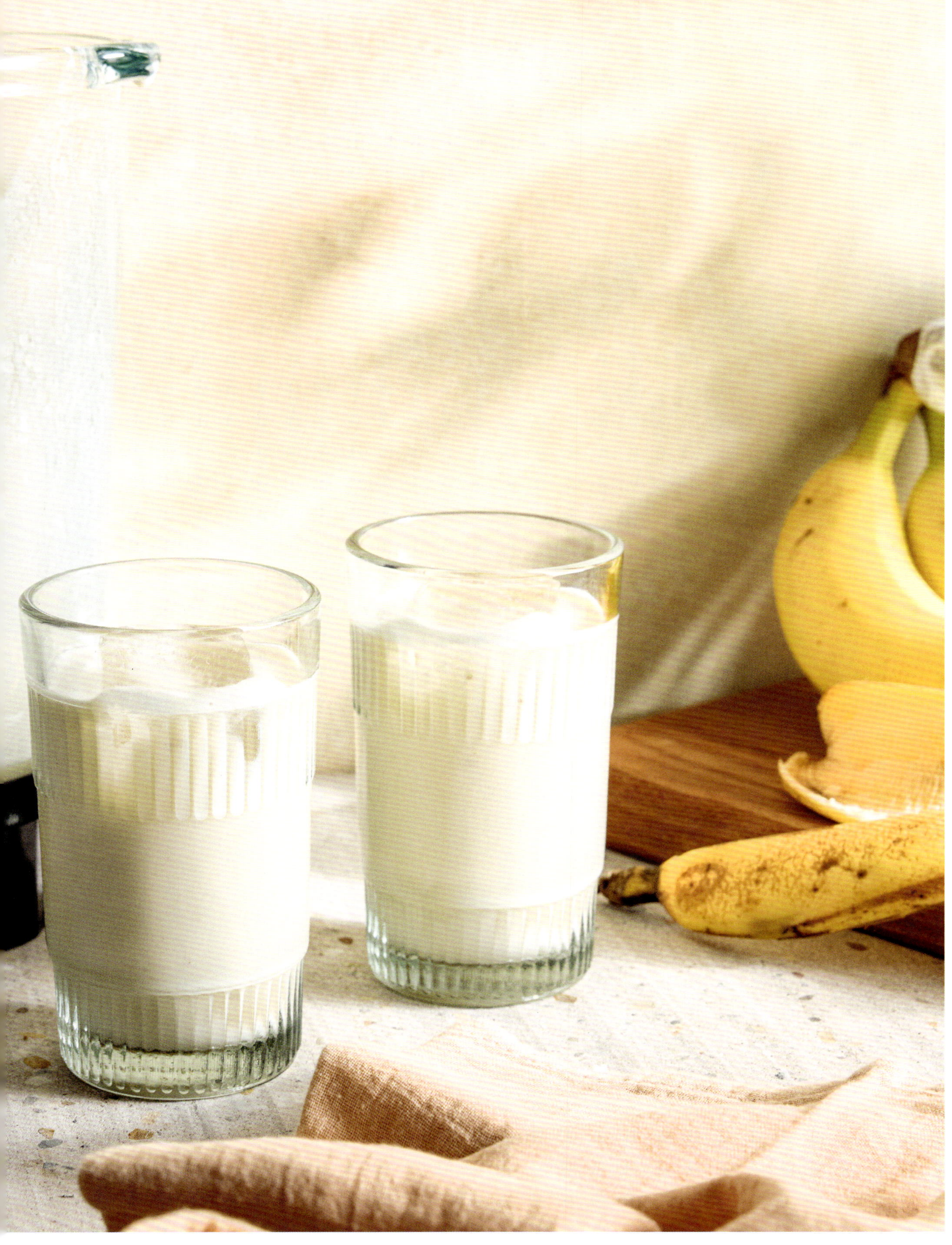

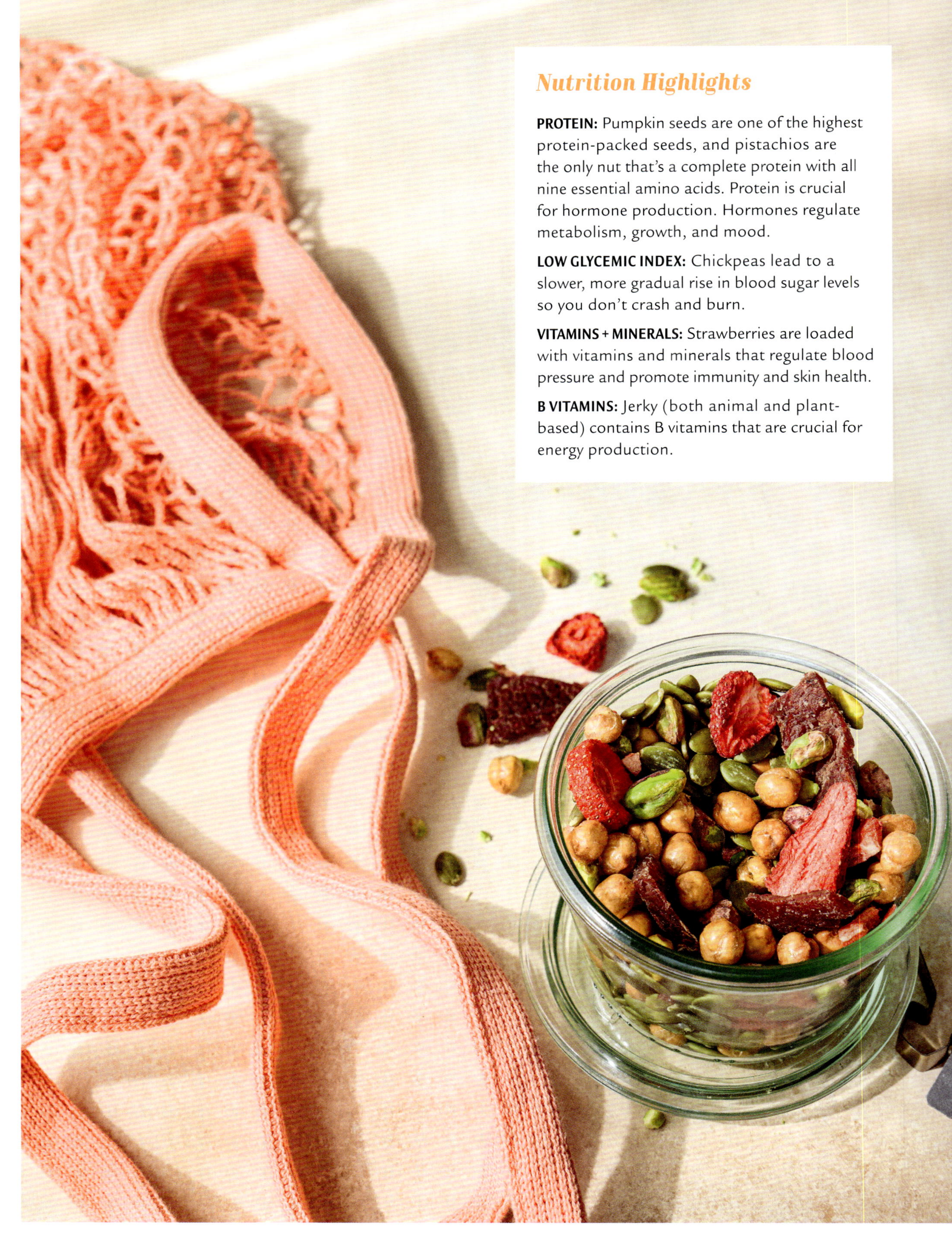

Nutrition Highlights

PROTEIN: Pumpkin seeds are one of the highest protein-packed seeds, and pistachios are the only nut that's a complete protein with all nine essential amino acids. Protein is crucial for hormone production. Hormones regulate metabolism, growth, and mood.

LOW GLYCEMIC INDEX: Chickpeas lead to a slower, more gradual rise in blood sugar levels so you don't crash and burn.

VITAMINS + MINERALS: Strawberries are loaded with vitamins and minerals that regulate blood pressure and promote immunity and skin health.

B VITAMINS: Jerky (both animal and plant-based) contains B vitamins that are crucial for energy production.

On-the-Go Trail Mix

MAKES 4½ CUPS | SERVES 6 TO 8
PREP TIME: 5 minutes

PER SERVING:	**CALORIES** 276 kcal	**PROTEIN** 17g	**FAT** 15g	**CARBOHYDRATE** 14g	**FIBER** 4g

6 ounces beef jerky (or whatever jerky you prefer, including veggie), chopped into bite-size pieces

1 cup lightly salted roasted pumpkin seeds, hulled or unhulled

1 cup lightly salted crunchy roasted chickpeas

1 cup freeze-dried strawberries

½ cup lightly salted roasted pistachios

I highly recommend prepping this yummy sweet-meets-savory trail mix once a week to bring with you while you're out and about. I drive a lot, so I often stash a bag in my car dashboard. It comes in handy when I'm really hungry but don't have time to stop for food. It can be tempting to cruise through a fast-food place in those situations (I'm not demonizing that; I hit up Taco Bell now and again), but this mix is an absolute flavor-bomb that won't make you feel like you're missing out.

The best thing about this trail mix is that you can customize it to your liking. Use your favorite freeze-dried fruit. Mix and match raw and toasted seeds. Just know that I have perfected the textures in this recipe, and the bite and flavor of crunchy and toasted seeds is much better than their raw counterparts.

In terms of pep in your step, the protein and fiber content of this mix slows down the digestion and absorption of the carbohydrates and helps stabilize your energy levels. This high-protein, high-fiber, and high-FLAVOR trail (or road!) mix will leave you feeling full, satiated, and pumped for your next destination.

In a large grab-and-go container with a tight lid, combine the jerky, pumpkin seeds, chickpeas, strawberries, and pistachios.

Close the lid and shake well to mix everything together. Keep the container in your car, in your backpack, clipped to your bike rack, etc., for a balanced snack on the go. It keeps for up to 1 week (see tip).

STEPH'S TIP

The freeze-dried strawberries will pick up residual moisture from the jerky, so they will likely become less crunchy and chewier. If you prefer them crunchy, simply store them separately and add while snacking.

Pick-Me-Up Pistachio Gelato

SERVES 4 TO 6
PREP TIME: 10 minutes
FREEZING TIME: 8 hours or overnight

PER SERVING:	CALORIES 275 kcal	PROTEIN 12g	FAT 14g	CARBOHYDRATE 27g	FIBER 2g

1 cup lightly salted roasted pistachios, divided

1½ cups nonfat or low-fat Greek yogurt

½ cup sweetened condensed milk

1 tablespoon fresh lime juice

This gelato is the perfect way to satisfy a nighttime sweet-tooth craving, because it's high in protein, so your blood sugar levels won't spike and crash. Plus, it doesn't require an ice cream maker. Pistachios are packed with protein, fiber, and healthy fats, making this gelato not only a treat but also a snack to keep you sated day or night.

Place ¾ cup of the pistachios in a blender. Blend on low speed, gradually increasing the speed to high, for 30 seconds to 1 minute, until the pistachios are finely ground. Add the yogurt, condensed milk, and lime juice and blend on low speed, gradually increasing the speed to high, for 1 to 2 minutes, until smooth.

Line a small 1- to 1½-quart baking dish or loaf pan with parchment paper. Pour the gelato mixture into the dish. Coarsely chop the remaining ¼ cup pistachios and sprinkle them evenly over the top. Freeze the gelato, uncovered, overnight (for 8 or more hours), until firm.

For serving, portion out whatever amount of the frozen gelato you want to enjoy, and allow to stand at room temperature for 20 to 40 minutes, until it is soft and scoops to your liking. It will be very firm straight out of the freezer (🍲), so if you aren't thawing all of it to enjoy right away, use a table knife or ice cream scoop to remove what you are eating. Tightly cover and freeze the rest for up to 2 weeks.

STEPH'S TIP

If you are in a rush or want your scoops to be fully formed and smooth, dip your scoop in hot water between scoops, so that it glides through the gelato more easily.

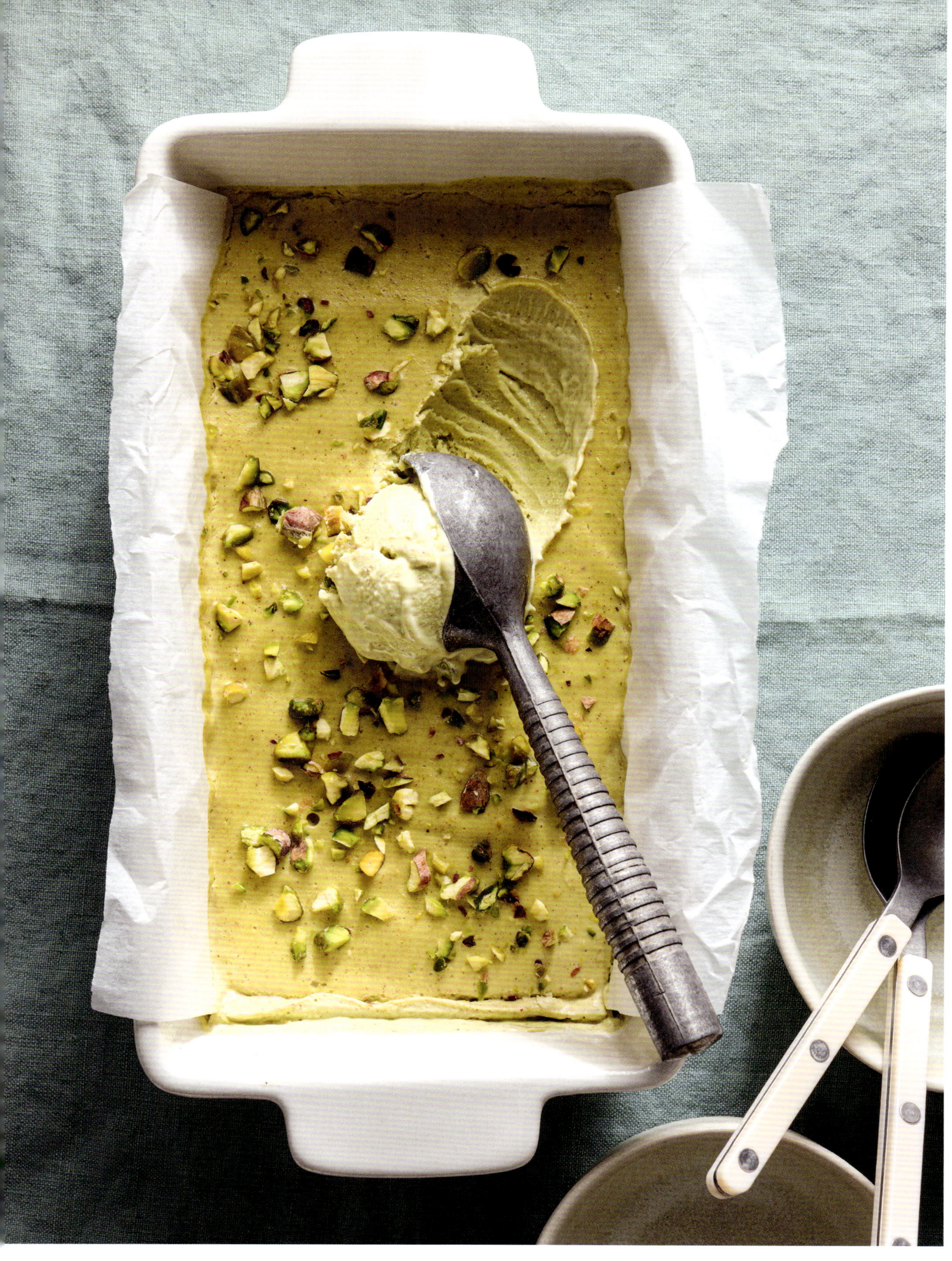

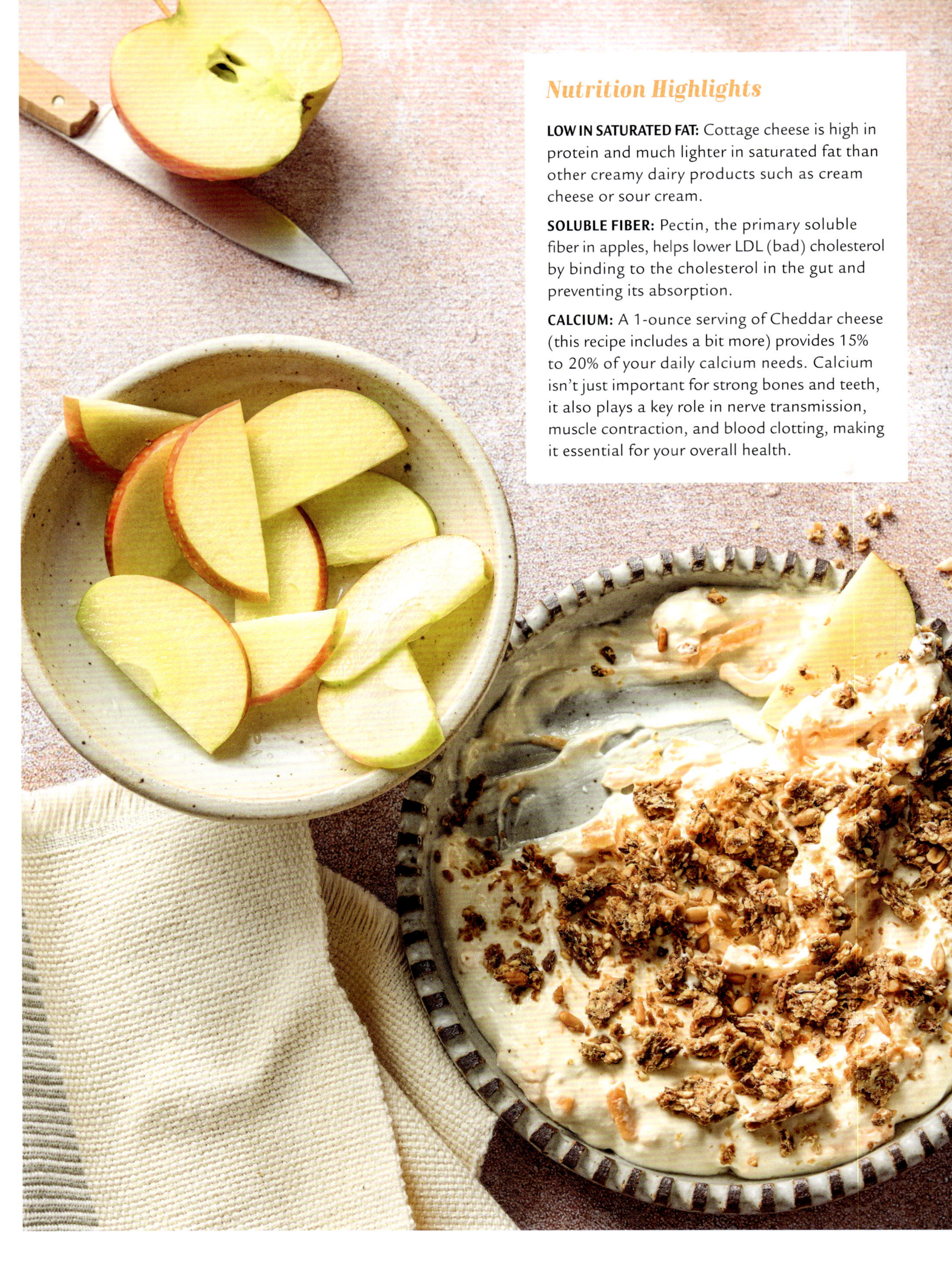

Nutrition Highlights

LOW IN SATURATED FAT: Cottage cheese is high in protein and much lighter in saturated fat than other creamy dairy products such as cream cheese or sour cream.

SOLUBLE FIBER: Pectin, the primary soluble fiber in apples, helps lower LDL (bad) cholesterol by binding to the cholesterol in the gut and preventing its absorption.

CALCIUM: A 1-ounce serving of Cheddar cheese (this recipe includes a bit more) provides 15% to 20% of your daily calcium needs. Calcium isn't just important for strong bones and teeth, it also plays a key role in nerve transmission, muscle contraction, and blood clotting, making it essential for your overall health.

Cheese & Crackers Remix *with* Apple Dippers

MAKES 1 HEAPING CUP DIP
SERVES 2 TO 4
PREP TIME: 10 minutes

PER SERVING:	CALORIES 200 kcal	PROTEIN 12g	FAT 9g	CARBOHYDRATE 18g	FIBER 2g

1 cup 2% cottage cheese (or whatever fat content you prefer)

2 tablespoons nonfat or low-fat Greek yogurt

1 tablespoon Dijon mustard

1½ teaspoons extra-virgin olive oil

⅛ teaspoon kosher salt

⅓ cup grated sharp Cheddar cheese

4 to 6 whole-grain crackers (I love garden veggie flavored crackers for this)

1 crisp, slightly tart, yet balanced apple, such as Braeburn, Fuji, Gala, or Honeycrisp, sliced vertically to resemble a cracker

I *really* love creamy and spreadable pimento cheese. I can eat a whole tub in one sitting. Unfortunately, the amount of saturated fat in that tub would change my whole blood panel, so I came up with a savory, spreadable, and dippable cheese that's loaded with protein and doesn't sacrifice big cheese flavor.

This snack is the perfect balance of sweet, salty, and tangy, plus you get that cracker-like crunch from the apple and crushed cracker topper. If you want to spice it up, add one to two tablespoons of minced pickled jalapeño or fresh jalapeño to the dip so that it tastes almost like a pepper Jack. I'm excited for you to make this.

In a food processor or blender, combine the cottage cheese, yogurt, mustard, olive oil, and salt. Blend until it is smooth and creamy, 30 to 40 seconds. Transfer the dip to a small bowl and stir in the Cheddar until fully incorporated.

Crunch and crumble your crackers! In a sturdy plastic bag, add the crackers. Leave a small opening at the top of the bag for air to escape and then cover the bag with a kitchen towel. Release any anger or irritation (*half* joking) by pounding the towel-covered bag with your fists, until you've coarsely crumbled the crackers to a granola-like texture.

Evenly sprinkle the crumbled crackers over the dip. Enjoy right away with sliced apple for dipping ( ).

STORAGE

Store airtight in the refrigerator for up to 1 week. For the best texture, add the crumbled crackers right before serving. If the dip separates at all or becomes watery while stored, simply give it a stir before serving.

STEPH'S TIP

If you want more or less cracker with your cheesy apple bites, keep the crumbs in the bag or transfer them to a small bowl, and dunk your cheese-coated apple slice directly in them. Yum!

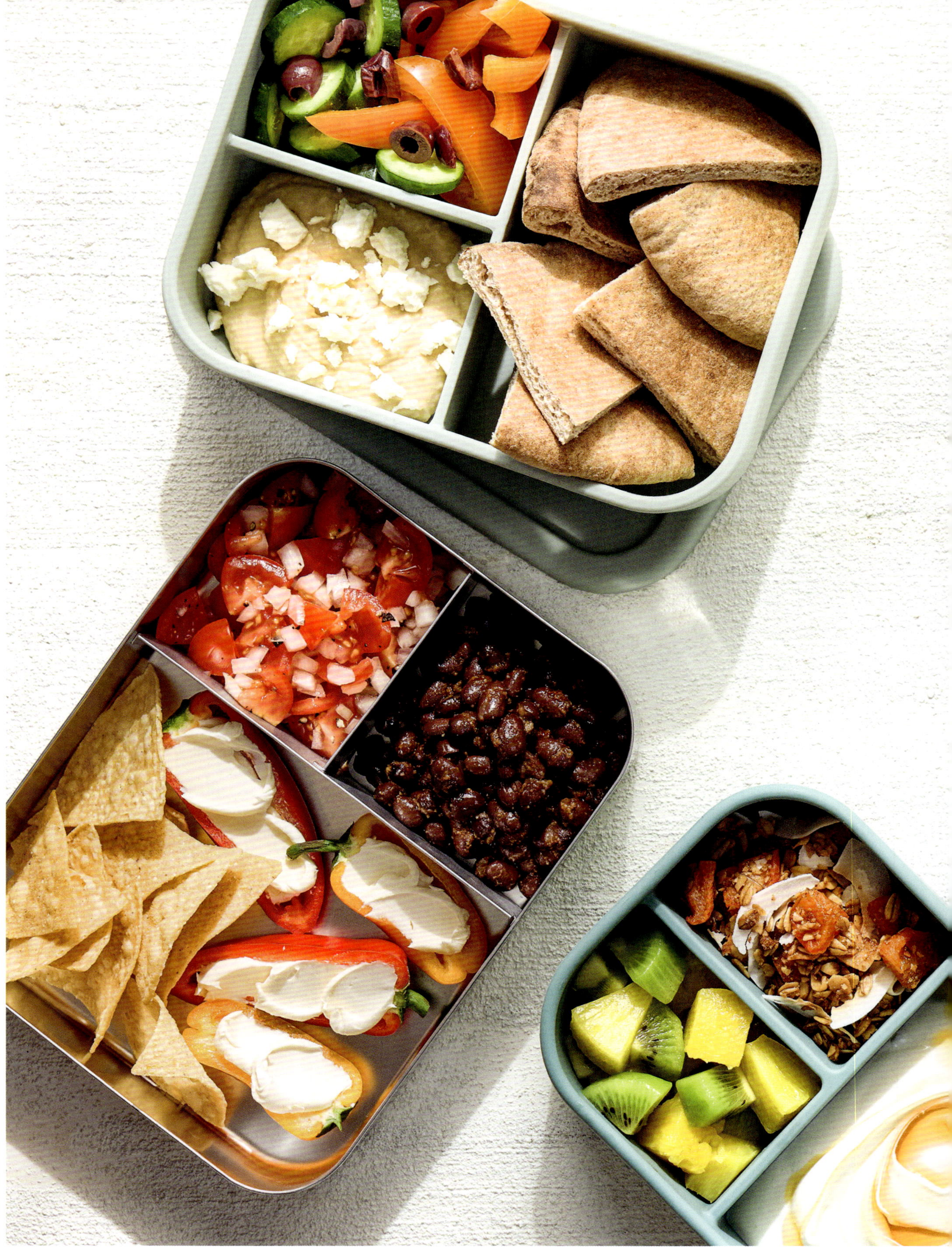

Bento Box Adult Snack Packers

These colorful good-for-you snack packs cover all your snacking needs in a healthy and satisfying way. They are loaded with energy-boosting foods and are meant to be snacked on all day.

If you don't have a bento box, simply arrange the components as you wish in another container or dish. I highly recommend getting one, though—they're so fun, and there are lots of options. Bento box recs: Choose one with multiple different-size compartments to keep snacks separate and fresh, leakproof sections to avoid spillage, and durable planet- and people-friendly materials like BPA-free plastic, stainless steel, or silicone.

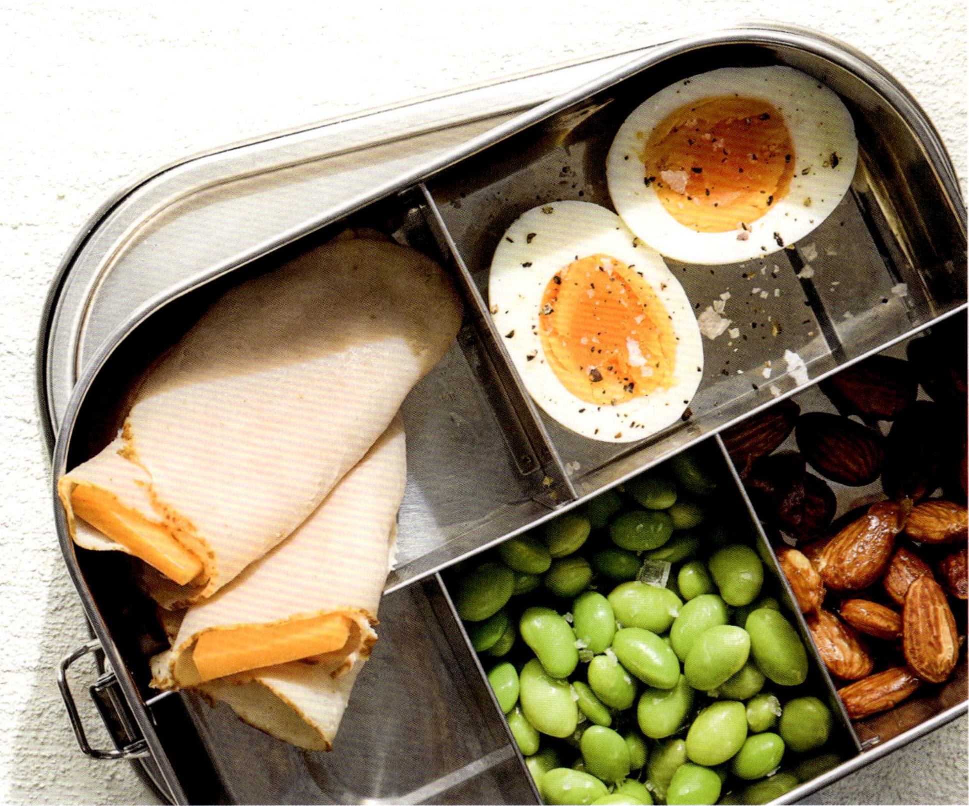

Hummus & Pita Bento Box

SERVES 1
PREP TIME: 10 minutes

PER SERVING:	**CALORIES** 415 kcal	**PROTEIN** 15g	**FAT** 21g	**CARBOHYDRATE** 48g	**FIBER** 7g

1 whole-grain pita, sliced into wedges

¼ cup hummus (whatever homemade or store-bought type you prefer)

¼ cup cubed feta cheese

⅓ cup diced English or salad cucumber

⅓ cup diced red bell pepper

1 tablespoon chopped Kalamata olives

This bento box is perfectly balanced with protein, healthy fats, and complex carbs for lasting energy. The chickpeas in the hummus equal plant-based protein and fiber that keeps you full and supports digestion. Kalamata olives are big on heart-healthy monounsaturated fats that help fight inflammation. And the whole-grain pita adds complex carbs for steady energy, plus B vitamins to support metabolism.

Place the pita wedges in the largest compartment. Arrange the hummus and feta in one of the smaller compartments. Arrange the cucumber, bell pepper, and olives in the other smaller compartment.

Dip the pita into the hummus, add toppings, and enjoy! This prepped and packed bento box can be refrigerated and enjoyed for up to 3 days.

Yogurt & Granola Parfait Bento Box

SERVES 1
PREP TIME: 10 minutes

PER SERVING:	**CALORIES** 449 kcal	**PROTEIN** 23g	**FAT** 8g	**CARBOHYDRATE** 75g	**FIBER** 7g

1 cup nonfat or low-fat Greek yogurt

1½ teaspoons honey

¼ cup granola

3 dried apricots or mango pieces, chopped

1 tablespoon shredded or flaked coconut, unsweetened or sweetened

1 kiwi, peeled and diced

½ cup chopped canned pineapple

This bento is simple, balanced, and perfect for when you need a quick snack that feels like a sweet treat but is quite nourishing. Greek yogurt provides protein to keep you full and satisfied while the granola and dried fruit add fiber and energy-boosting carbs. The coconut flakes add a touch of healthy fat, and kiwi and pineapple brighten everything up with their burst of vitamin C and antioxidants.

In the largest compartment or small bowl, stir together the yogurt and honey until the honey is fully incorporated.

In a smaller compartment, stir together the granola, dried fruit, and coconut. In the other smaller compartment, combine the kiwi and pineapple.

When ready to eat, mix the toppings into the yogurt. The prepped and packed bento box can be refrigerated and enjoyed for up to 3 days.

Southwest Black Beans Bento Box

SERVES 1
PREP TIME: 10 minutes

PER SERVING:	**CALORIES** 398 kcal	**PROTEIN** 13g	**FAT** 18g	**CARBOHYDRATE** 50g	**FIBER** 12g

2 mini sweet peppers, halved and seeded

2 tablespoons cream cheese

Handful of tortilla chips, broken in half if large

½ cup canned black beans (or ½ cup cooked), drained and rinsed if canned

¼ teaspoon ground cumin

⅛ teaspoon garlic powder

⅛ teaspoon smoked paprika

Kosher salt

1½ teaspoons fresh lime juice, divided

½ cup diced cherry tomatoes

1 tablespoon finely chopped white onion

I think of this box as a mini "build-your-own" healthy nachos kit. Top the tortilla chips with each of the components for fun, layered bites and dunk the cream cheese–stuffed peppers into the black beans and salsa. The black beans are a powerhouse of plant-based protein, fiber, iron, and magnesium, all which help keep you full, energized, and satisfied. The cream cheese–stuffed mini peppers add creaminess and a vitamin C boost. The salsa adds a pop of fresh spiced flavor, antioxidants, and hydration.

Using a spoon or a table knife, fill the bell pepper halves evenly with the cream cheese (about 1½ teaspoons per) and place them in the larger compartment along with the tortilla chips if eating immediately (if not, store the tortilla chips in a small separate bag or container to stay crunchy).

In one of the smaller compartments of the bento box or in a small bowl, stir together the black beans, cumin, garlic powder, smoked paprika, a pinch of salt, and ¾ teaspoon of the lime juice. In the other small compartment or a small bowl, stir together the tomatoes, onion, a pinch of salt, and the remaining ¾ teaspoon lime juice. The prepped and packed bento box can be refrigerated and enjoyed for up to 3 days.

Protein-Packed Bento Box

SERVES 1
PREP TIME: 10 minutes

PER SERVING:	**CALORIES** 586 kcal	**PROTEIN** 42g	**FAT** 40g	**CARBOHYDRATE** 25g	**FIBER** 8g

2 ounces sliced deli turkey

1 ounce slice Cheddar cheese, cut into 2 rectangles

1 hard-boiled egg (store-bought is fine), peeled and halved

Kosher salt and freshly ground black pepper

½ cup shelled edamame, cooked (I use frozen and follow package cooking directions) and cooled

1 teaspoon unseasoned rice vinegar

¼ teaspoon flaky sea salt or a pinch of kosher salt

¼ cup Honey & Spice Roasted Almonds (recipe follows)

This is my go-to box to curb mindless snacking. It's got a little bit of everything—turkey, Cheddar, roasted almonds, hard-boiled egg—with a perfect balance of protein, fiber, and healthy fats. It's ideal for grazing between meetings, post-gym refueling, or when you need an afternoon pick-me-up. I love prepping this box on days I know I'll be too busy to sit down for a proper breakfast or lunch.

Fold and wrap the turkey slices around the middle of the Cheddar cheese rectangles and arrange them in the largest compartment along with the hard-boiled egg halves. Season the egg to taste with salt and pepper.

In one of the smaller compartments or in a small bowl, combine the edamame, rice vinegar, and flaky salt and toss gently to coat. Add the almonds to the other smaller compartment. The prepped and packed bento box can be refrigerated and enjoyed for up to 3 days.

Honey & Spice Roasted Almonds

MAKES 2 CUPS
PREP TIME: 5 minutes
COOK TIME: 13 minutes

PER ¼ CUP:	**CALORIES** 246 kcal	**PROTEIN** 8g	**FAT** 20g	**CARBOHYDRATE** 14g	**FIBER** 4g

2 cups whole almonds
1 tablespoon extra-virgin olive oil
1½ tablespoons honey
½ teaspoon kosher salt, divided
2 tablespoons sugar
¼ to ½ teaspoon cayenne pepper

I like to roast a pan of these sweet and spiced almonds on Sundays so I have something quick and satisfying to graze on throughout the week. They're not just great for snacking. I often chop and toss them into salads, sprinkle them over yogurt, or package them into cute little jars for homemade gifts. My friends and family all love it when they get a jar. Almonds are a wonderful source of healthy fats, fiber, and protein, making them a very satisfying and good-for-you snack.

Preheat the oven to 350°F. Line a sheet pan with parchment paper.

In a medium bowl, combine the almonds, olive oil, honey, and ¼ teaspoon of the salt. Stir well until the almonds are evenly coated. Spread the almond mixture in an even layer on the prepared sheet pan. Roast for 13 minutes.

Meanwhile, in a small bowl, stir together the sugar, cayenne pepper to taste, and the remaining ¼ teaspoon salt.

Remove the almonds from the oven and sprinkle them evenly right away with the sugar/salt/cayenne mixture. Using two spoons, carefully toss the almonds until they are evenly coated and in a single layer on the pan.

Cool completely, then transfer to an airtight jar or container, leaving behind and discarding any excess sugar mixture. Store the almonds in an airtight container at room temperature for up to 2 weeks.

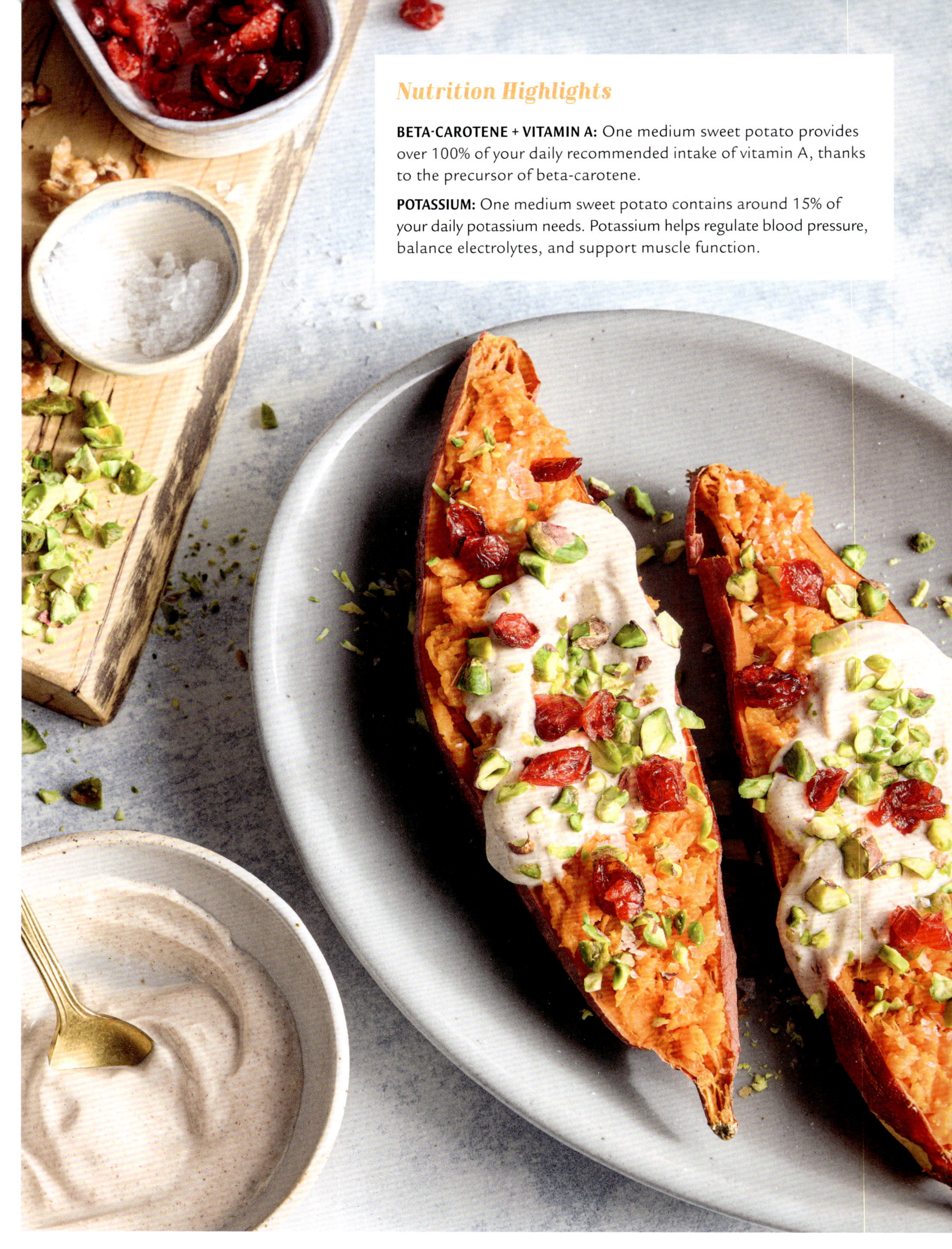

Nutrition Highlights

BETA-CAROTENE + VITAMIN A: One medium sweet potato provides over 100% of your daily recommended intake of vitamin A, thanks to the precursor of beta-carotene.

POTASSIUM: One medium sweet potato contains around 15% of your daily potassium needs. Potassium helps regulate blood pressure, balance electrolytes, and support muscle function.

Quick Sweet Potato Snack

SERVES 1 OR 2
PREP TIME: 5 minutes
COOK TIME: 10 minutes

PER SERVING:	**CALORIES** 128 kcal	**PROTEIN** 5g	**FAT** 0g	**CARBOHYDRATE** 27g	**FIBER** 3g

1 (12- to 16-ounce) sweet potato, rinsed and patted dry

½ cup nonfat or low-fat Greek yogurt

1½ teaspoons honey

½ teaspoon ground cinnamon

Pinch of kosher salt

Toppings (optional): chopped nuts such as walnuts or pecans, granola, or dried fruit such as raisins or cranberries

My fiancé, Miles, is as in love with sweet potatoes as he is with me. Just kidding. Sort of. He ate them for lunch every day for an *entire year*! And that's why I've included his microwave technique for cooking them. As for nutrition, you get complex carbs plus a bunch of vitamins. I love all the optional toppings, depending on my mood, but I most often sprinkle the steamy potato halves with chopped nuts.

Pierce the sweet potato 10 to 12 times with a fork. Place it on a microwave-safe plate and microwave on high, turning it about halfway through, until it is tender and easy to pierce with a fork all the way to the center, 7 to 10 minutes (microwave power varies widely). Slice the potato in half lengthwise and set it aside until it is cool enough to handle, about 15 minutes.

Meanwhile, in a small bowl, stir together the yogurt, honey, and cinnamon.

Once cool enough to handle, fluff the potato flesh with a fork and add a pinch of salt as you fluff. Top each potato half evenly with the yogurt mixture.

Serve the potato halves in a bowl. For added texture and flavor, top with nuts, granola, and/or dried fruit (if using).

STORAGE + REHEAT

Once cooled, store the potatoes airtight in the refrigerator for up to 3 days. Store the yogurt mixture and any optional toppings separately in an airtight container in the refrigerator for up to 3 days. To reheat, warm in a pan over medium heat until heated through, or microwave.

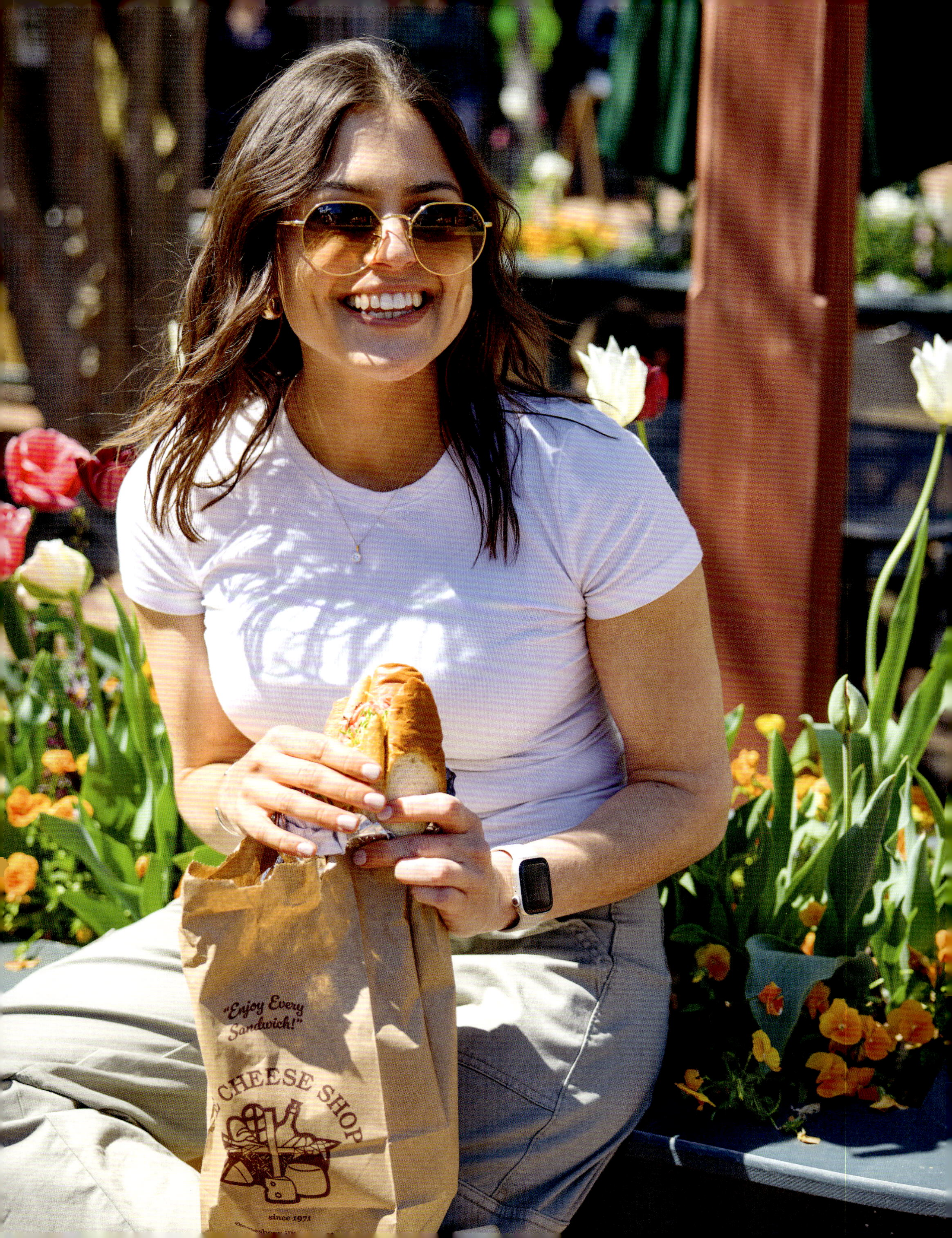
"Enjoy Every Sandwich!"
CHEESE SHOP
since 1971

Salads, Bowls, Wraps & Sandwiches

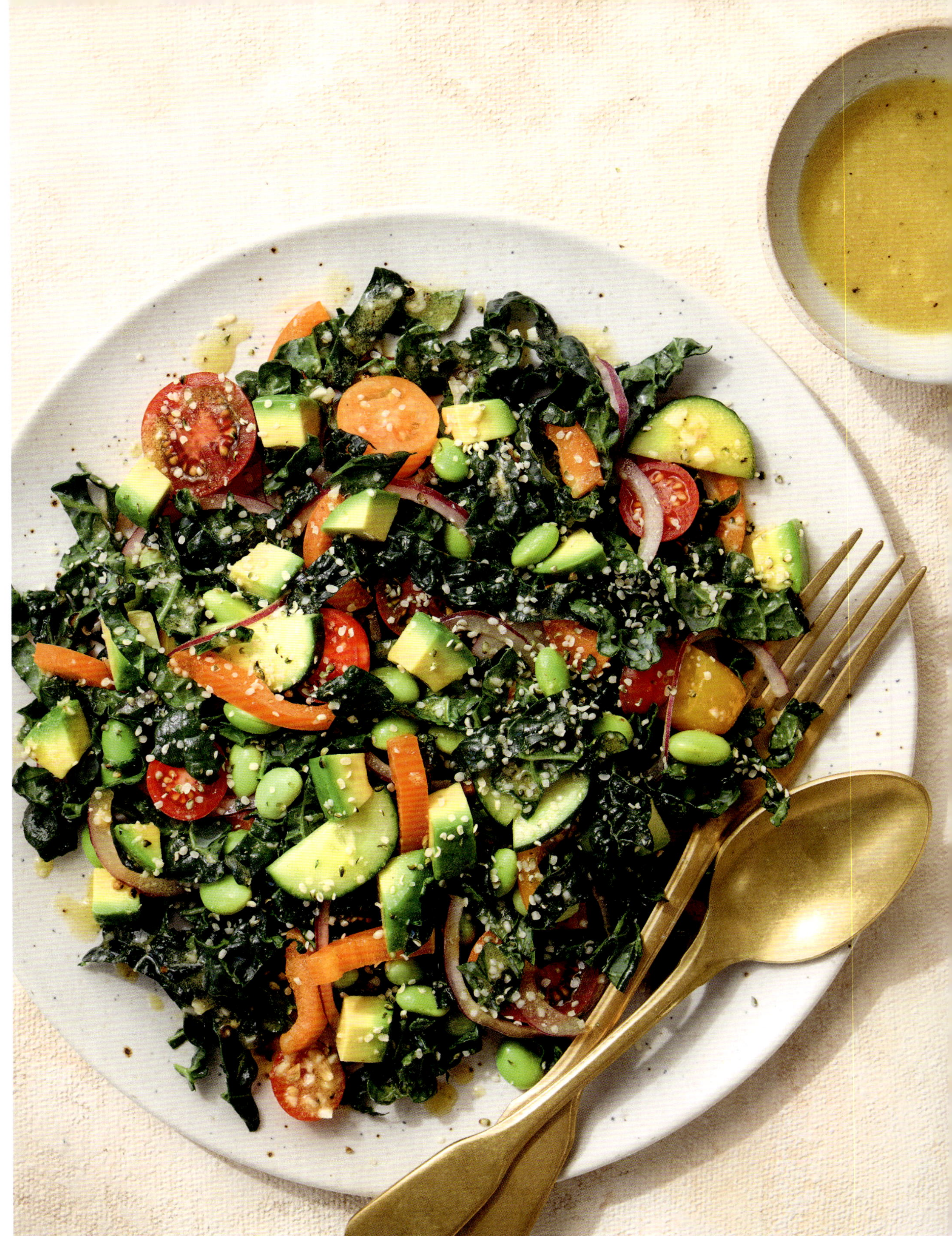

Lizzo Salad

SERVES 2
PREP TIME: 15 minutes

PER SERVING SALAD:	**CALORIES** 492 kcal	**PROTEIN** 25g	**FAT** 24g	**CARBOHYDRATE** 40g	**FIBER** 18g
VINAIGRETTE (PER 2 TBSP):	**CALORIES** 131 kcal	**PROTEIN** 0g	**FAT** 14g	**CARBOHYDRATE** 3g	**FIBER** 0g

1 bunch kale, stemmed and finely chopped (about 6 cups lightly packed; ½ pound)

1½ cups shelled edamame, cooked (I use frozen and follow package cooking directions) and cooled

1 red or orange bell pepper, quartered and thinly sliced

1 English or large salad cucumber, diced

1 avocado, diced

½ cup thinly sliced red onion

½ cup halved or quartered cherry tomatoes

3 tablespoons hemp hearts (hulled hemp seeds)

Garlicky Vinaigrette

¼ cup plus 2 tablespoons extra-virgin olive oil

¼ cup fresh lemon juice (about 1 lemon)

1 tablespoon Dijon mustard

1½ teaspoons honey, plus more to taste

1½ teaspoons minced garlic (1 or 2 cloves)

½ teaspoon kosher salt, plus more to taste

⅛ teaspoon freshly ground black pepper, plus more to taste

I'll never forget the day Lizzo duetted my video on TikTok in early 2022 and gave this veggie-amped salad of mine her stamp of approval. An absolute honor. Lizzo is a rapper, singer, flutist superstar, and an all-around badass. This salad is perfect for her and you when you crave something meatless and packed with protein for a tasty side. It's Lizzo-approved, so you know it's gonna be a hit.

The hemp hearts here are filled with high-quality plant-based protein, omega-3 and omega-6 fatty acids, as well as minerals like magnesium, potassium, iron, and zinc. They are super tasty and versatile and can be sprinkled on just about everything, including salads, soups, pasta, yogurt, oatmeal, and more.

So, get out those salad bowls and start chop, chop, chopping! Pump up Lizzo's "Good as Hell" song when you do or "About Damn Time"—the one that we played on TikTok for this.

In a large bowl, massage the kale by hand for about 3 minutes until it softens and wilt; this breaks down the fibers and mellows the flavor.

Add the edamame, bell pepper, cucumber, avocado, onion, tomatoes, and hemp hearts to the bowl, gently toss, and set aside.

Make the garlicky vinaigrette: In a medium bowl, whisk together the olive oil, lemon juice, mustard, honey, garlic, salt, and pepper until the dressing comes together and emulsifies. Taste and add more honey, salt, or pepper to taste. Makes about ¾ cup.

Drizzle the dressing over the salad and gently toss until everything is evenly coated. Serve immediately. This salad is best enjoyed day of.

STORAGE

Store the salad and dressing in separate airtight containers in the refrigerator for up to 1 day.

Warm Lentil Salad *with* Roasted Veggies

SERVES 1 OR 2
PREP TIME: 10 minutes
COOK TIME: 45 minutes

PER SERVING:	**CALORIES** 532 kcal	**PROTEIN** 27g	**FAT** 28g	**CARBOHYDRATE** 47g	**FIBER** 16g

½ cup green or brown lentils, rinsed

2½ cups water

½ teaspoon kosher salt, divided

3 cups (about 12 ounces) precut frozen broccoli/cauliflower/carrot mix (or use whatever mix you like)

Half a 14- to 16-ounce block extra-firm tofu, prepressed (not packed in water) if available, cut into ½-inch cubes

2 tablespoons extra-virgin olive oil, divided

2 tablespoons soy sauce, divided

1 teaspoon finely grated or minced peeled fresh ginger

1 tablespoon honey or maple syrup

1 garlic clove, minced

Cooking spray or neutral oil, for greasing

Sesame seeds (optional), for garnish

This warm savory salad is full of big-flavor soy sauce umami plus fiber-loaded lentils, and it's another quick and easy roasted frozen veggies dish, like the Sheet-Pan Smashed Brussels Sprouts (page 212). Same technique. I prefer this salad warm, but it's great at any temperature.

Preheat the oven to 450°F. Place a sheet pan in it to warm.

In a medium pot, combine the lentils, water, and ¼ teaspoon of the salt. Bring to a boil over high heat. Once boiling, decrease the heat to low and simmer uncovered until the lentils are tender but not mushy, 20 to 30 minutes. (Most brown lentils cook faster than green lentils.)

Meanwhile, in a large bowl, combine the mixed frozen vegetables (don't thaw!), tofu, 1 tablespoon of the olive oil, 1 tablespoon of the soy sauce, and the remaining ¼ teaspoon salt and stir to combine.

In a small bowl, whisk together the remaining 1 tablespoon soy sauce, remaining 1 tablespoon olive oil, the ginger, honey, and garlic to make the dressing.

Drain and discard any excess water from the cooked lentils, transfer them to a large bowl, add half of the dressing, and gently stir to combine.

Once the oven is preheated, carefully remove the hot sheet pan. Lightly grease it with cooking spray or oil (). Carefully transfer the seasoned tofu and frozen vegetables to the sheet pan in a single, even layer. Roast until both are cooked through and lightly browned, about 20 minutes.

Transfer the roasted vegetables and tofu to the lentil bowl, add the remaining dressing, and gently stir to combine. Garnish with sesame seeds (if using) and serve warm.

NUTRITION PSA

Tofu myth debunk: The naturally occurring phytoestrogens in tofu *are not* the same as human estrogen! That misinformation has been buzzing around for a while. Let's please move on. I love tofu—it's high in protein plus unsaturated fats and super-duper tasty in this 100 percent plant-based dish.

STORAGE + REHEAT

Once cooled, store airtight in the refrigerator for up to 3 days. To reheat, warm in a pan over medium heat until heated through, or microwave.

STEPH'S TIP

It's important not to line the sheet pan because you want the frozen veggies and tofu to sizzle, sear, and brown right when they hit the just-out-of-the-oven hot sheet pan.

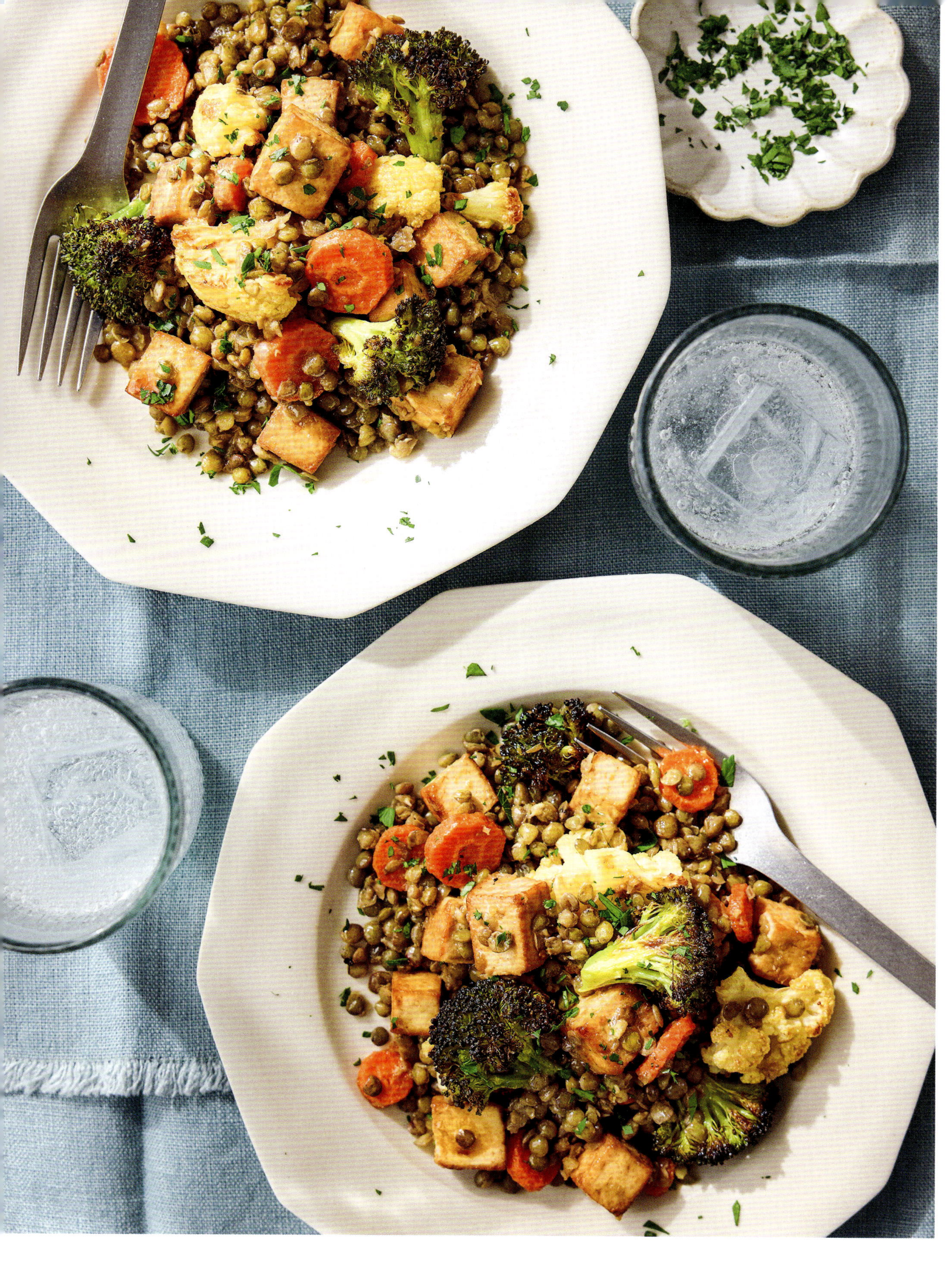

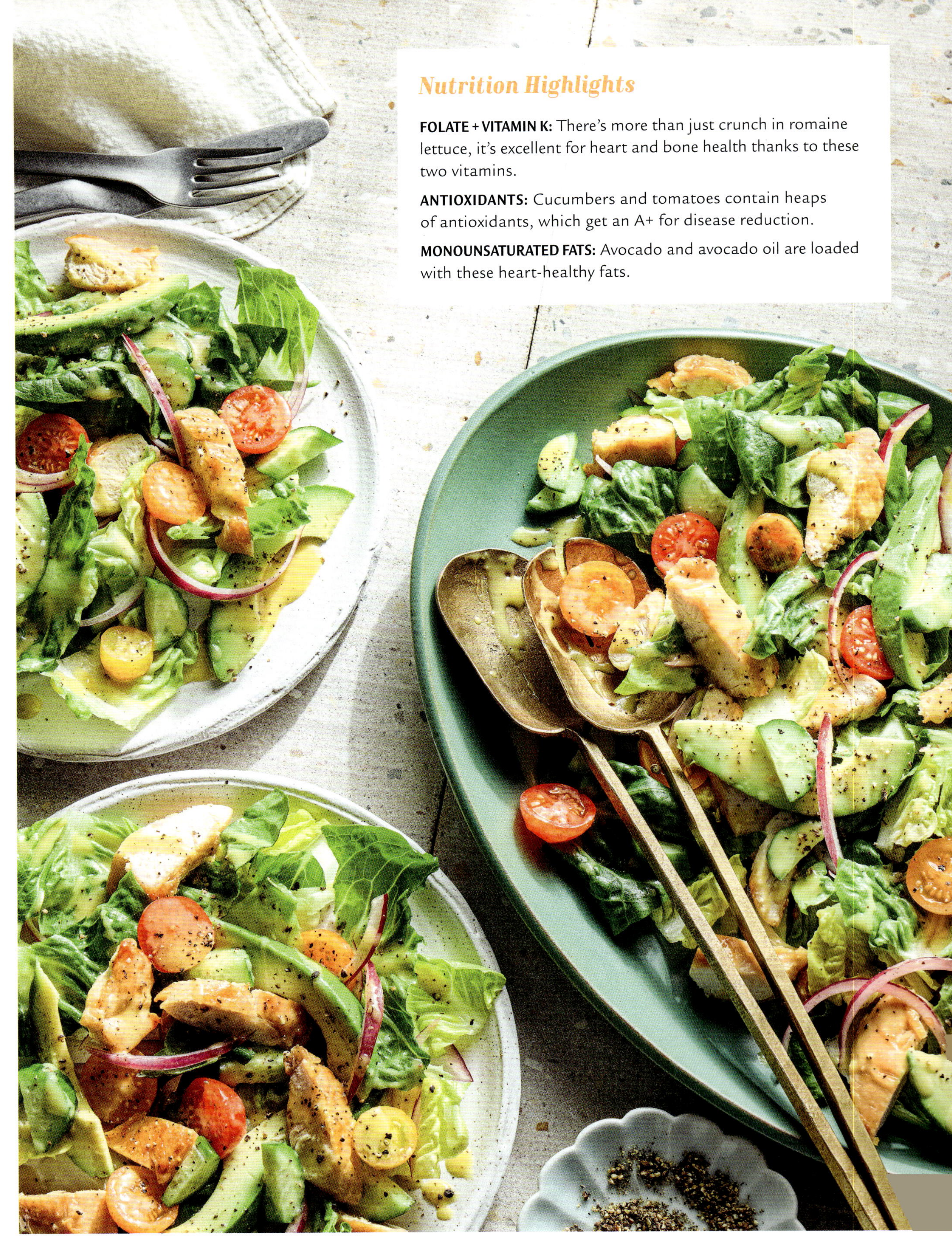

Nutrition Highlights

FOLATE + VITAMIN K: There's more than just crunch in romaine lettuce, it's excellent for heart and bone health thanks to these two vitamins.

ANTIOXIDANTS: Cucumbers and tomatoes contain heaps of antioxidants, which get an A+ for disease reduction.

MONOUNSATURATED FATS: Avocado and avocado oil are loaded with these heart-healthy fats.

Chicken Tender Salad *with* Honey Mustard Dressing

SERVES 4
PREP TIME: 10 minutes
COOK TIME: 10 minutes

PER SERVING:	CALORIES 325 kcal	PROTEIN 30g	FAT 12g	CARBOHYDRATE 13g	FIBER 6g

- 1 pound chicken tenderloins or 2 large chicken breasts sliced into 8 to 10 pieces
- ½ teaspoon kosher salt
- 1 tablespoon avocado oil
- 1 head romaine lettuce, chopped
- 1 English or large salad cucumber, halved lengthwise and sliced into ¼-inch-thick half-moons
- 1 cup halved or quartered cherry tomatoes
- 1 avocado, sliced
- ½ red onion, thinly sliced
- 1 cup Honey Mustard Dressing (recipe follows)
- Freshly ground black pepper (optional)

This fresh salad is the perfect blend of crispy-crunchy greens, savory chicken, creamy avocado, and sweet cherry tomatoes, all tossed in a generous amount of my addictive honey mustard dressing. I typically make this one for a quick weeknight dinner or prep it for weekday lunches.

Preheat the oven to 400°F.

Pat the chicken dry with a paper towel and season with the salt. In a large ovenproof pan, heat the avocado oil over medium heat. When the oil is hot, sear the chicken on one side for about 5 minutes without moving it, for a golden-brown sear. Carefully flip the chicken pieces, then immediately transfer the pan to the oven.

Bake until the internal temperature reaches 165°F, about 2 minutes. Set aside to cool for a few minutes.

In a large bowl, gently toss the lettuce, cucumber, tomatoes, avocado, and red onion. Slice the chicken into bite-size pieces and add them to the bowl.

Drizzle the salad with the honey mustard dressing, toss gently to combine, season with pepper, if desired, and serve immediately.

STORAGE

Store the salad (without dressing) in an airtight container in the refrigerator for up to 2 days. Store the dressing separately in an airtight container in the refrigerator for up to 1 week.

Honey Mustard Dressing

MAKES 1 HEAPING CUP

PER 2 TABLESPOONS:	CALORIES 131 kcal	PROTEIN 0g	FAT 14g	CARBOHYDRATE 3g	FIBER 0g

- ¼ cup apple cider vinegar
- ¼ cup Dijon mustard
- 2 tablespoons honey
- ½ teaspoon garlic powder
- ¼ teaspoon kosher salt
- ⅛ teaspoon freshly ground black pepper
- ¼ cup extra-virgin olive oil

In a small bowl, whisk together the vinegar, mustard, honey, garlic powder, salt, and pepper until the honey and mustard are fully combined. Slowly whisk in the olive oil, so that the dressing comes together and emulsifies.

Tunacado Toasties

SERVES 1 OR 2
PREP TIME: 5 minutes
COOK TIME: 5 minutes

PER SERVING:	**CALORIES** 379 kcal	**PROTEIN** 23g	**FAT** 9g	**CARBOHYDRATE** 22g	**FIBER** 8g

½ large avocado

One 5- to 6-ounce can solid white albacore tuna in water, drained and flaked

¼ cup 2% cottage cheese (or whatever fat content you prefer)

2 cups microgreens (or any greens of choice, finely chopped), divided

2 tablespoons finely chopped pickled banana pepper or pepperoncini

2 tablespoons fresh dill, finely chopped

1 tablespoon finely chopped green onions (white and green parts)

1 tablespoon fresh lemon juice (about ½ small lemon)

⅛ teaspoon kosher salt

2 slices whole-wheat bread

If you're a fan of tuna salad, I can't wait for you to try this! It takes tuna salad to the next level with a bunch of fresh ingredients in the mix—avocado, microgreens, green onions, lemon—and it's a breeze to make. Eat it straight-up, scooped over a salad, in a sandwich or wrap, or as I most like to, spread on sliced whole-wheat toasties (toast triangles).

As far as nutrition goes, it doesn't get more balanced. The tuna is your lean protein loaded with omega-3 fatty acids, which are great for your heart. Cottage cheese piles on even more protein plus calcium for bone health. And as for the avocado—hello healthy monounsaturated fats! The microgreens deliver vitamins C, E, and K, all of which support immune health and reduce inflammation. And you can thank the whole-wheat bread for its digestion-aiding and energy-sustaining fiber.

In a medium bowl, mash the avocado with a fork or spoon until fairly smooth. Add the tuna and cottage cheese and stir until well combined. Add 1 cup of the microgreens, the banana pepper, dill, green onions, lemon juice, and salt. Stir to combine.

In a medium serving bowl, place the remaining 1 cup microgreens (). Top them with the prepared tuna mixture.

Toast the bread until golden brown and nicely crisped. Slice each piece of toasted bread diagonally into 2 triangles and serve alongside the tuna mixture. Refrigerate leftover tuna salad for up to 3 days.

STEPH'S TIP

I like having the microgreens on the bottom because it's easier to eat them that way, but you can also first top the toast with them and then spread on the tuna mix.

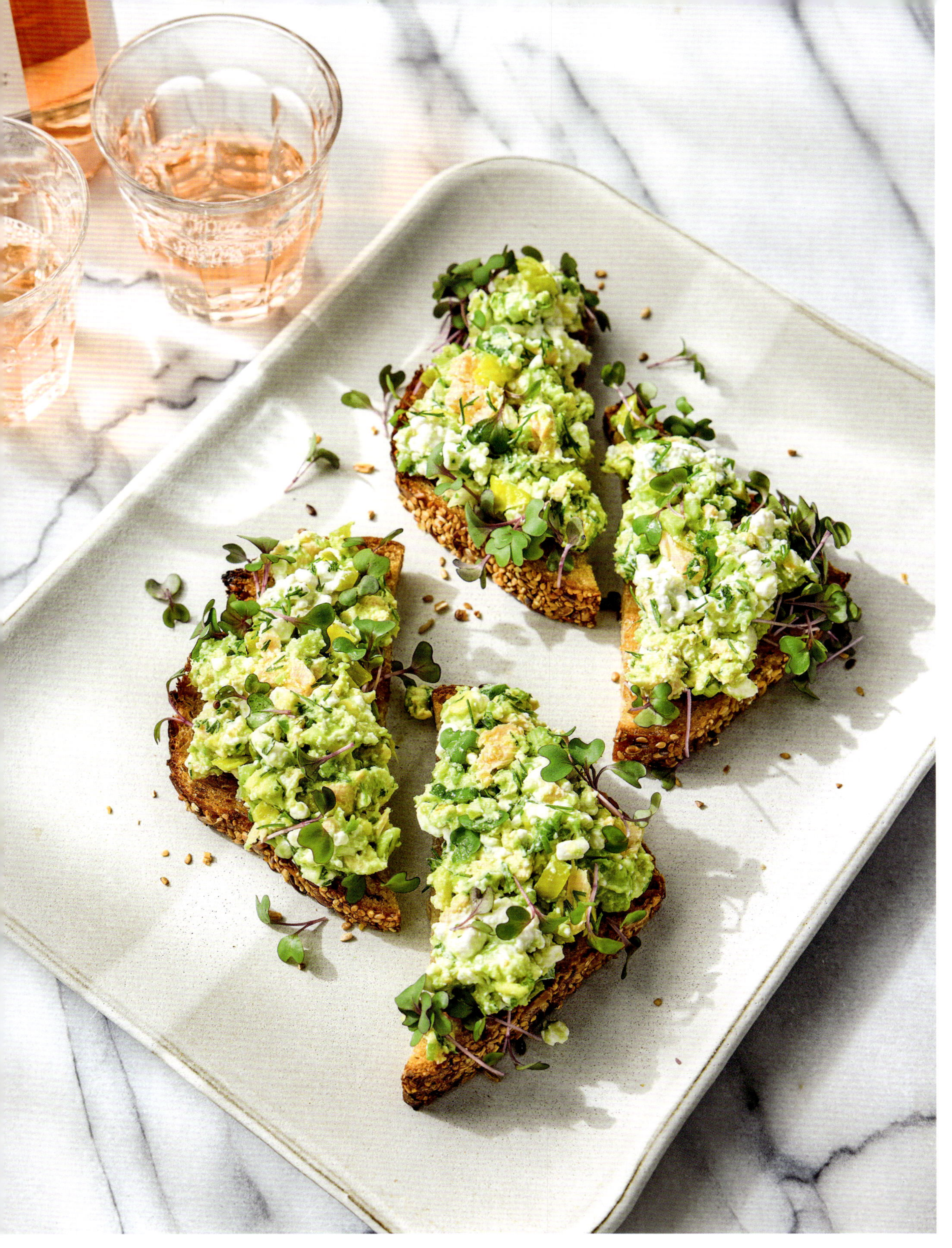

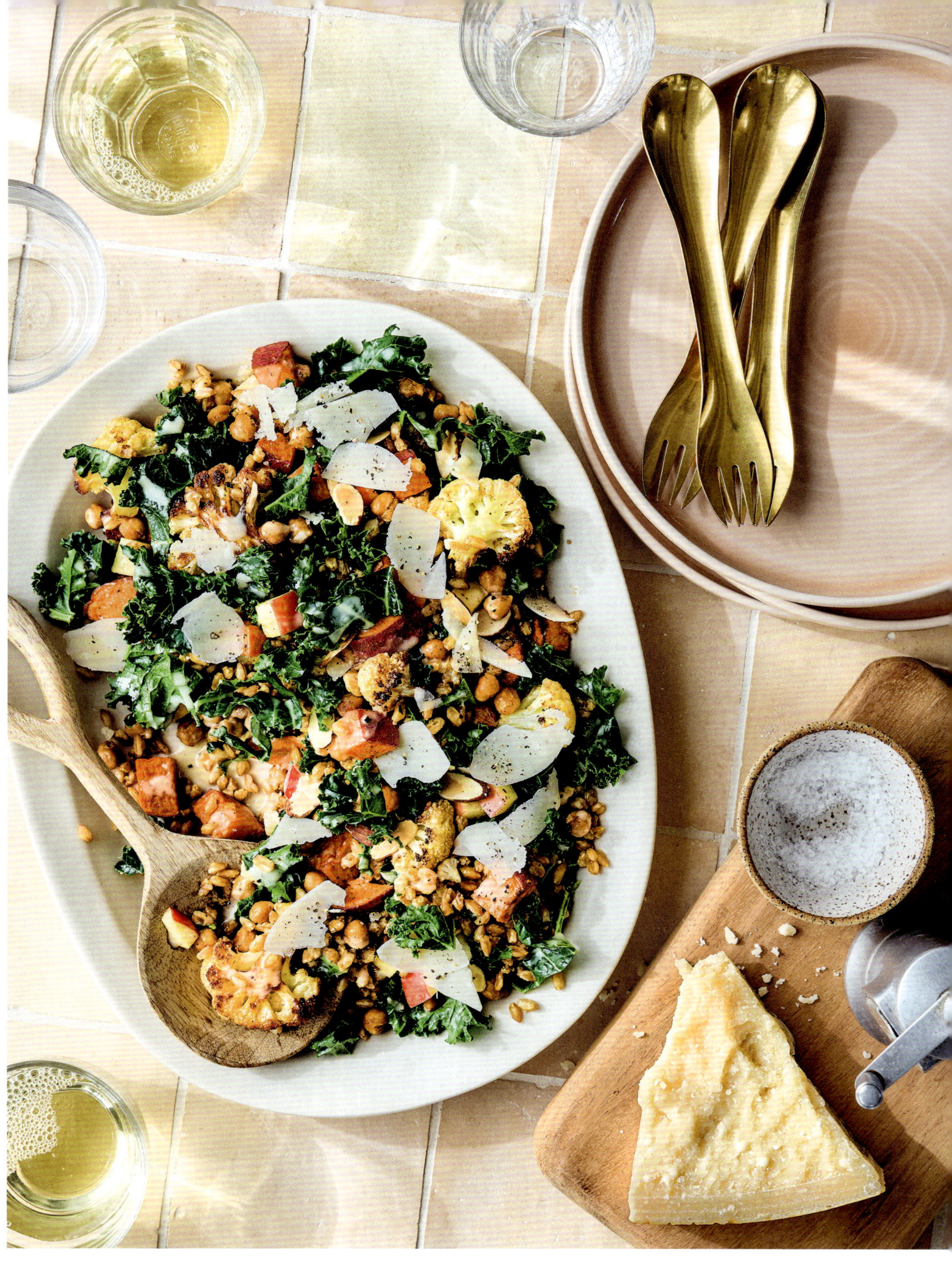

Roasted Veggie Harvest Bowls

SERVES 4 TO 6
PREP TIME: 25 minutes
COOK TIME: 45 minutes

PER SERVING:	CALORIES 391 kcal	PROTEIN 15g	FAT 19g	CARBOHYDRATE 46g	FIBER 11g

1¾ cups vegetable broth (or preferred broth)

1 cup farro

Roasted Veggies

3 tablespoons extra-virgin olive oil

1 teaspoon ground cumin

1 teaspoon sweet paprika

½ teaspoon ground nutmeg

½ teaspoon kosher salt, plus more to taste

1 (12- to 16-ounce) sweet potato, unpeeled and cut into ½-inch cubes

1 head cauliflower, cut into florets

One 15-ounce can chickpeas (or 1½ cups cooked chickpeas), drained and rinsed if canned, patted dry

Lemon-Tahini Dressing

3 tablespoons fresh lemon juice (about ½ large lemon)

2 tablespoons tahini

1 tablespoon maple syrup

¼ teaspoon kosher salt

¼ teaspoon freshly ground black pepper

Salad

3 cups (about ½ bunch, or ¼ pound) firmly packed finely chopped kale

1 apple, cored and cut into ½-inch cubes

⅓ cup sliced almonds, toasted

⅓ cup shaved Parmesan cheese

I often prepare this roasty, toasty bowl when I'm entertaining or need to bring a dish to any gathering involving food. Everyone loves it. It's special because of all the different bite-size textures and flavors, and it works well as both a main or hearty side with something like grilled steak or roasted fish. In terms of nutrition, the bowl combines complex carbohydrates, plant-based proteins, and healthy fats—in other words, it's really good for you.

I especially love making this in September and October, when fall sets in. The ingredients are in season then, so they're at their peak and easier on the wallet. Due to its many components, this one is perfect for weekend meal prep.

Keep in mind that the lemon-tahini dressing here can be doubled or tripled—it scales up perfectly—and keeps for up to a week in the fridge. It's great for all sorts of salads, especially ones with kale or cabbage, this bowl and others, and as a veggie dip. And, if you want a saucier bowl, as I often do, you can always up the dressing.

In a medium pot, bring the broth to a boil over high heat. Add the farro, decrease the heat to low, cover, and simmer until the farro is tender with a slight bite and most of the broth is absorbed, 25 to 45 minutes ( ). If necessary, drain off excess broth. Set aside.

Meanwhile, make the roasted veggies: Preheat the oven to 425°F. Line a sheet pan with parchment paper, a silicone baking mat, or aluminum foil (you'll thank yourself when you clean up after!).

In a large bowl (large enough to hold all of the roasted veggies and cooked farro later), whisk together the olive oil, cumin, paprika, nutmeg, and salt. Add the sweet potato, cauliflower, and chickpeas to the bowl and toss to combine. Transfer this mix evenly to the prepared sheet pan and reserve the bowl for tossing and serving.

Roast for 20 minutes. Remove the sheet pan from the oven and flip, toss, and move the veggies and chickpeas around the pan. Then return to the oven and roast until everything is a bit crisped and nicely browned, another 15 to 20 minutes. Season with additional salt to taste.

Make the lemon-tahini dressing: In a small bowl, whisk together the lemon juice, tahini, maple syrup, salt, and pepper until smooth. Adjust the seasoning if necessary.

Continued

Assemble the salad: When the roasted veggies and chickpeas are done, transfer them to the large bowl you oiled and seasoned them in. Add the cooked farro (it's great in here at any temperature, but I prefer it warm), kale, apple, and almonds and toss to combine. Add the dressing and toss until it's fully incorporated.

Evenly divide among serving bowls and top each serving evenly with the Parmesan.

NUTRITION PSA

Keep the skins on the sweet potatoes (all potatoes!) to save time and add more nutrients. The skin of sweet potatoes is rich in fiber, vitamins (especially vitamin C and several B vitamins), and minerals such as potassium and manganese.

STORAGE + REHEAT

If you don't plan to eat all the bowls at once, keep the dressing and Parmesan separate and dress and garnish the bowls before serving. Leftovers can be cooled and refrigerated airtight for up to 4 days. To reheat, warm in a pan over medium heat until heated through, or microwave. For best results, add the Parmesan right before serving.

STEPH'S TIP

Farro has a wide range in terms of cooking time, depending on whether you are using whole grain, semi-pearled, or pearled (the latter two cook faster), so taste it at 25 minutes, and in 5-minute increments after that if you need to cook it longer.

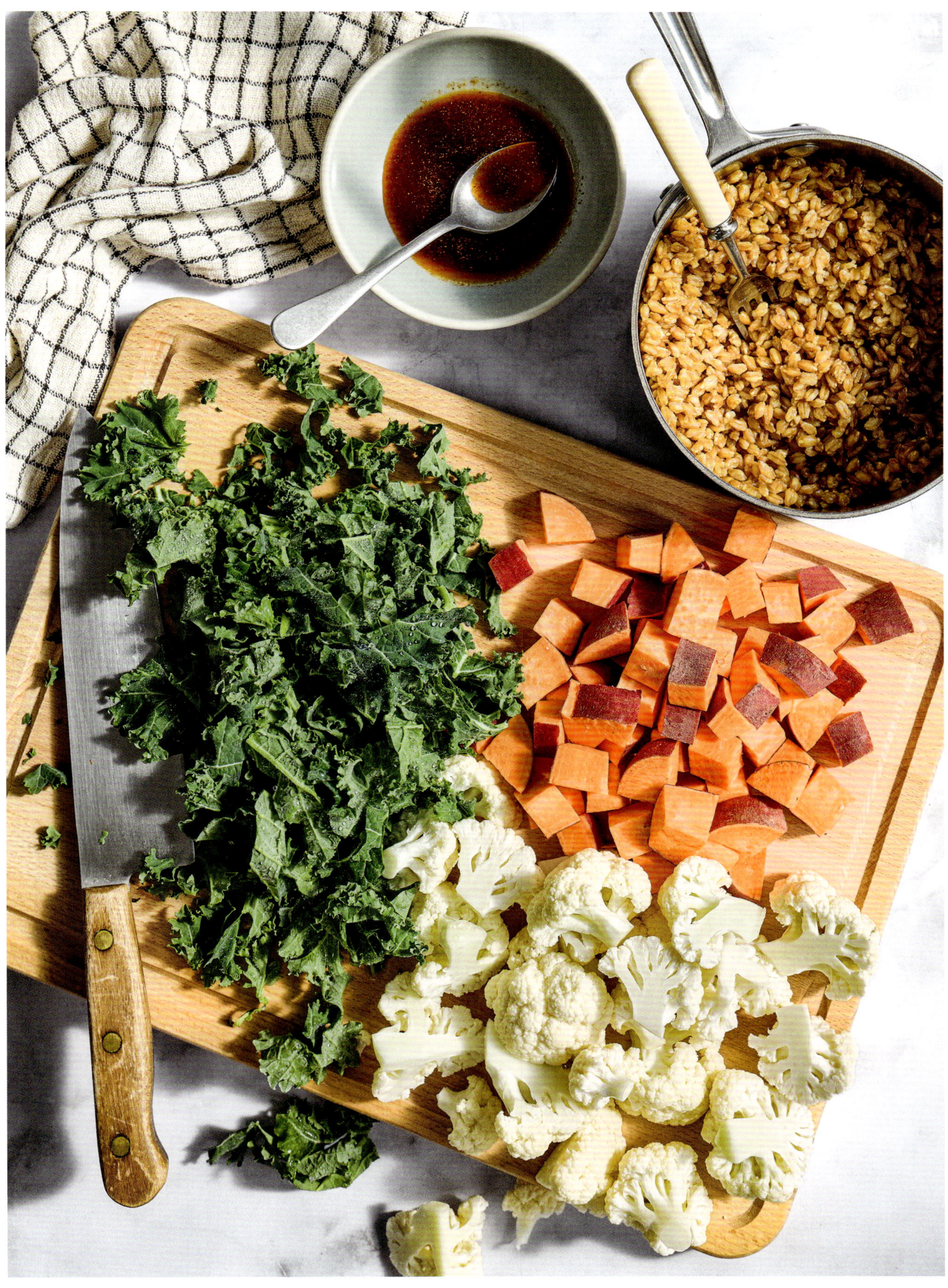

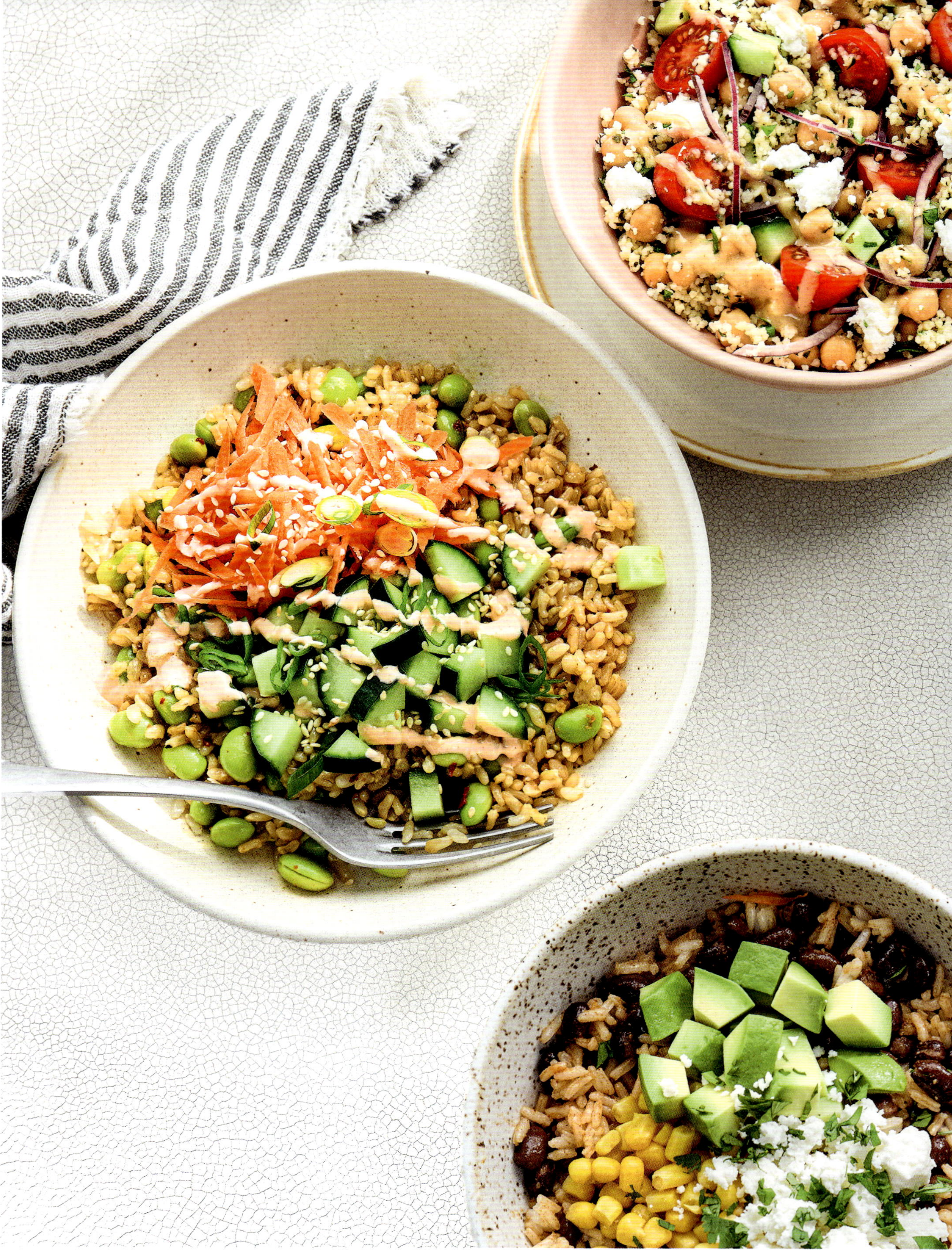

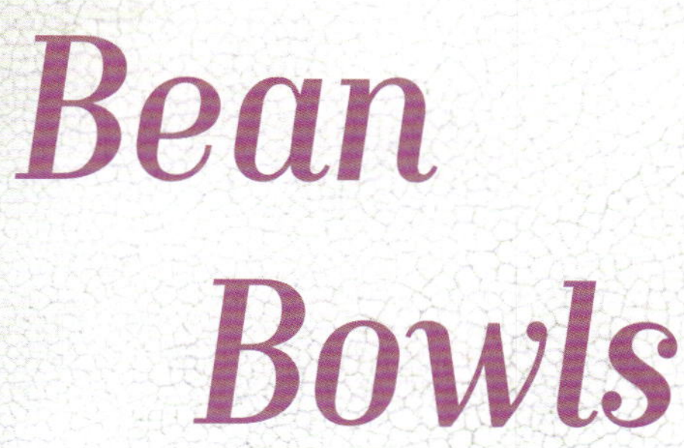

Bean Bowls

These recipes showcase my undying love for beans. Greens, rice, or other grains are usually the base of bowls, why not beans? According to the National Institutes of Health, 95 percent of Americans are not meeting their fiber needs. With rising rates of colorectal cancer, this deficit is no surprise. An easy way to up your fiber game: Eat more beans!

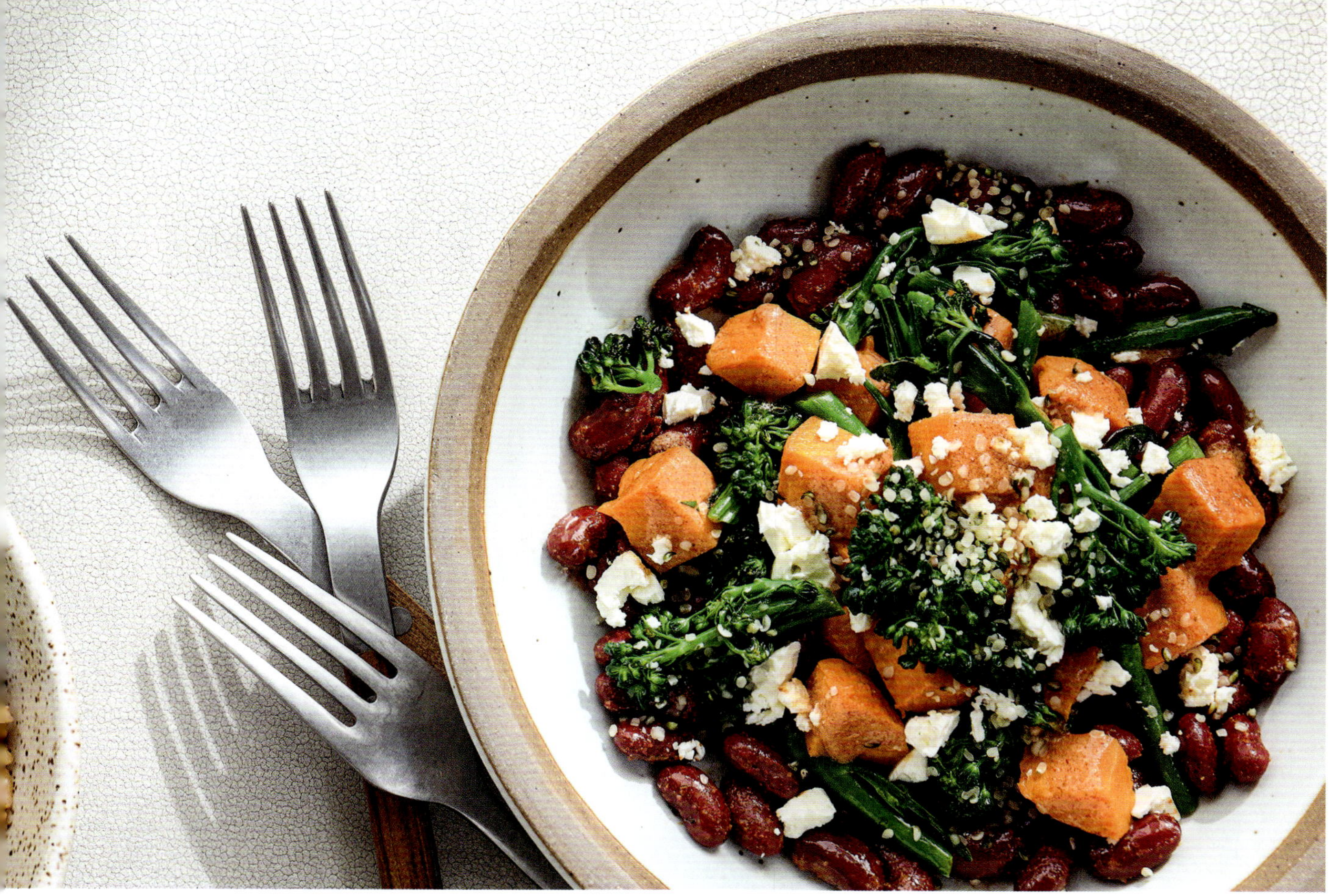

Edamame Bowl

SERVES 1
PREP TIME: 10 minutes

PER SERVING: | **CALORIES** 400 kcal | **PROTEIN** 24g | **FAT** 19g | **CARBOHYDRATE** 36g | **FIBER** 12g

1 cup shelled edamame, cooked (I use frozen and follow package cooking directions)

1 tablespoon reduced-sodium soy sauce

1½ teaspoons extra-virgin olive oil

¼ teaspoon red pepper flakes

¼ teaspoon garlic powder

¼ cup cooked brown rice (follow package cooking directions; or use precooked)

¼ cup grated carrots

⅓ cup diced English or salad cucumber

1 tablespoon sliced green onions (white and green parts)

1½ teaspoons toasted sesame seeds

Yogurt-Sriracha Dressing

2 tablespoons nonfat or low-fat Greek yogurt

1 tablespoon water

1 teaspoon Sriracha sauce

½ teaspoon fresh lemon juice

⅛ teaspoon garlic powder

1 or 2 pinches of kosher salt

When you think of beans you might not immediately think of edamame, but they're one of my favorites and so good for you. Just 1 cup of cooked edamame contains 17 grams of protein—and not just any protein, a complete protein with all nine essential amino acids! I always keep a bag of frozen shelled edamame in my freezer. Simply pop them in the microwave (or in a pot on a stovetop) to thaw and cook. The texture and flavors of this bowl with its grated and diced veggies, sesame seeds, and yogurt-Sriracha dressing are 100 percent YUM!

In your serving bowl, stir together the edamame, soy sauce, olive oil, pepper flakes, and garlic powder until the edamame are fully coated. Add the brown rice and stir to combine. Top the edamame and rice with the carrots, cucumber, green onions, and sesame seeds.

Make the yogurt-Sriracha dressing: In a small bowl, quickly stir the yogurt, water, Sriracha, lemon juice, garlic powder, and salt. Drizzle it over the bowl or serve it on the side. Enjoy right away.

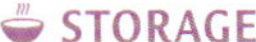

STORAGE

Store the bowl ingredients and dressing separately in airtight containers in the refrigerator for up to 3 days and drizzle when serving.

Hearty Kidney Beans & Sweet Potato Bowl

SERVES 1
PREP TIME: 10 minutes
COOK TIME: 10 minutes

PER SERVING:	CALORIES 561 kcal	PROTEIN 28g	FAT 31g	CARBOHYDRATE 83g	FIBER 19g

1 (12- to 16-ounce) sweet potato

Smoky Maple Dijon Vinaigrette

1 tablespoon Dijon mustard

1 tablespoon apple cider vinegar

2 teaspoons maple syrup

1½ teaspoons extra-virgin olive oil

¼ teaspoon smoked paprika

Pinch of kosher salt

Bowl

1½ teaspoons extra-virgin olive oil

1 cup bite-size pieces broccoli or Broccolini

⅛ teaspoon kosher salt

1 cup canned or cooked kidney beans, drained and rinsed if canned

½ teaspoon ground cumin

½ teaspoon smoked paprika

¼ teaspoon cayenne pepper

2 tablespoons crumbled goat cheese or feta cheese

1 tablespoon hemp hearts (hulled hemp seeds)

When I'm craving a warm, comforting meal but I'm short on time, this bowl is my friend. And now, it's yours! It's hearty, big flavored, and it comes together in no time thanks to the microwave sweet potato tip. Thank you for that, Miles! It's a lifesaver on busy days—steamy sweet potato, smoky savory beans, vibrant broccoli or Broccolini, all drizzled in a smoky maple Dijon vinaigrette.

Pierce the sweet potato 10 to 12 times with a fork. Place it on a microwave-safe plate and microwave on high, turning it about halfway through, until it is tender and easy to pierce with a fork all the way to the center, 7 to 10 minutes (microwave power varies widely). Slice the potato in half lengthwise and set it aside until it is cool enough to handle, about 15 minutes.

In a small bowl, scoop the flesh out of one half of the cooked sweet potato (save the other half and the skin for another use). Mash the potato with a potato masher, fork, or spoon until smooth.

Make the smoky maple Dijon vinaigrette: In a small bowl, stir together the mustard, vinegar, maple syrup, olive oil, smoked paprika, and salt.

Assemble the bowl: In a small pan, heat the olive oil over medium heat. Once hot, sauté the broccoli until tender, 3 to 5 minutes. Sprinkle with the salt and set aside.

In your serving bowl, stir together the kidney beans, cumin, smoked paprika, and cayenne until well combined. Top with the mashed sweet potato, goat cheese, hemp hearts, and cooked broccoli. Drizzle the vinaigrette over the bowl or serve it on the side. Enjoy right away.

YOU DO YOU

Most of these bowls call for 1 cup of canned beans, which leaves about ½ cup of beans in the can. Refrigerate leftover beans in an airtight container and use them as a quick meal topping for extra fiber or a protein boost.

STORAGE

Store the bowl ingredients and dressing separately in airtight containers in the refrigerator for up to 3 days and drizzle when serving.

Chickpea, Couscous & Feta Bowl

SERVES 1
PREP TIME: 10 minutes
COOK TIME: 5 minutes

PER SERVING:	**CALORIES** 599 kcal	**PROTEIN** 23g	**FAT** 18g	**CARBOHYDRATE** 78g	**FIBER** 15g

½ cup water

¼ cup couscous

1 cup canned or cooked chickpeas, drained and rinsed if canned

1 teaspoon dried oregano

1 teaspoon fresh lemon juice

½ teaspoon extra-virgin olive oil

¼ teaspoon garlic powder

¼ teaspoon kosher salt

½ cup diced English or salad cucumber

¼ cup halved or quartered cherry tomatoes

2 tablespoons crumbled goat or feta cheese

2 tablespoons thinly sliced red onion

1 tablespoon chopped fresh flat-leaf parsley leaves

Lemon Tahini Sauce

1 tablespoon tahini

1 tablespoon fresh lemon juice (about ½ small lemon)

2 teaspoons water

1 teaspoon honey

¼ teaspoon ground cumin

⅛ teaspoon kosher salt

This bowl is a sunny trip to the Mediterranean with its vibrant lemony and olive oil–coated chickpeas, couscous, tomatoes, goat cheese, and more. And like many of my bean bowls, it's vegan if you ditch the cheese. When it comes to couscous, there are many types to choose from. I prefer the tiny-grain couscous that this recipe calls for, most often referred to as Moroccan—as opposed to the larger pearl varieties—because of its delicate texture and also how quick and easy it is to prepare. Combine it with boiled water, cover it, and 5 minutes later it's ready to eat!

In a small pot, bring the water to a boil over high heat. Once boiling, add the couscous, stir quickly, cover, remove from the heat, and let steam for about 5 minutes until all the water is absorbed. Fluff with a fork and set aside.

In your serving bowl, stir together the chickpeas, oregano, lemon juice, olive oil, garlic powder, and salt until evenly coated. Add the couscous and stir to combine. Top the couscous and chickpeas with the cucumber, tomatoes, goat cheese, red onion, and parsley.

Make the lemon tahini sauce: In a small bowl, stir together the tahini, lemon juice, water, honey, cumin, and salt. Drizzle the sauce over the bowl or serve it on the side. Enjoy right away.

STORAGE

Store the bowl ingredients and sauce separately in airtight containers in the refrigerator for up to 3 days and drizzle when serving.

Southwest Black Bean Bowl

SERVES 1
PREP TIME: 15 minutes

PER SERVING:	**CALORIES** 531 kcal	**PROTEIN** 29g	**FAT** 13g	**CARBOHYDRATE** 78g	**FIBER** 19g

1 cup canned or cooked black beans, drained and rinsed if canned

¼ teaspoon ground cumin

¼ teaspoon smoked paprika

¼ teaspoon garlic powder

⅛ teaspoon kosher salt

½ cup cooked white rice (follow package directions; or use precooked)

¼ cup canned corn, drained

¼ avocado, diced

¼ cup halved or quartered cherry tomatoes

¼ cup cubed queso fresco or Mexican cheese

1½ tablespoons chopped fresh cilantro

Lime Crema Dressing

2 tablespoons nonfat or low-fat Greek yogurt

Grated zest of ¼ lime

1½ teaspoons fresh lime juice

¼ teaspoon honey

⅛ teaspoon ground cumin

1 to 2 pinches of kosher salt

I'm a big fan of Chipotle's burrito bowl. It's one of those on-the-go meals that hits the spot for me every time. This bowl is my take on it, with the beans as the base, rather than rice. More plant-based protein and fiber, please! If you have any leftover meat—grilled chicken, shredded beef—or roasted veggies, add them to the bowl, too, if it sounds good.

In your serving bowl, combine the black beans, cumin, smoked paprika, garlic powder, and salt. Stir until the beans are evenly coated. Add the rice and stir to combine. Top the beans and rice with the corn, avocado, tomatoes, queso fresco, and cilantro.

Make the lime crema dressing: In a small bowl, stir together the yogurt, lime zest, lime juice, honey, cumin, and salt.

Drizzle the dressing over the bowl or serve it on the side. Enjoy right away.

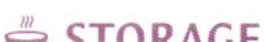

Store the bowl ingredients and sauce separately in airtight containers in the refrigerator for up to 3 days and drizzle when serving.

Ranch Smash Burger Bowls

SERVES 4
PREP TIME: 15 minutes
COOK TIME: 10 to 15 minutes

PER SERVING:	CALORIES 436 kcal	PROTEIN 33g	FAT 24g	CARBOHYDRATE 21g	FIBER 8g

4 cups chopped, lightly packed mixed greens lettuce (about 3 ounces)

1 cup halved or quartered cherry tomatoes

¾ cup thinly sliced red onion

2 tablespoons extra-virgin olive oil

3 cups sliced white or cremini mushrooms (or 8-ounce package sliced mushrooms)

1 pound ground beef (10% to 15% fat)

1½ teaspoons kosher salt, divided

¼ teaspoon freshly ground black pepper

One 15-ounce can black beans (or 1½ cups cooked black beans), drained and rinsed

1 avocado, sliced

⅓ cup diced sour dill pickles (about 1 pickle)

¼ cup chopped pickled banana peppers or pepperoncini

Yogurty Ranch Dressing

½ cup nonfat or low-fat Greek yogurt

1 tablespoon water

2 teaspoons ranch dip or dressing seasoning

You might be surprised to learn that I eat a burger at least once a week. Growing up, I often left the bun behind. I wasn't scared of carbs (little me had zero idea what they were), I just loved the ground beef on its own. To this day, I tend to only eat about half of the bun. When the craving hits, I make this bowl, loaded with toppings, flavor, and nutrients. I replace the bun with another carb—beans, which are packed with nutrients. I top it with my delicious high-protein yogurty ranch. I pretty much drench my burgers and fries in ranch when eating out.

In a large bowl, toss the lettuce, tomatoes, and onion. Set aside.

In a large pan, heat the olive oil over medium-high heat. When hot, add the mushrooms and stir until they start to soften, about 3 minutes. Push the mushrooms to one side of the pan and add the beef. Keep the mushrooms on the side of the pan as you cook the beef, and stir them occasionally throughout.

Using a spatula, press down on the beef so that it fills nearly three-quarters of the pan. Season with ½ teaspoon of the salt. Cook the beef until it is fairly browned, 2 to 3 minutes, and then flip it. Using your spatula, press down on the beef again. Season the browned side with ½ teaspoon of the salt, and cook until the other side is browned, 2 to 3 minutes.

Using your spatula in the pan, coarsely chop the beef into 2-inch chunks and combine it with the mushrooms. Season with the remaining ½ teaspoon salt and all the pepper. Stir occasionally until the beef is cooked through and everything is nicely browned, 3 to 4 more minutes. Add the black beans and cook until they are warmed through, about 1 minute. Remove the pan from the heat.

Make the yogurty ranch dressing: In a small bowl, stir together the yogurt, water, and ranch seasoning. If you like a thinner dressing, add a little bit of water until it gets to your desired consistency.

Evenly divide the lettuce mixture among four bowls. Top with the hot beef/mushroom/bean mixture, finishing with the avocado, pickles, and banana peppers. Drizzle the bowls evenly with the yogurt ranch dressing and enjoy.

STORAGE

Store the bowl ingredients and dressing separately in airtight containers in the refrigerator for up to 3 days and drizzle when serving.

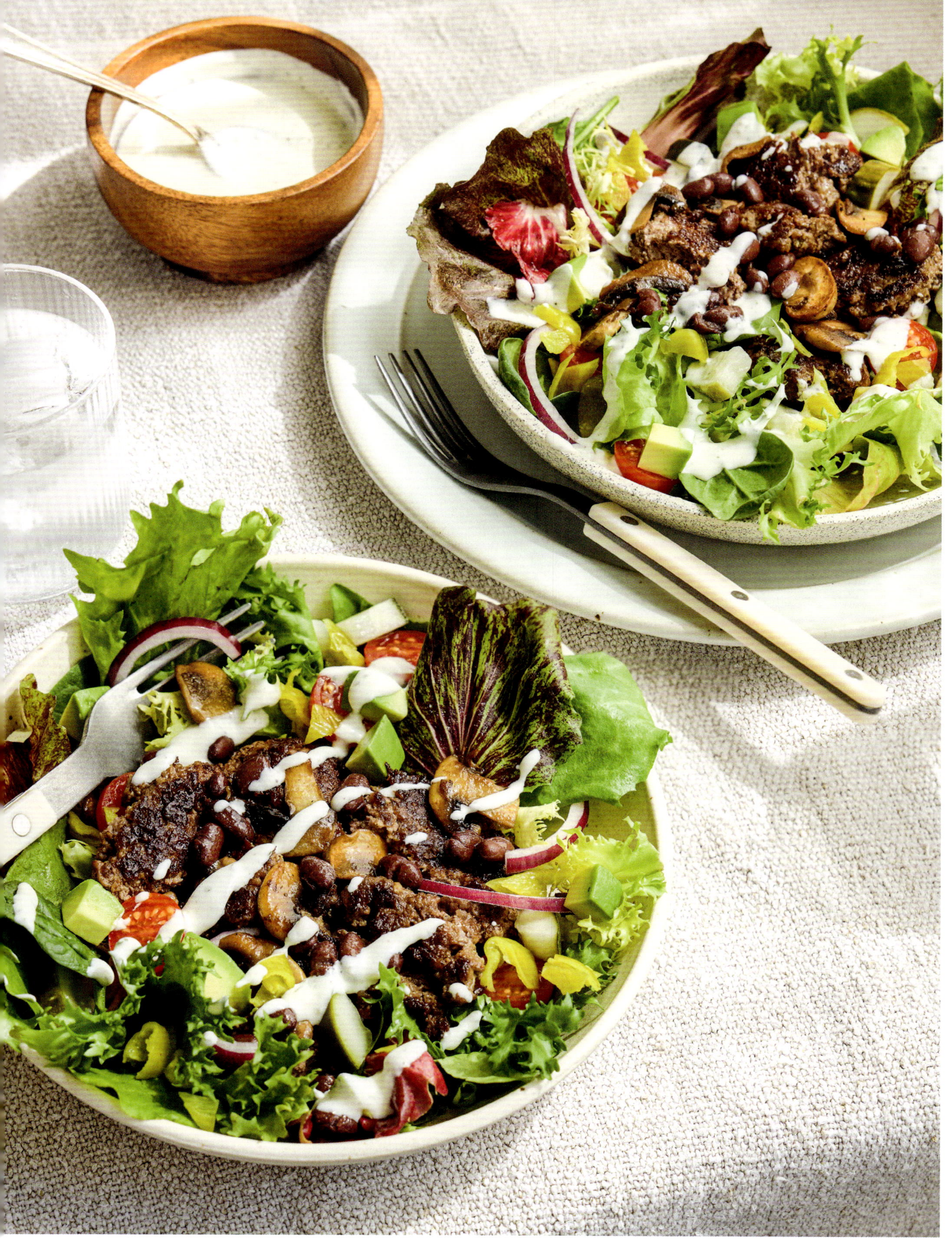

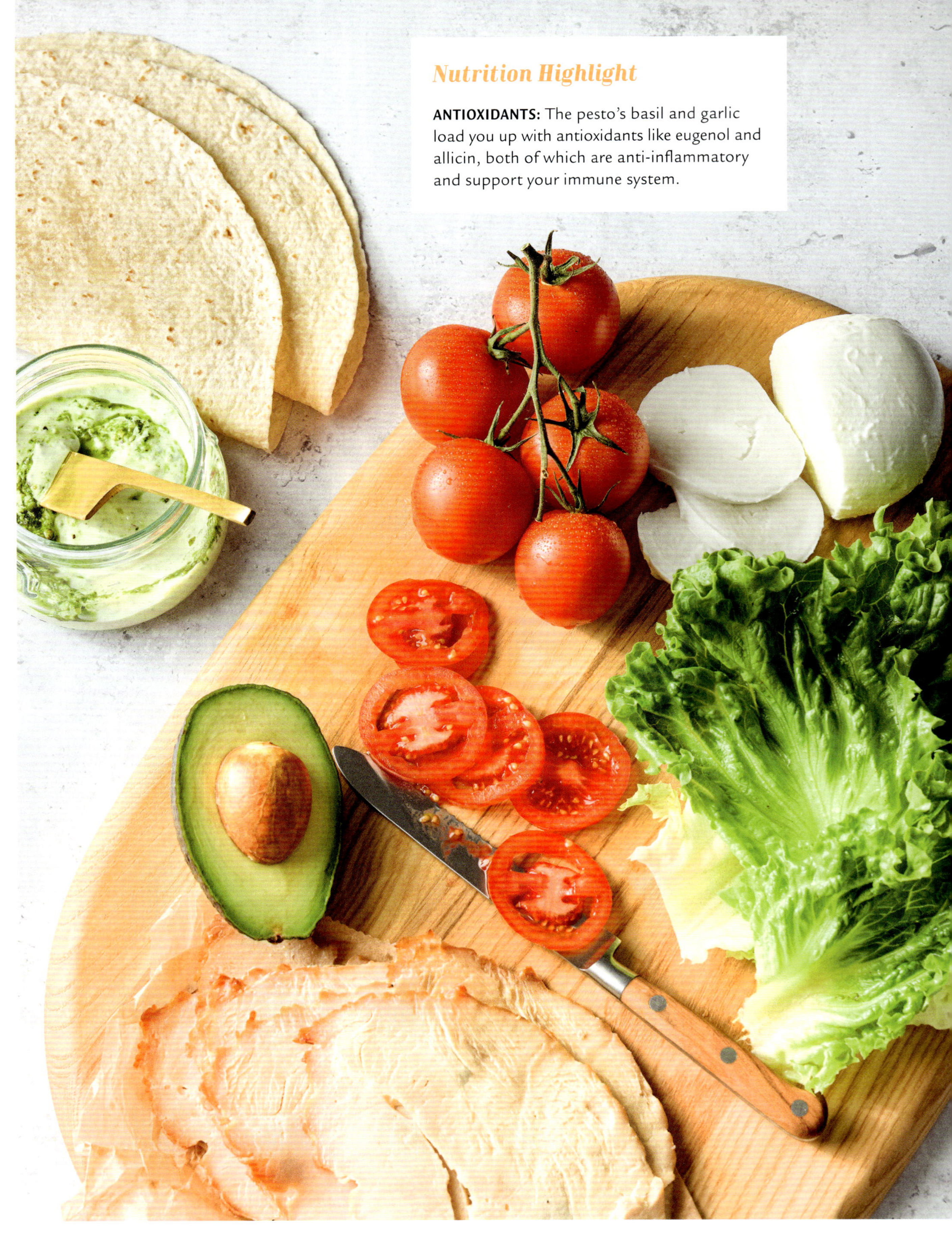

Nutrition Highlight

ANTIOXIDANTS: The pesto's basil and garlic load you up with antioxidants like eugenol and allicin, both of which are anti-inflammatory and support your immune system.

Turkey Pesto Wrap

SERVES 1
PREP TIME: 10 minutes

PER SERVING:	**CALORIES** 605 kcal	**PROTEIN** 33g	**FAT** 32g	**CARBOHYDRATE** 44g	**FIBER** 5g

¼ cup nonfat or low-fat Greek yogurt

1 tablespoon pesto, homemade (page 46) or store-bought

1 tablespoon light mayonnaise

1 large burrito-size flour tortilla

3 slices deli turkey

3 slices part-skim or whole milk mozzarella cheese

2 slices tomato

½ cup lightly packed thinly sliced green leaf lettuce

¼ avocado, sliced

Turkey sandwiches were often in my lunchbox growing up—simple and classic deli turkey slices plus lettuce on soft white bread with the crust sliced off. I love you, Mom! This wrap is a grown-up version of that childhood favorite layered with more flavor and nutrition thanks to the mozz, avocado, and tomato. The creamy pesto sauce is really yummy and my quick-easy pesto recipe is on page 46 if you want to start with homemade pesto. Maybe you double or triple it and use it for other wraps and sammies? If so, store it in an airtight container in the refrigerator for up to 3 days.

In a small bowl, stir together the yogurt, pesto, and mayonnaise. Set the creamy pesto sauce aside.

Warm the tortilla for 10 to 15 seconds in the microwave, or 10 to 20 seconds in a dry pan over a burner, until warm and pliable.

Place the tortilla flat on a clean surface. Spread three-quarters (about ¼ cup) of the creamy pesto sauce evenly onto the middle of the wrap, leaving about a 1-inch border clear all around. Layer the fillings over it in this order: turkey, mozzarella, tomato, and lettuce. Top the lettuce evenly with the remaining pesto sauce and the avocado.

Carefully fold the tortilla up from the bottom over the filling, then fold in the sides, and roll the wrap up until it is snug and sealed. For easier handling, and to prevent filling from falling out, wrap it in parchment paper or waxed paper, tucking in the ends as you roll the same way that you rolled up the wrap. Slice the wrap in half diagonally and enjoy! This wrap is best enjoyed day of.

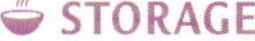

STORAGE

Store airtight in the refrigerator for up to 1 day.

Veggie "Tuna" Salad

SERVES 2 OR 3
PREP TIME: 10 minutes

PER SERVING:	**CALORIES** 333 kcal	**PROTEIN** 14g	**FAT** 18g	**CARBOHYDRATE** 31g	**FIBER** 12g

One 15-ounce can chickpeas (or 1½ cups cooked), drained and rinsed

1 avocado, halved and pitted

½ cup diced celery (1 to 2 stalks)

⅓ cup diced dill pickles (I prefer baby dills here for their crunch!)

⅓ cup nonfat or low-fat Greek yogurt

⅓ cup finely diced white onion

¼ cup crumbled feta cheese

2 tablespoons fresh lemon juice (about ½ lemon)

1 tablespoon nutritional yeast flakes

½ teaspoon garlic powder

¼ teaspoon kosher salt

⅛ teaspoon freshly ground pepper

While canned tuna is a go-to budget-friendly protein that I certainly enjoy, some people hesitate, or even steer entirely clear of it, due to its mercury levels. That's why I came up with this easy swap with another affordable, tasty option: chickpeas! Not only are chickpeas packed with protein, they're also loaded with fiber. Tuna is also known for its energizing vitamin B_{12}, which helps us metabolize fats and carbohydrates, so we can efficiently convert food into energy. Since chickpeas lack B_{12}, simply stir in some B_{12}-rich nutritional yeast and you're good to go.

I love this recipe because it's quick and easy to prep throughout the week and it's so versatile. Load it into delicious sandwiches and wraps, top a salad with a healthy scoop of it, or grab some crackers and dip in. This ready-to-go weekday "tuna" salad checks all the boxes and keeps you fueled and energized.

In a large bowl, use a potato masher or the bottom of a canning jar or sturdy cup to mash the chickpeas until they are fairly smooth. Scoop the avocado in and mash it into the chickpeas until the mixture is fairly smooth like guacamole.

Add the celery, pickles, yogurt, onion, feta, lemon juice, nutritional yeast, garlic powder, salt, and pepper and stir until well combined. Serve and enjoy!

STORAGE

Store airtight in the refrigerator for up to 3 days.

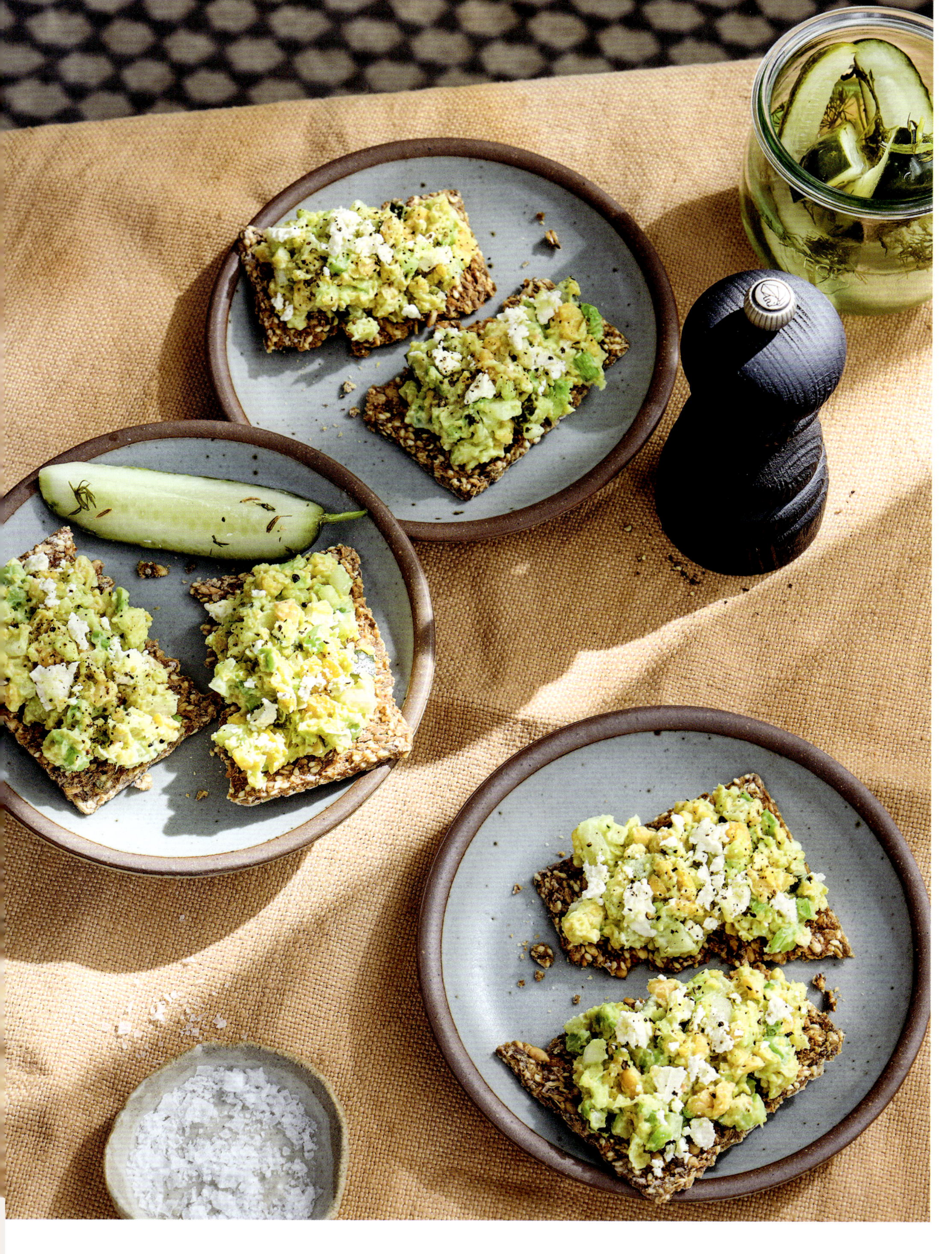

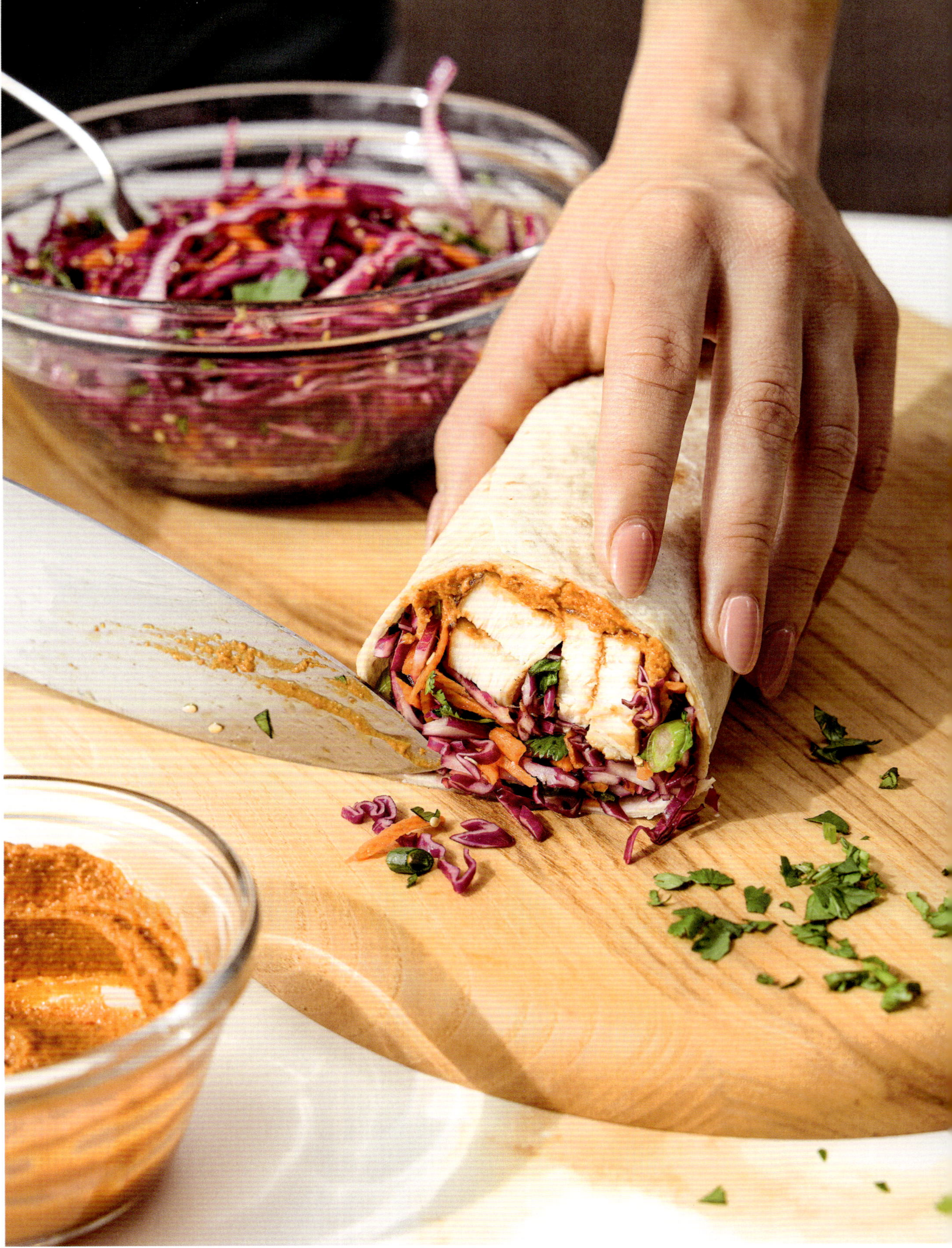

Grilled Chicken Slaw Wrap *with* Curried Peanut Sauce

SERVES 4
PREP TIME: 20 minutes
MARINATING TIME: 2 hours
COOK TIME: 15 minutes

PER SERVING:	**CALORIES** 634 kcal	**PROTEIN** 45g	**FAT** 34g	**CARBOHYDRATE** 50g	**FIBER** 8g

Chicken & Marinade

3 boneless, skinless chicken breasts (about 8 ounces each), halved crosswise

¾ cup reduced-sodium soy sauce

5 garlic cloves, minced

1 tablespoon finely grated or minced peeled fresh ginger

1 tablespoon brown sugar

Sesame Slaw

6 cups thinly sliced red cabbage (about 12 ounces)

½ cup grated carrots

½ cup sliced almonds

½ cup thinly sliced green onions (white and green parts)

½ cup chopped fresh cilantro (leaves and stems)

2 tablespoons toasted sesame seeds

2½ tablespoons unseasoned rice vinegar

1 tablespoon honey

1 teaspoon toasted sesame oil

½ teaspoon kosher salt

⅓ cup extra-virgin olive oil

My fiancé, Miles, made me a version of this delicious and colorful wrap on one of our first dates. Although it's not quite the same, the inspiration comes from his mom's recipe, so, this one is dedicated to Miles's loving mom.

Cabbage is incredibly nutritious, and red cabbage contains anthocyanins, water-soluble plant pigments known for reducing inflammation and lowering heart disease risk. Its high water content (nearly 92 percent!) supports hydration and healthy skin. It's also packed with B vitamins, including folate—vital for DNA synthesis and cell function, particularly during pregnancy. *And* it contains potassium, calcium, and magnesium, which support overall health and well-being. Go, cabbage!

I like to prep this over the weekend for the week. Make and refrigerate everything separately. When it's time, simply warm the tortilla and grilled chicken (or add it cold) and assemble.

Marinate the chicken: In a zip-top bag or medium bowl, combine the chicken, soy sauce, garlic, ginger, and brown sugar. Make sure all chicken pieces are submerged in the marinade. Seal the bag or cover the bowl and refrigerate for about 2 hours.

Meanwhile, make the sesame slaw: In a large bowl, combine the cabbage, carrots, almonds, green onions, cilantro, and sesame seeds. In a small bowl, whisk together the rice vinegar, honey, sesame oil, and salt. Slowly whisk in the olive oil, so that the dressing emulsifies. Drizzle the vinaigrette over the slaw and toss well.

Make the curried peanut sauce: In a small pot, combine the water, peanut butter, curry paste, and barbecue sauce, stirring until smooth. Cook over medium-low heat until warm, 2 to 3 minutes. Remove from the heat and set aside.

To finish: Brush or scrape the grill grates and lightly oil them. Light or heat your grill to medium-high.

Once the grill is fully heated, remove the chicken from the marinade (shake off and discard excess marinade), place on the grates, and grill, turning once, until the pieces have reached an internal temperature of 165°F, 3 to 5 minutes per side. Transfer the chicken to a clean plate or platter. Once cool enough to handle, slice into ½- to 1-inch-thick pieces.

Continued

Curried Peanut Sauce

2 tablespoons water

1½ tablespoons unsalted peanut butter

1 tablespoon Thai red curry paste

1½ teaspoons barbecue sauce

To Finish

Neutral oil, for grill grates

4 large burrito-size tortillas (whatever type you prefer)

Heat each tortilla for 10 to 15 seconds in the microwave, or 10 to 20 seconds in a dry pan over a burner, until warm and pliable.

Place the tortillas flat on a clean surface. Top them with the cabbage slaw (about 1½ cups each) and then evenly divide the grilled chicken among them, leaving about a 1-inch border clear all around. Top each evenly with peanut sauce (about 1 heaping teaspoon).

To roll the wraps, carefully fold the tortilla up from the bottom over the filling, then fold in the sides, and roll the wraps up until they are snug and sealed. These are pretty full wraps, so you'll want to squeeze them and carefully roll them so that the filling doesn't fall out. For easier handling, and to prevent filling from falling out, wrap the wraps in parchment paper or waxed paper, tucking in the ends as you roll the same way that you rolled up the wrap. Slice them in half diagonally and enjoy! These wraps are best enjoyed day of.

STORAGE

Store the dressed slaw, grilled chicken, and peanut sauce separately in airtight containers and refrigerate for up to 2 days.

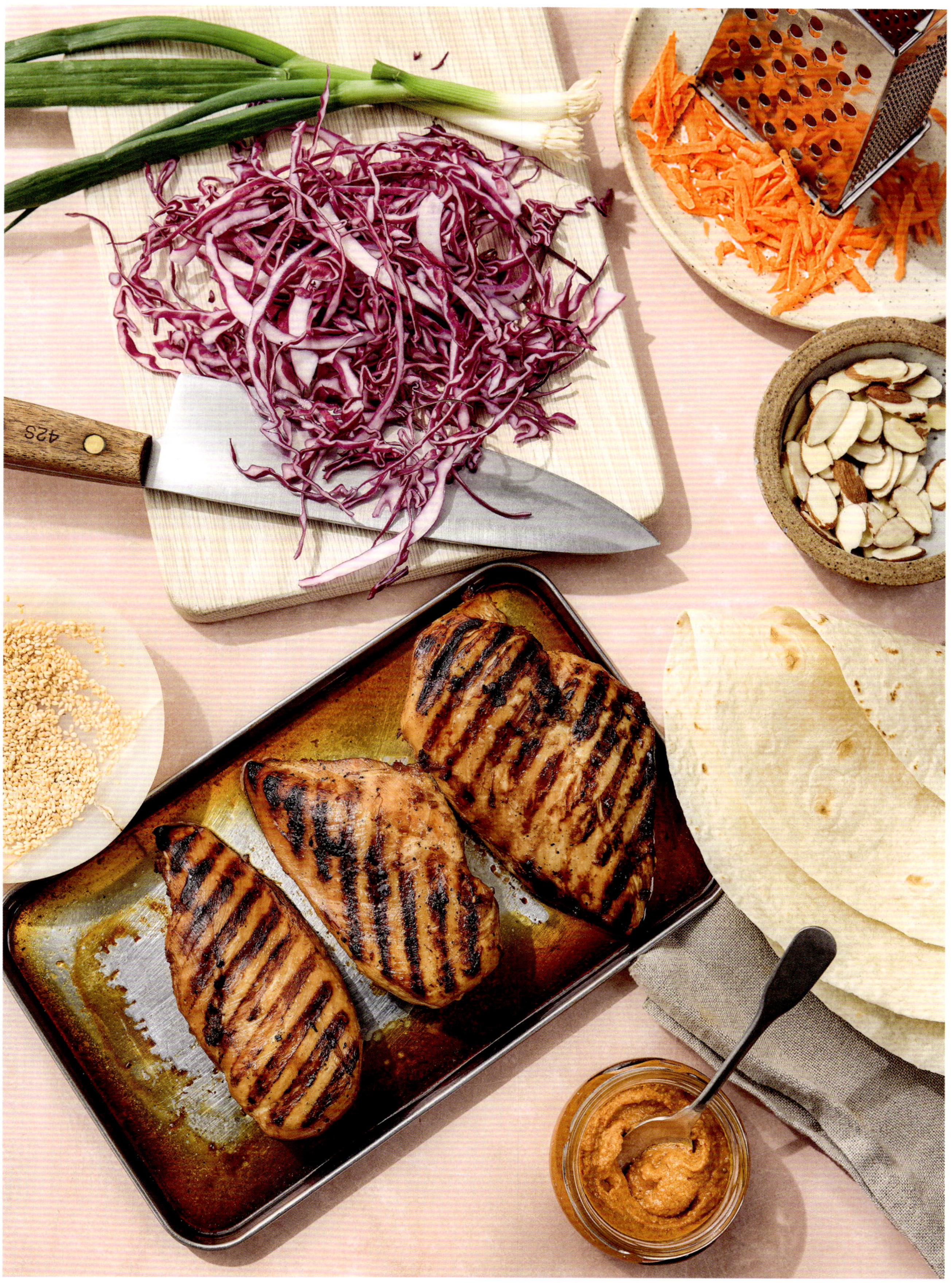

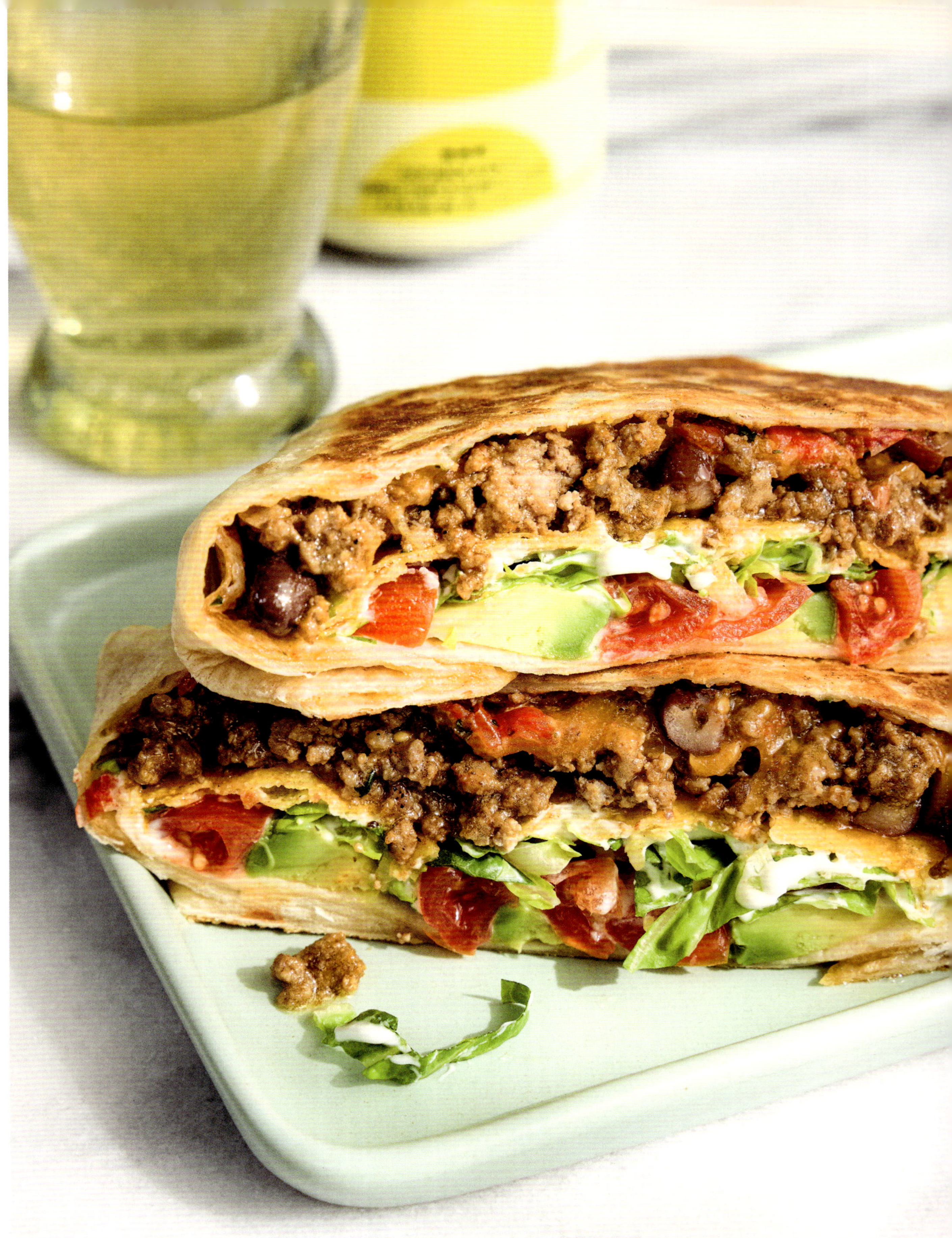

Stephwrap Supreme

SERVES 1
PREP TIME: 10 minutes
COOK TIME: 10 minutes

PER SERVING:	**CALORIES** 652 kcal	**PROTEIN** 43g	**FAT** 34g	**CARBOHYDRATE** 56g	**FIBER** 9g

4 ounces lean (preferably 7% fat) ground turkey, lean ground beef, or plant-based meat or sausage

¼ cup canned or cooked black beans, drained and rinsed if canned

2 tablespoons salsa (whatever type and heat you prefer), divided

2 tablespoons water

2 teaspoons taco seasoning mix

2 burrito-size flour tortillas, divided

1 corn tostada shell or a few baked tortilla chips

2 tablespoons nonfat or low-fat Greek yogurt

¼ avocado, sliced

¼ cup chopped cherry tomatoes

¼ cup lightly packed thinly sliced green leaf lettuce

2 tablespoons grated Cheddar cheese

Cooking spray or neutral oil, for greasing

My favorite fast food hands down is Taco Bell—its Crunchwrap Supreme is so good! It's a pretty balanced meal, too, with the protein-rich beef, fiber-full beans, and veg. My version is way better for you than fast food, of course, and calls for Greek yogurt rather than sour cream, lean meat, and avocado for even more fiber and healthy fats. Mastering the folding technique might feel intimidating, but I promise it's easy. After you make one, you'll feel like a pro.

Heat a small pan over medium heat. Once hot, add the turkey and cook for about 4 minutes, stirring occasionally, breaking up the meat as you do, until it is nicely browned. Add the black beans, 1 tablespoon of the salsa, the water, and taco seasoning and cook, stirring once or twice, until the beans are heated through, 1 to 2 minutes. Remove from the heat and set aside.

Warm one of the tortillas for 10 to 15 seconds in the microwave, or 10 to 20 seconds in a dry pan over a burner, until warm and pliable. Place the warmed tortilla flat on a clean surface. In the center of the tortilla, layer and/or spread the following to roughly the size and shape of the tostada shell: the remaining 1 tablespoon salsa, browned turkey and beans, tostada, yogurt, avocado, tomatoes, lettuce, and Cheddar.

Slice the second tortilla into 4 same-sized wedges (you'll only use one). Take one wedge and place it in the middle on top of the cheese.

Using both hands, tuck and fold the edges of the bottom tortilla into pleats over the top tortilla wedge in order to enclose and seal the wrap. I tuck while turning the entire wrap counterclockwise with one hand, and hold the wrap together, on the top, with the other hand, until I have folded all of the pleats, usually 7 or 8. Lightly press down on the crunch wrap and put a small plate or bowl on top to secure it.

Lightly grease a medium pan with cooking spray or oil over medium heat. Once the pan is hot, carefully place the wrap pleated-side down in the pan. Cook for 2 to 3 minutes on each side, adding more oil as needed when you flip it, until it is golden and crisp. Slice in half and enjoy! This wrap is best enjoyed day of.

Turkey, Pear & Whipped Cottage Cheese Sammy

SERVES 1
PREP TIME: 10 minutes

PER SERVING:	**CALORIES** 395 kcal	**PROTEIN** 38g	**FAT** 7g	**CARBOHYDRATE** 49g	**FIBER** 10g

¼ cup 2% cottage cheese (or whatever fat content you prefer)

1½ teaspoons honey

2 thick slices whole-grain or sourdough bread (or sandwich bread of choice)

2 teaspoons Dijon mustard

4 ounces sliced deli turkey breast

½ cup lightly packed fresh arugula

½ ripe pear, thinly sliced

Pears don't get enough attention and this sandwich is in their honor. It stacks them with turkey, peppery arugula, and a creamy whipped cottage cheese spread. I love the flavor and texture of a good ripe pear. So sweet and special. Fully ripe pears have a somewhat buttery texture. They're also lovely grilled or roasted and yummy in all sorts of salads and smoothies. One pear contains 6 to 8 grams of fiber. That's a lot. I recommend keeping the skin on for added antioxidants.

In a small bowl, stir the cottage cheese and honey together. Mash the cottage cheese against the side of the bowl with the spoon to crush the curds, and then quickly stir and almost whip it until it's fairly smooth and creamy. Since it's such a small amount, a hand mixer or whisk won't work.

Toast the bread until golden brown and nicely crisped. Evenly spread the mustard on one slice of the bread and spread the whipped cottage cheese/honey on the other slice. Evenly layer the turkey over the mustard slice. Top it with the arugula and then the pear. Place the cottage cheese–topped slice on top, and gently press down on the sandwich to bring it all together.

Slice the sandwich in half and serve immediately. It's best enjoyed day of.

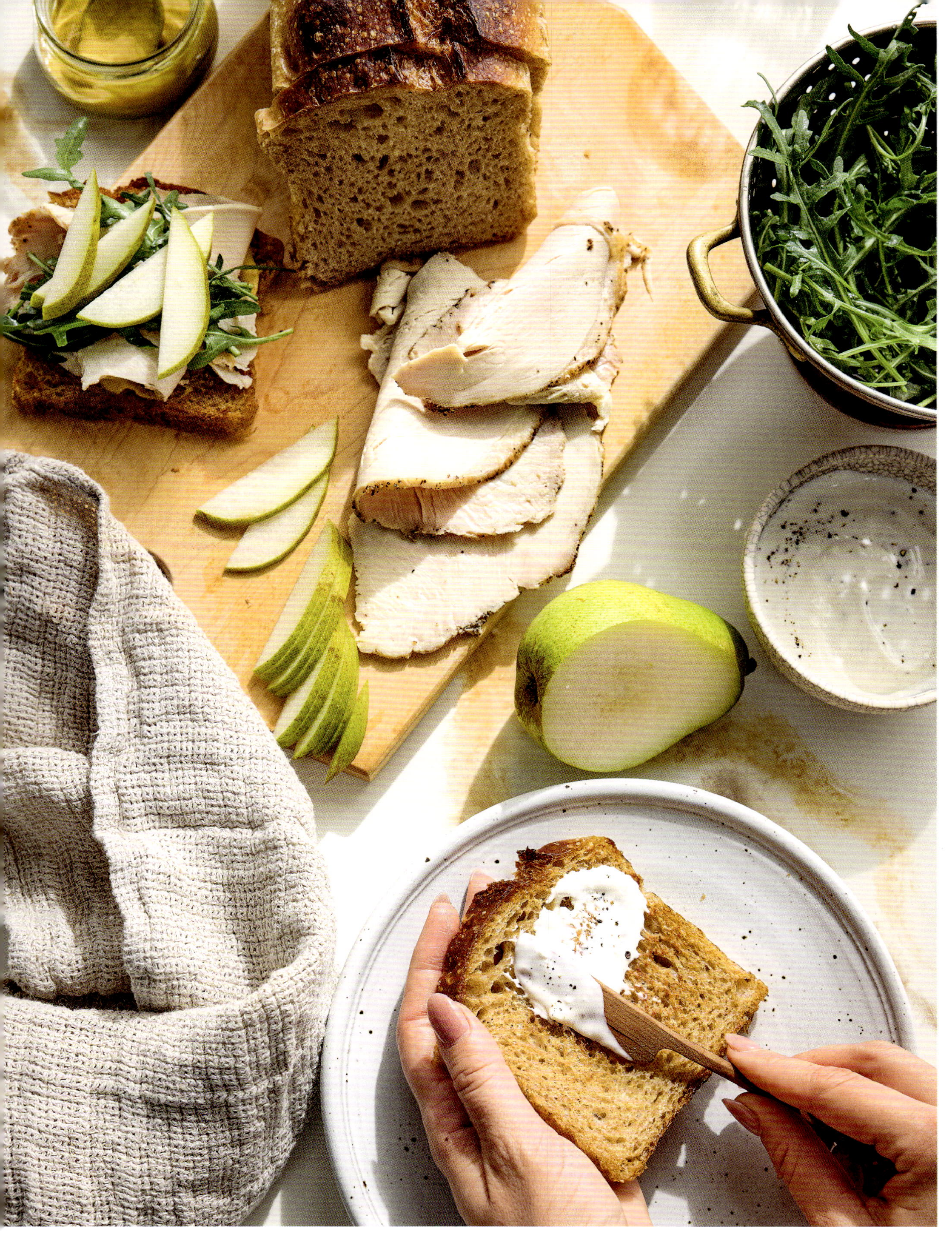

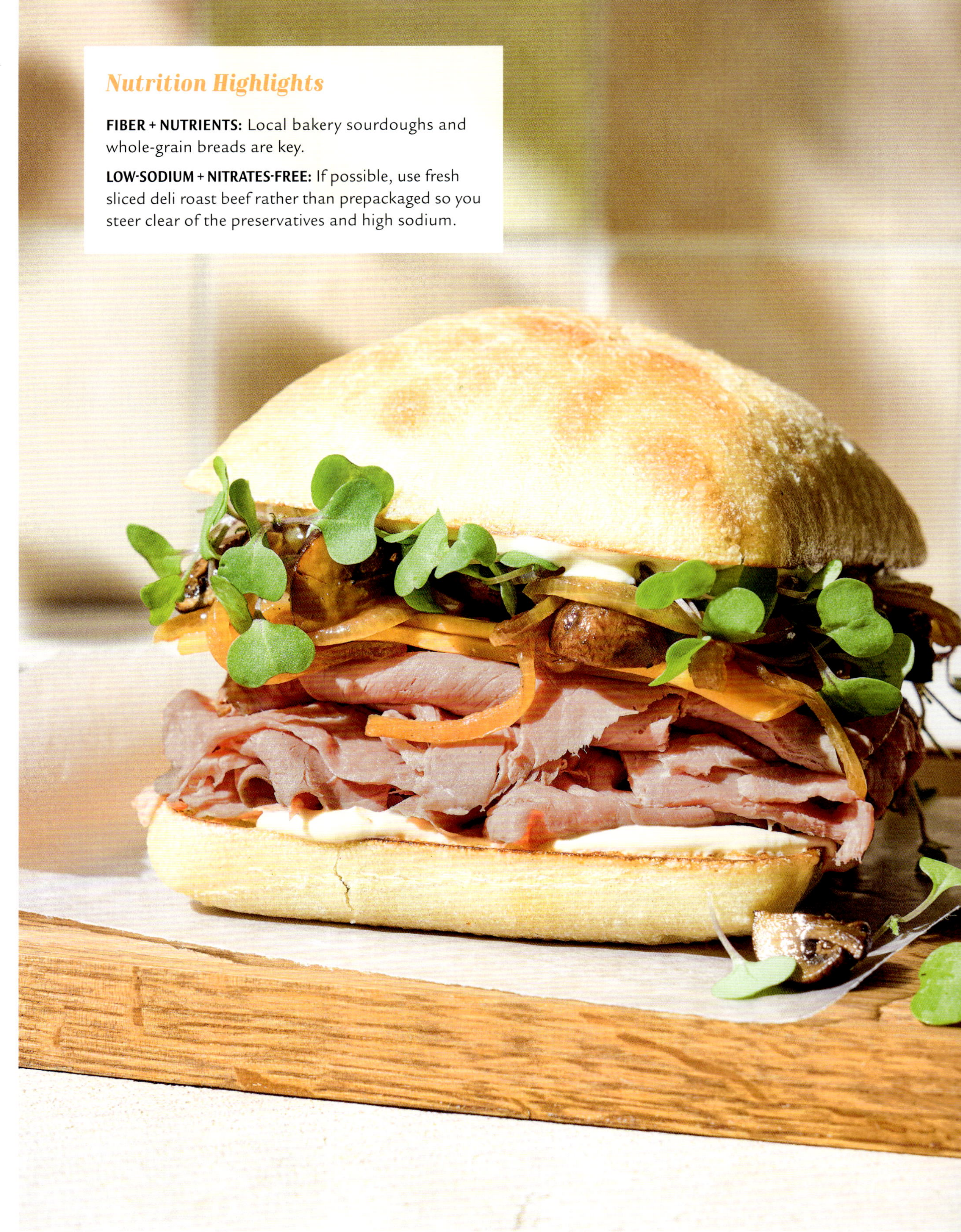

Nutrition Highlights

FIBER + NUTRIENTS: Local bakery sourdoughs and whole-grain breads are key.

LOW-SODIUM + NITRATES-FREE: If possible, use fresh sliced deli roast beef rather than prepackaged so you steer clear of the preservatives and high sodium.

Roast Beef–Cheddar Sandwich *with* Onions & Mushrooms

SERVES 1
PREP TIME: 5 minutes
COOK TIME: 10 minutes

PER SERVING:	CALORIES 530 kcal	PROTEIN 40g	FAT 32g	CARBOHYDRATE 38g	FIBER 3g

1½ teaspoons extra-virgin olive oil

⅓ cup sliced white or cremini mushrooms

⅓ cup thinly sliced yellow onion

Kosher salt

2 tablespoons nonfat or low-fat Greek yogurt

1 teaspoon Worcestershire sauce

½ teaspoon honey

¼ teaspoon Dijon mustard

1 ciabatta roll or sandwich bread of choice, halved

4 ounces roast beef

1 to 2 slices Cheddar cheese

¼ cup lightly packed microgreens

My favorite lunch spot in Williamsburg, Virginia, where I live, is The Cheese Shop. I stop in at least once a week for my go-to order: roast beef sandwich with Cheddar and microgreens. This is my take on it.

Of course, the dietitian in me saw an opportunity to sneak in even more nutrition here with a quick mushroom and onion sauté. Yum!

In a large pan, heat the oil over medium heat until hot. Add the mushrooms and sauté, stirring occasionally, until they begin to soften, about 2 minutes. Add the onion and cook, stirring occasionally, until it begins to soften and gain a little color, 3 to 4 minutes. Add a pinch of salt, stir to incorporate, remove from the heat, and set aside.

In a small bowl, stir together the yogurt, Worcestershire sauce, honey, mustard, and a pinch of salt.

Lightly toast the ciabatta roll halves, if desired. Spread about 2 tablespoons of the yogurt sauce (most of it) on the bottom half of the roll, and the remaining sauce on the top half. Layer the sliced roast beef over the bottom half, followed by the Cheddar, sautéed onions and mushrooms, and microgreens. Place the other lightly dressed ciabatta roll half on top, and gently press down on the sandwich to bring it all together.

Slice the sandwich in half and serve immediately. It's best enjoyed day of.

YOU DO YOU

Feel free to add other sautéed veggies like bell peppers, spinach, or tomatoes for even more nutrients, texture, and flavor.

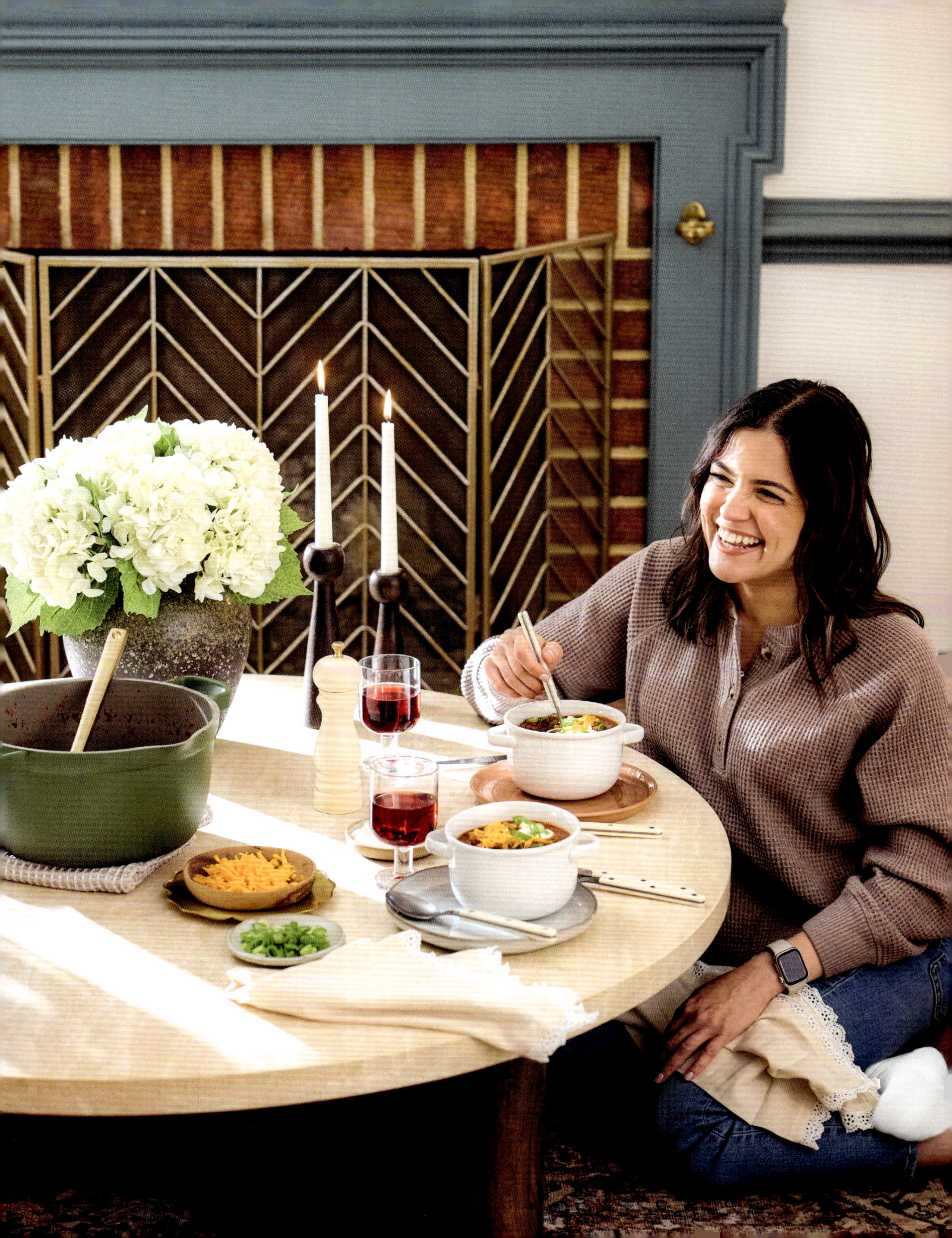

Nourishing Mains

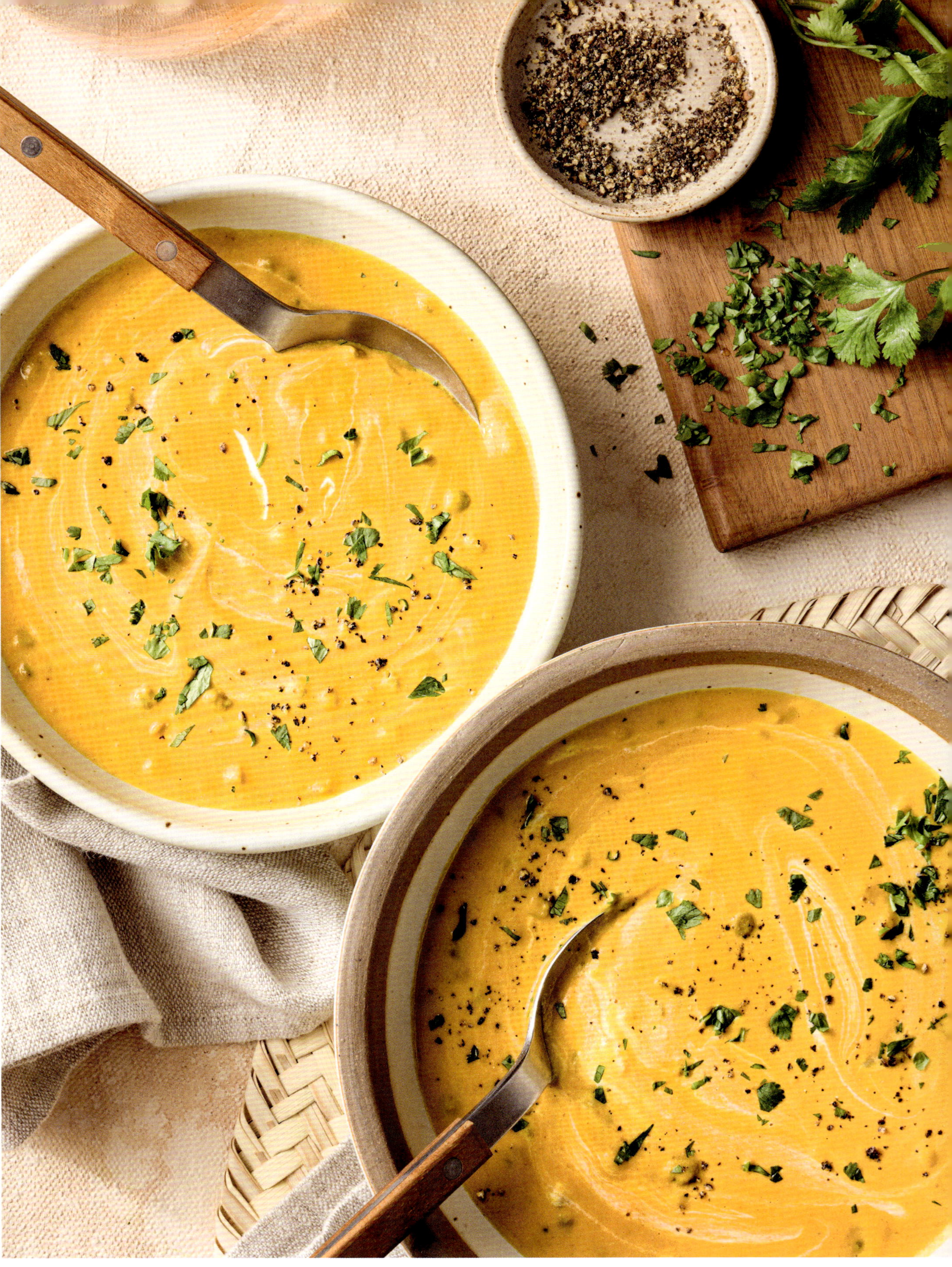

Curried Pumpkin–Lentil Soup

SERVES 4 TO 6
PREP TIME: 10 minutes
COOK TIME: 40 minutes

PER SERVING:	CALORIES 434 kcal	PROTEIN 18g	FAT 19g	CARBOHYDRATE 46g	FIBER 12g

- 2 tablespoons extra-virgin olive oil
- 1 large yellow onion, diced
- 1 red bell pepper, diced
- 2 carrots, diced
- 1 tablespoon plus 1 teaspoon curry powder
- 2 teaspoons ground cumin
- 2½ cups vegetable broth (or preferred broth)
- One 15-ounce can pumpkin puree
- One 15-ounce can cannellini beans (or 1½ cups cooked beans), drained and rinsed
- 1 teaspoon kosher salt, plus more to taste
- ¼ teaspoon freshly ground black pepper, plus more to taste
- 1 cup nonfat or low-fat Greek yogurt (optional, for extra protein)
- Two 14.5-ounce cans lentil-vegetable soup (I love Amy's Kitchen Organic Soups) or two 15-ounce cans canned lentils plus ½ cup water
- One 13.5-ounce can full-fat coconut milk
- Stemmed and chopped fresh cilantro or parsley (optional), for garnish

The warmth, spice, and comforting curry creaminess of this soup is like a thick, cozy quilt or a crackling midwinter fire. The best. We tend to love canned pumpkin in the fall and then give it the cold shoulder the rest of the year. It deserves more! It's packed with fiber, potassium, and vitamins A and C. I love it in this soup simmered with lentils (high in protein and fiber), veggies, and coconut milk.

I often pair curried dishes like this one with tangy Greek yogurt because it melds well with, and slightly mellows, the heat and bold spices. I also often blend white beans into my canned soups, as I do here, to make soups "creamier" without adding a drop of heavy cream.

In a large pot or Dutch oven, warm the olive oil over medium heat until hot. Add the onion and bell pepper and cook, stirring occasionally, until they begin to soften, about 5 minutes. Add the carrots and cook, stirring occasionally, until slightly tender, 3 to 4 minutes. Stir in the curry powder and cumin and cook for about 1 minute, until fragrant.

Add the broth, pumpkin puree, beans, salt, and pepper and stir well to combine. Increase the heat to high and bring to a boil. Once boiling, decrease the heat to low and simmer, uncovered, until the vegetables soften and everything melds, 15 to 20 minutes. Remove the pot from the heat.

With a ladle, carefully transfer the soup to a blender or use an immersion blender directly in the pot. Add the yogurt if using. You might need to blend the soup in batches depending on the size of your blender. Puree on low speed, gradually increasing the speed to high, for 1 to 2 minutes until smooth.

Return the pureed soup to the pot and place over medium-high heat. Add the lentil soup and coconut milk and stir to incorporate. Season with salt and pepper to taste. Cook, stirring occasionally, until the soup is hot and almost simmering, 4 to 5 minutes.

Serve and garnish with cilantro or parsley, if desired.

STORAGE + REHEAT

Once cooled, store airtight in the refrigerator for up to 4 days, or in the freezer for up to 3 months. To reheat, gently warm in a pan over medium-low heat until heated through, or microwave. Add a little water or broth if needed to loosen the soup. For best results, garnish with the cilantro or parsley right before serving.

One-Pan Shakshuka *with* Lentils & Eggplant

SERVES 3 OR 4
PREP TIME: 10 minutes
COOK TIME: 40 minutes

PER SERVING:	CALORIES 252 kcal	PROTEIN 14g	FAT 13g	CARBOHYDRATE 22g	FIBER 9g

1 tablespoon extra-virgin olive oil

1 red bell pepper, chopped

1 small eggplant (about 12 ounces), diced

2 tablespoons tomato paste

1 teaspoon sweet paprika

1 teaspoon chili powder

1 teaspoon dried oregano

¼ teaspoon kosher salt, plus more to taste

⅛ teaspoon freshly ground black pepper, plus more to taste

2 cups vegetable broth (or preferred broth)

One 14.5-ounce can diced tomatoes, undrained

½ cup dried green or brown lentils, rinsed

6 large eggs

Pita bread (optional), warmed, for serving

Shakshuka is a traditional savory Middle Eastern dish that's served morning, noon, and night. It has warm spices, is saucy with tomato and red peppers, and is typically nestled with eggs. I add lentils and eggplant for an extra protein and fiber boost that makes it a satisfying, wholesome meal. Add pita, and you're in business.

Lentils are a great plant-based, fiber-full protein source. If you're not a fan of eggplant, try using zucchini or mushrooms.

In a large pan, warm the olive oil over medium heat until hot. Add the bell pepper and eggplant and cook, stirring occasionally, until they have softened and slightly browned, 5 to 7 minutes. Stir in the tomato paste, paprika, chili powder, oregano, salt, and pepper. Cook for 1 to 2 minutes until fragrant.

Add the broth, tomatoes with their juices, and lentils. Stir to combine and bring to a simmer. Decrease the heat to low, cover, and cook until the lentils are tender and a lot of the liquid has been absorbed, 20 to 30 minutes (most brown lentils cook faster than green lentils). You want the shakshuka to be thick and saucy like a meaty red sauce. If it becomes too dry at any point, add more broth or water. Once the lentils are cooked, season with salt and pepper to taste.

Use a spoon or spatula to create 6 small wells or pockets in the shakshuka. Gently crack an egg into each well. Increase the heat to medium-low, cover the pan, and cook until the egg whites are set but the yolks are still runny, 4 to 5 minutes ( ). For firmer yolks, cook a bit longer.

Remove the pan from the heat. Serve hot with warm pita bread for dipping, if desired.

STORAGE + REHEAT

Once cooled, store airtight in the refrigerator for up to 3 days. To reheat, warm in a pan over medium heat until heated through, or microwave. For best results, remove the eggs while reheating, and add them, to warm them, at the end, right before serving. If overcooked, the eggs can become dense and rubbery.

STEPH'S TIP

If you prefer sunny-side up eggs with golden yolks, don't cover the pan, and continue to cook the shakshuka and eggs for about the same amount of time, carefully nudging the whites down and into the shakshuka, and breaking them up gently, so as not to pierce the yolks, as the eggs set.

YOU DO YOU

In a rush? Replace the dried lentils with canned (and rinsed!) lentils or white beans and halve the broth and simmer time.

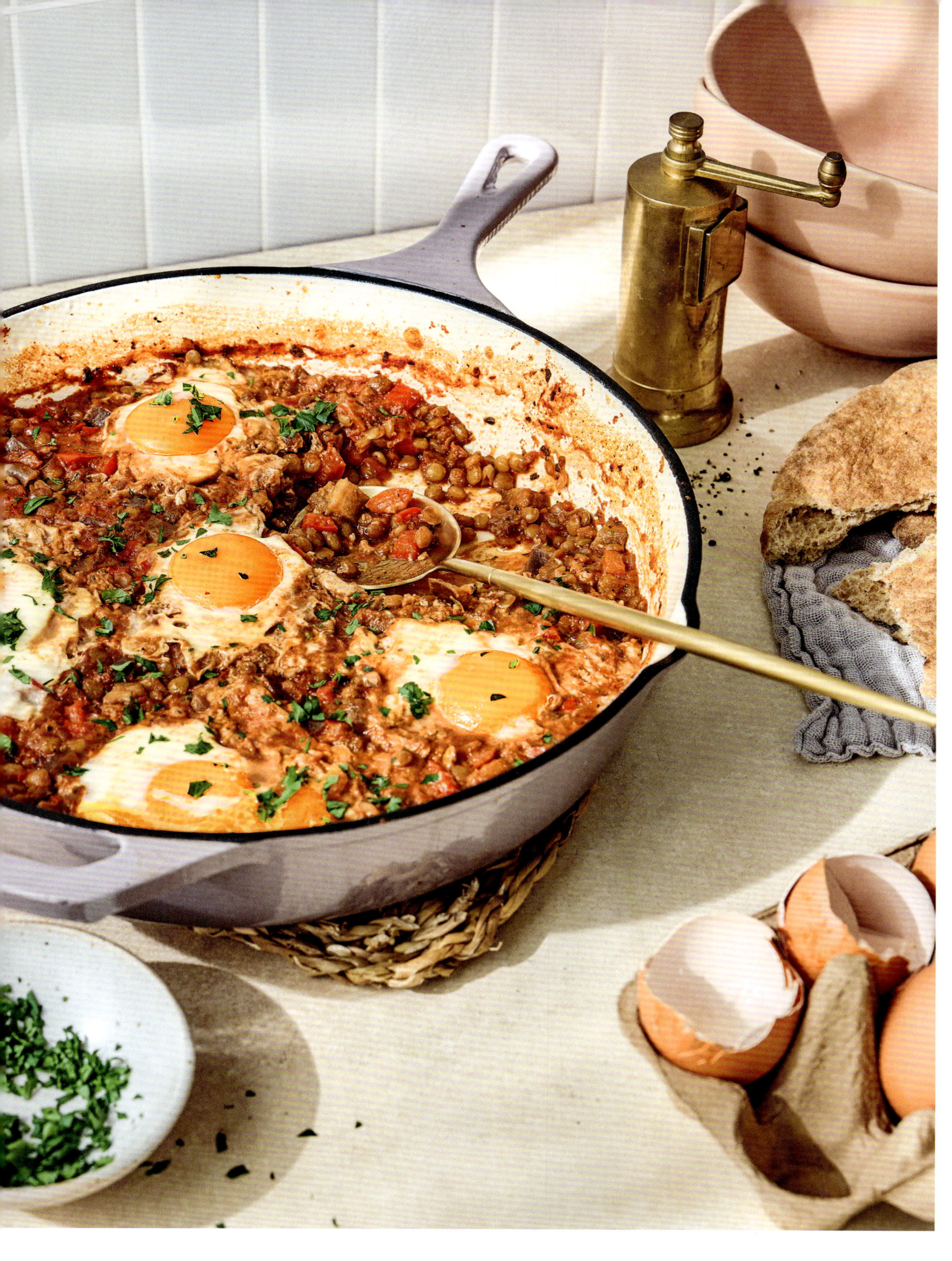

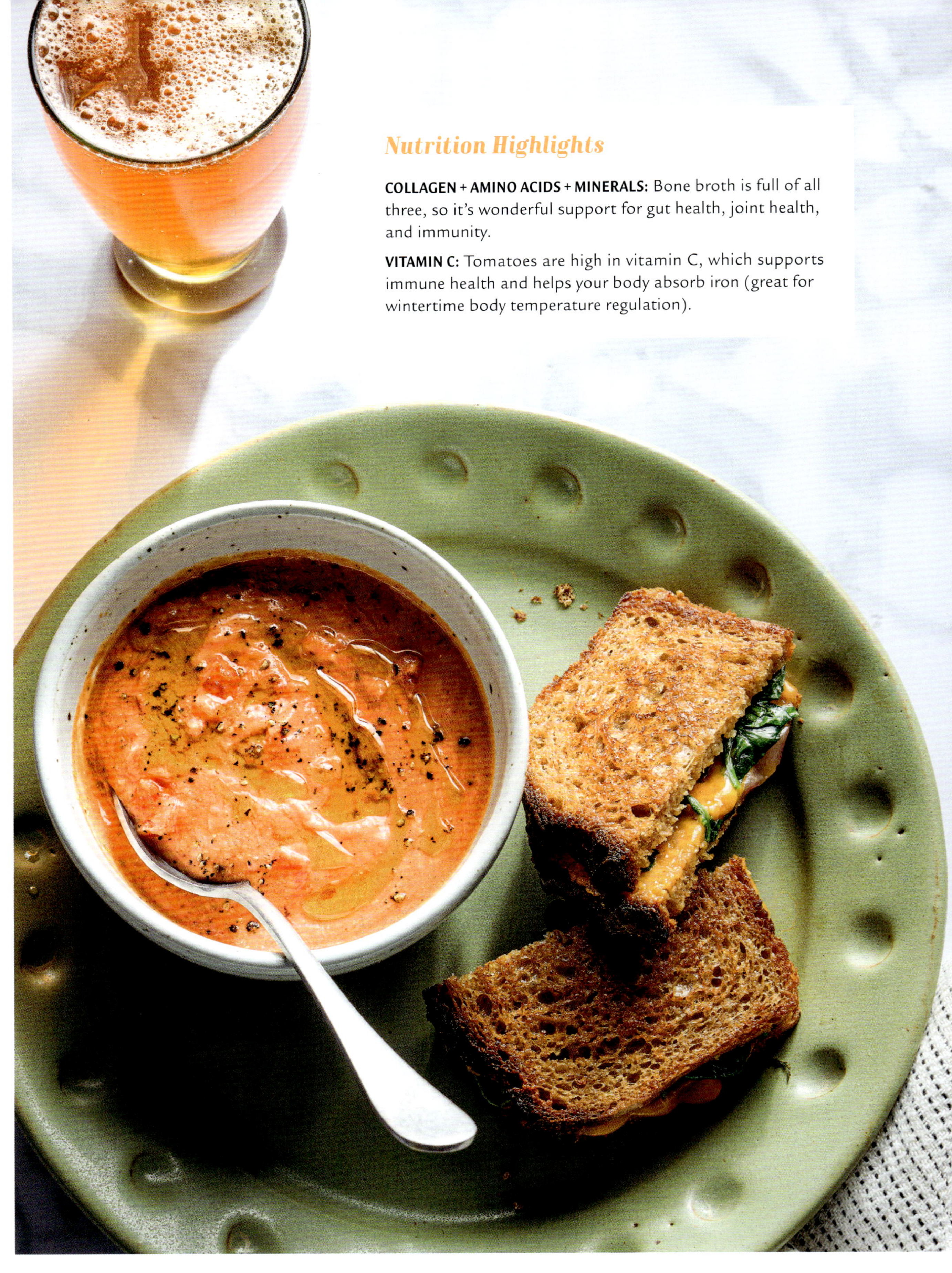

Nutrition Highlights

COLLAGEN + AMINO ACIDS + MINERALS: Bone broth is full of all three, so it's wonderful support for gut health, joint health, and immunity.

VITAMIN C: Tomatoes are high in vitamin C, which supports immune health and helps your body absorb iron (great for wintertime body temperature regulation).

High-Protein Tomato Soup

SERVES 1
PREP TIME: 5 minutes
COOK TIME: 15 minutes

PER SERVING:	CALORIES 454 kcal	PROTEIN 20g	FAT 24g	CARBOHYDRATE 48g	FIBER 10g

1½ tablespoons extra-virgin olive oil

½ white onion, finely chopped

1 tablespoon tomato paste

One 15-ounce can crushed tomatoes

1 cup bone broth

1 teaspoon Italian seasoning

¼ teaspoon kosher salt

½ cup 2% cottage cheese (or whatever fat content you prefer)

I crave tomato soup and grilled cheese throughout the winter. It's a classic and comforting combo, and I know I'm not alone. By blending creamy cottage cheese into my one-serving tomato soup, you get a lovely velvety texture and protein boost with zero heavy cream. A veggie-loaded grilled cheese is packed with protein, carbs, fats, fiber, and vitamins. So, pair this soup with one for a quick and satisfying solo lunch, or easy weeknight dinner.

In a medium pot, warm the olive oil over medium-low heat until hot. Add the onion and cook, stirring occasionally, until it begins to soften, 4 to 5 minutes. Add the tomato paste and cook, breaking it up with a spoon as it cooks, for about 1 minute. Stir in the tomatoes, bone broth, Italian seasoning, and salt.

Using a ladle, transfer about ½ cup of the soup mixture to a blender or food processor and add the cottage cheese. Blend, starting at low and slowly increasing to high, for about 1 minute until smooth. Set aside ( ).

Meanwhile, bring the soup to a simmer. Once simmering, partially cover, decrease the heat to low, and cook, stirring occasionally, until the soup is hot and the flavors melded, 6 to 8 minutes.

Remove the soup pot from the heat, uncover, and let the soup cool for about 5 minutes. This way, the cottage cheese puree doesn't separate when you add it to the soup. Once slightly cooled, add the blended cottage cheese mixture to the soup and stir until fully combined.

Return the pot to the stovetop over low heat and simmer for about 5 minutes. Don't worry if the cottage cheese mixture separates, it will come back together while simmering! This soup is best enjoyed day of.

STORAGE + REHEAT

Once cooled, store airtight in the refrigerator for up to 2 days. To reheat, gently warm in a pot over medium-low heat until heated through, or microwave.

YOU DO YOU

If you want an even smoother soup, blend all of the soup mixture with the cottage cheese once cooled.

Creamy Chickpea Curry

SERVES 4 TO 6
PREP TIME: 15 minutes
COOK TIME: 45 minutes

PER SERVING:	**CALORIES** 492 kcal	**PROTEIN** 23g	**FAT** 19g	**CARBOHYDRATE** 62g	**FIBER** 17g

2 tablespoons extra-virgin olive oil

1 yellow onion, finely chopped

3 garlic cloves, minced

2 teaspoons curry powder

½ teaspoon ground cumin

3 cups vegetable broth or water (or preferred broth)

One 14.5-ounce can diced tomatoes, undrained

1½ cups dried green or brown lentils, rinsed

1 cup quinoa, rinsed

2 cups water

Three 15-ounce cans chickpeas (or 4½ cups cooked chickpeas), drained and rinsed

2 cups lightly packed chopped spinach or kale

Once 13.5-ounce can full-fat coconut milk

1 teaspoon ground turmeric

½ teaspoon kosher salt

1 cup nonfat or low-fat Greek yogurt

¼ cup chopped fresh cilantro (optional)

Get cozy and make a big pot of this feel-good curry when you want to warm up yourself and your loved ones inside and out. It's loaded with protein, essential amino acids, and fiber thanks to the chickpeas, lentils, and quinoa. Fiber supports digestive health, stabilizes blood sugars, and keeps you satiated. The combination of iron-rich lentils and vitamin C–rich tomatoes does wonders for iron absorption, as well.

In a large pot or Dutch oven, heat the olive oil over medium heat until hot. Add the onion and cook, stirring occasionally, until it begins to soften, 5 to 7 minutes. Stir in the garlic, curry powder, and cumin and cook until fragrant, 1 to 2 minutes.

Stir in the broth, diced tomatoes with their juices, and the lentils. Increase the heat to high and bring the curry to a boil. Once boiling, decrease the heat to low, cover the pot, and simmer, stirring occasionally, until the lentils are tender and have absorbed most of the liquid, 25 to 35 minutes (most brown lentils cook faster than green lentils).

Meanwhile, in a medium pot, combine the quinoa and water. Bring it to a boil over high heat. Decrease the heat to medium-low, cover the pot, and simmer until the quinoa is fully cooked and tender and all of the water has been absorbed, 12 to 15 minutes. Fluff it with a fork, cover, and set aside.

Add the chickpeas, spinach, coconut milk, turmeric, and salt to the curry and stir to incorporate. Increase the heat to high, bring the curry to a boil for 2 to 3 minutes, then remove the pot from the heat.

If serving four people, spoon 1 cup of quinoa in each bowl and top with 2 cups of curry. If you're serving six, spoon a heaping ½ cup of quinoa into each bowl and top with 1⅓ cups of curry. Divide the Greek yogurt evenly among the bowls for a cool, creamy protein boost, and top evenly with the cilantro (is using).

STORAGE + REHEAT

Cool and store the yogurt, quinoa, and curry in separate airtight containers in the refrigerator for up to 4 days. The quinoa and curry can be frozen for up to 3 months. To reheat, gently warm in a pot over medium-low heat until heated through, or microwave.

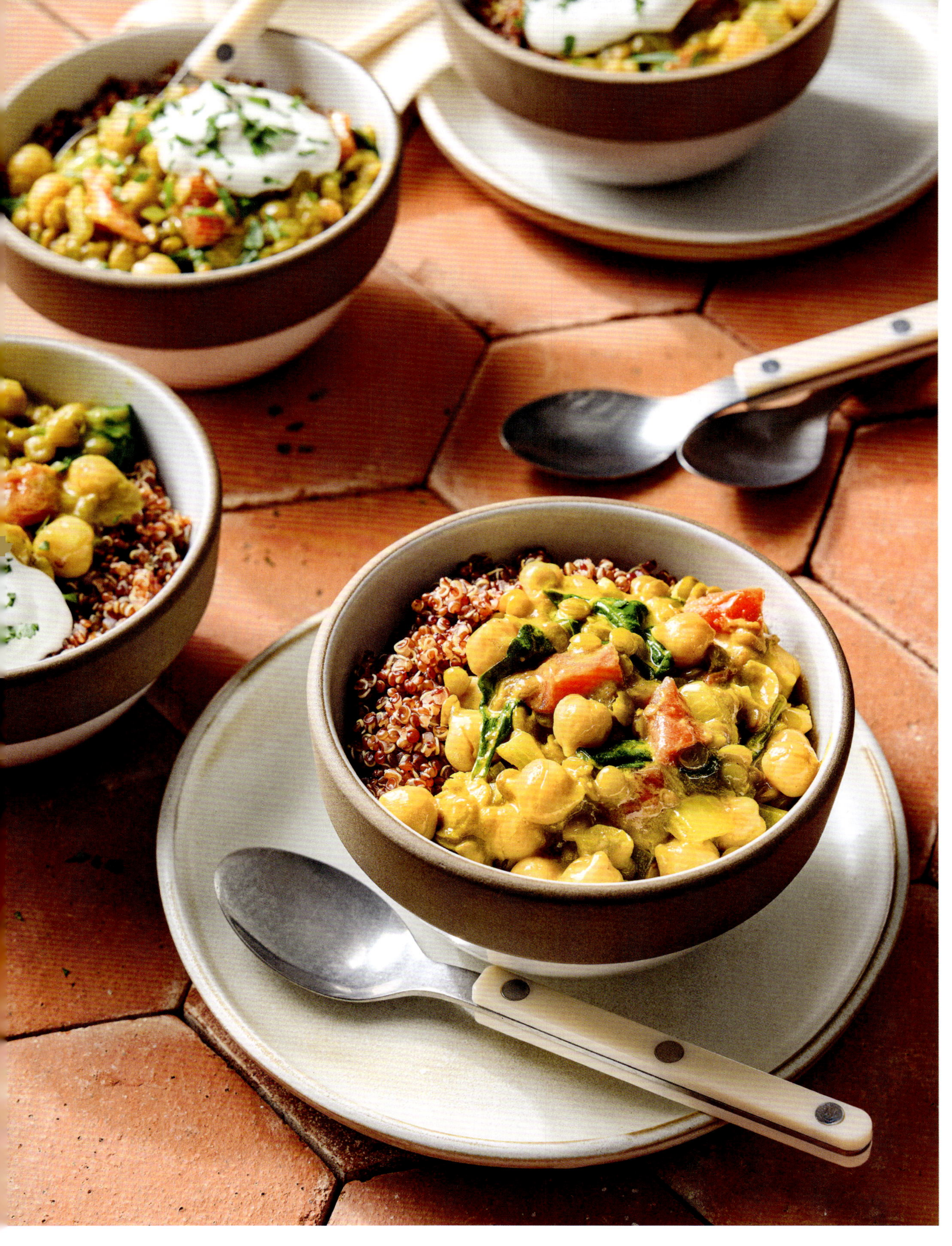

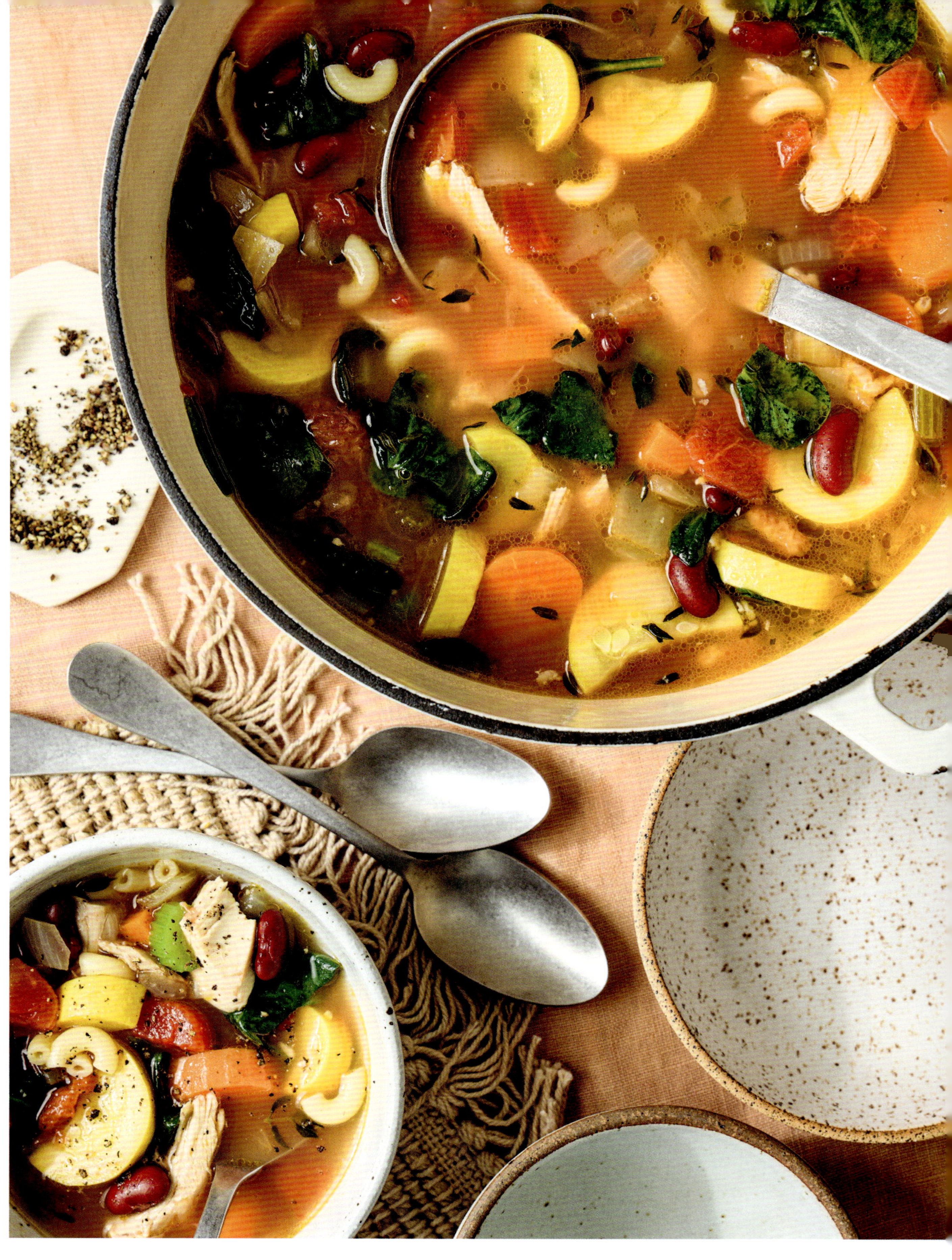

Kitchen Sink Soup

SERVES 4 TO 6
PREP TIME: 15 minutes
COOK TIME: 25 to 50 minutes

PER SERVING:	CALORIES 279 kcal	PROTEIN 21g	FAT 7g	CARBOHYDRATE 39g	FIBER 9g

1 tablespoon extra-virgin olive oil

1 white onion, chopped

3 garlic cloves, minced

2 carrots, peeled and chopped

2 celery stalks, chopped

1 yellow squash, chopped

6 cups chicken broth (or preferred broth)

One 14.5-ounce can diced tomatoes, undrained

1 tablespoon fresh lemon juice (about ½ small lemon)

1 teaspoon dried basil

1 teaspoon dried oregano

1 teaspoon dried thyme

½ teaspoon red pepper flakes

¼ teaspoon kosher salt, plus more to taste

½ cup uncooked or 1 cup cooked grain or pasta, such as rice, quinoa, farro, or elbow macaroni

One 15-ounce can preferred beans (or 1½ cups cooked), drained and rinsed

1 to 2 cups cooked protein (rotisserie chicken works well)

2 cups lightly packed fresh spinach

Whether you're cleaning out the fridge or doing weekly meal prep, Kitchen Sink Soup tackles food waste and makes quick work of leftover veggies, grains, and proteins. Use what you have and feel free to substitute to your heart's desire. This soup is loaded with fiber with all the beans, grains, and veggies, so you're taking good care of your digestive health when you eat it. The carrots, squash, and leafy greens provide vitamins A, C, and iron, all of which support immune health, eye health, and energy levels. The best part? No pot of Kitchen Sink Soup is ever the same! I highly recommend keeping a small container in your fridge to collect leftover veggies throughout the week.

In a large pot or Dutch oven, heat the olive oil over medium heat until hot. Add the onion and garlic and cook, stirring occasionally, until it begins to soften, 3 to 4 minutes. Add the carrots and celery and cook, stirring occasionally, until they begin to soften, 5 to 7 minutes. Add the squash and cook until it begins to soften, 2 to 3 more minutes.

Add the broth, diced tomatoes with their juices, lemon juice, basil, oregano, thyme, pepper flakes, and salt. Increase the heat to high and bring the soup to a boil. Stir in the uncooked grains or pasta (if you're using cooked grains or pasta, add them in the next step with the beans and protein and proceed accordingly), then decrease the heat to low. Cover, and simmer until the grains or pasta are tender, 10 to 30 minutes. If it is not soupy enough, add more water or broth until it's the desired consistency.

Once the grains or pasta are cooked, add the beans and cooked protein and cook for 3 to 4 minutes to warm them through. Season with salt to taste.

Stir in the spinach. Once it has wilted, about 1 minute, ladle the soup into bowls and serve hot.

STORAGE + REHEAT

Once cooled, store airtight in the refrigerator for up to 4 days, or frozen for up to 3 months. To reheat, gently warm in a pot over medium heat until heated through, or microwave. Add a splash of broth or water if you'd like to thin it.

Sheet-Pan Salmon & Veggies

SERVES 4
PREP TIME: 10 minutes
COOK TIME: 15 minutes

PER SERVING:	CALORIES 320 kcal	PROTEIN 28g	FAT 19g	CARBOHYDRATE 7g	FIBER 3g

1 bunch of asparagus, ends trimmed and halved

1 pint cherry tomatoes, on the vine if possible (removed from the vine or left on the vine for roasting, your preference!)

1 tablespoon plus 1½ teaspoons extra-virgin olive oil, divided

1½ teaspoons Italian seasoning

1 teaspoon garlic powder

½ teaspoon kosher salt, divided

¼ teaspoon freshly ground black pepper, divided

4 skin-on salmon fillets (3 to 4 ounces each)

1 lemon, halved

Balsamic Glaze (optional), homemade (recipe follows) or store-bought

Chopped fresh parsley leaves (optional), for garnish

This is a busy weeknight go-to for me. It comes together quickly, it's colorful, and it's loaded with nutrients. I love how perfectly the salmon cooks when you wrap the fillets in the foil just so. It's also easy to customize. Don't want fish? Use another meat or veg protein. Want more herbs and spices in the mix? Add them!

Salmon is one of the best sources of omega-3s, especially EPA and DHA, which are both great for brain and heart health and for keeping inflammation in check. It's also packed with vitamin D, which contributes to bone health, and B vitamins, especially B_{12}, which is essential for energy, brain function, and red blood cell production.

Preheat the oven to 450°F.

On one half of a sheet pan, combine the asparagus and cherry tomatoes. Drizzle them with 1 tablespoon of the olive oil and sprinkle with the Italian seasoning, garlic powder, ¼ teaspoon of the salt, and ⅛ teaspoon of the pepper. Toss gently until evenly coated.

Pat the salmon fillets dry with a paper towel and place them skin-side down on a piece of aluminum foil large enough to loosely wrap them. The foil should be roughly 24 inches long. This will keep the fillets from drying out. Place them in the foil on the sheet pan next to the vegetables.

Drizzle the fillets evenly with the remaining 1½ teaspoons olive oil and sprinkle them evenly with the remaining ¼ teaspoon salt and ⅛ teaspoon pepper. Take one of the lemon halves and cut it into slices. Top each fillet with 1 lemon slice. Lightly crimp and close the foil over the top of the salmon fillets so they are covered, but with some gaps for steam to escape. Roast until the salmon is fully cooked (check the middle) and flakes easily, 12 to 14 minutes. The asparagus should be tender and the tomatoes lightly blistered.

If desired, drizzle the vegetables with balsamic glaze to taste and garnish with fresh parsley. Squeeze the remaining lemon half over the veggies before serving.

STORAGE + REHEAT

Once cooled, store airtight in the refrigerator for up to 3 days. To reheat, warm in a pan over medium heat until heated through, or heat in the oven at 350°F for 5 to 10 minutes. Store any garnish separately.

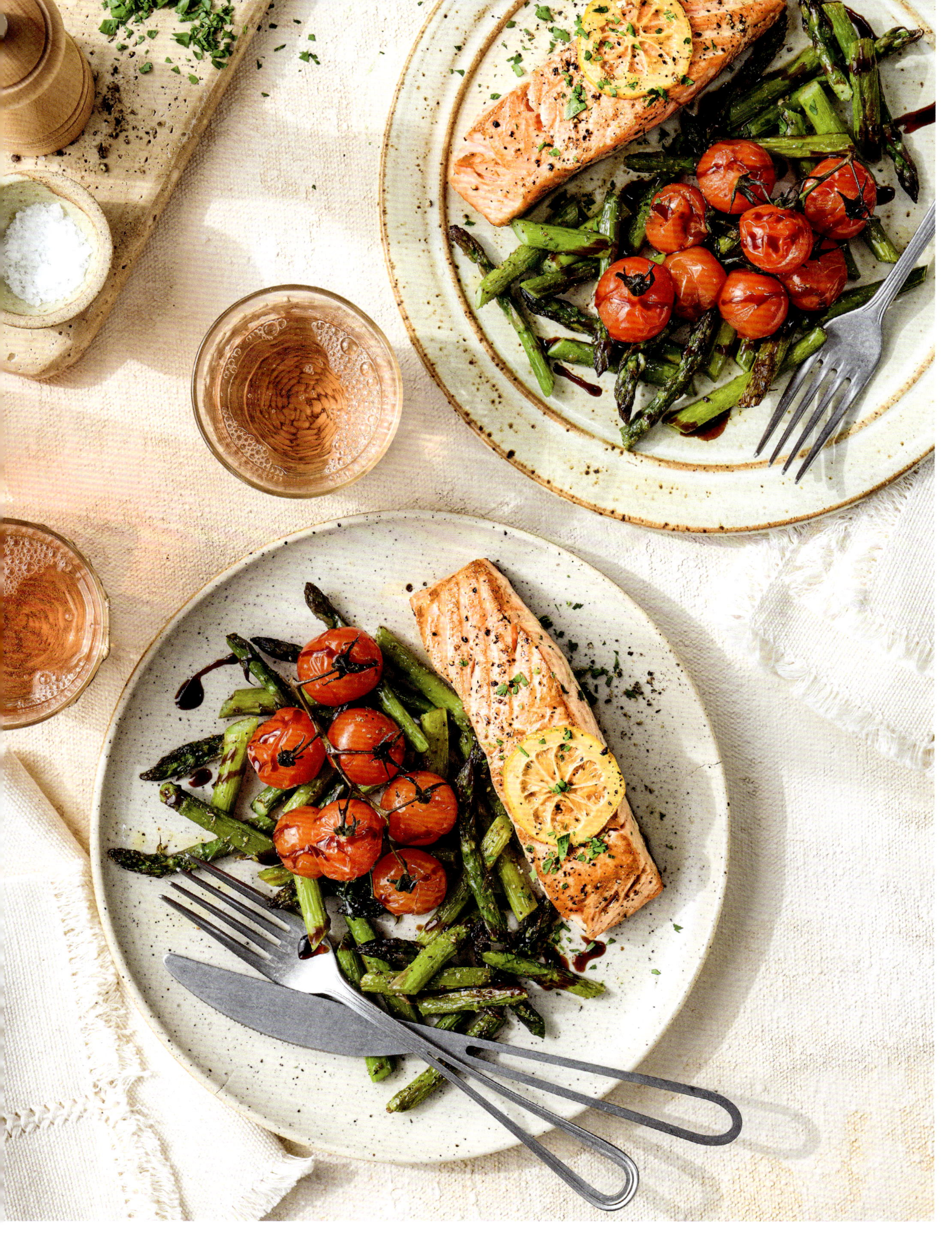

Balsamic Glaze

MAKES ½ CUP
COOK TIME: 45 minutes

PER TABLESPOON:	**CALORIES** 82 kcal	**PROTEIN** 0g	**FAT** 0g	**CARBOHYDRATE** 18g	**FIBER** 0g

2 cups balsamic vinegar

¼ cup lightly packed brown sugar or honey

In a small pot, stir together the vinegar and brown sugar. Bring to a boil over high heat, then decrease the heat to low and simmer until reduced to ½ cup, 45 minutes to 1 hour. You want the glaze to coat the back of a spoon when hot, and to be the consistency of syrup once cooled. Store airtight in the refrigerator for up to 1 month.

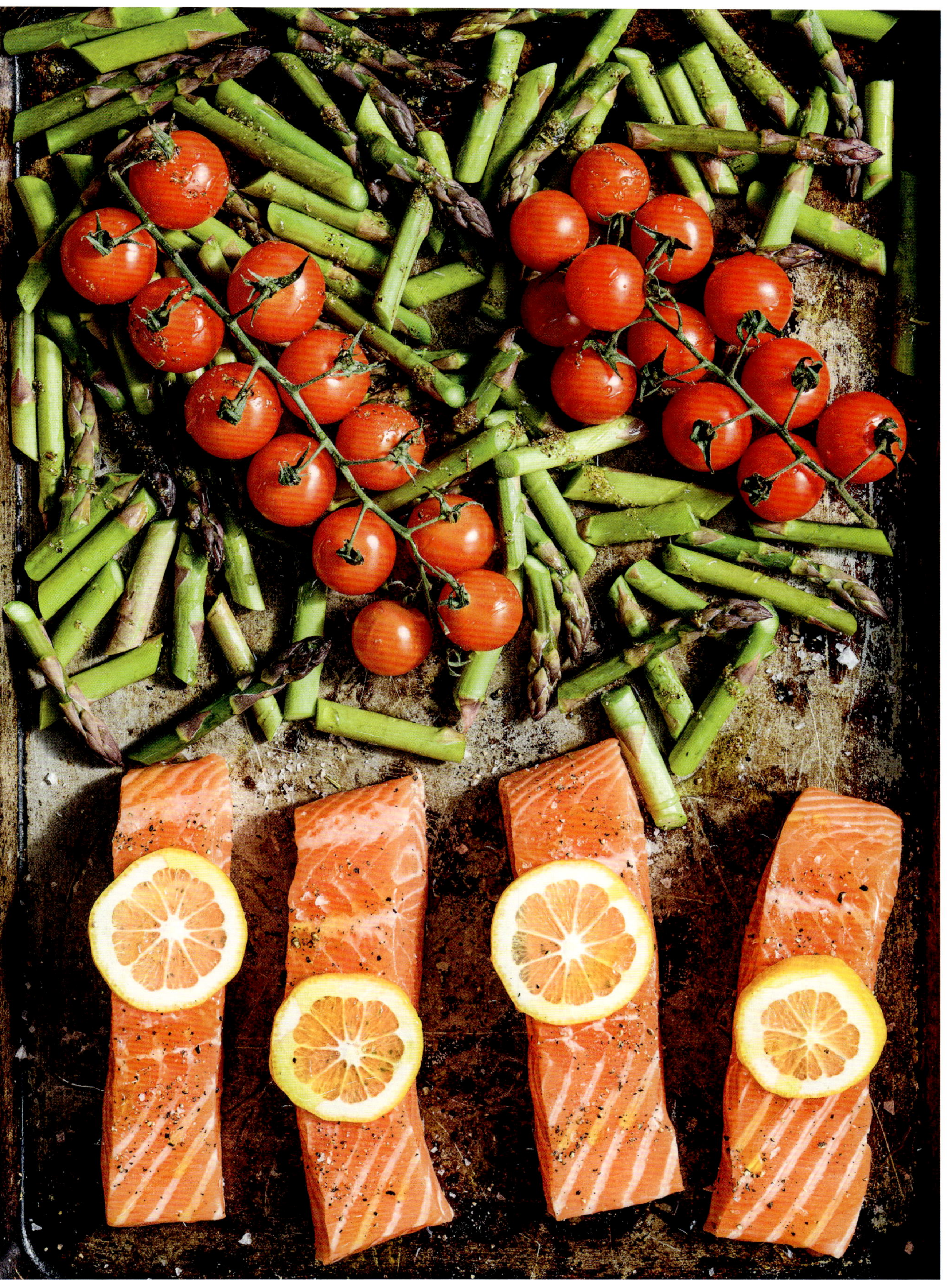

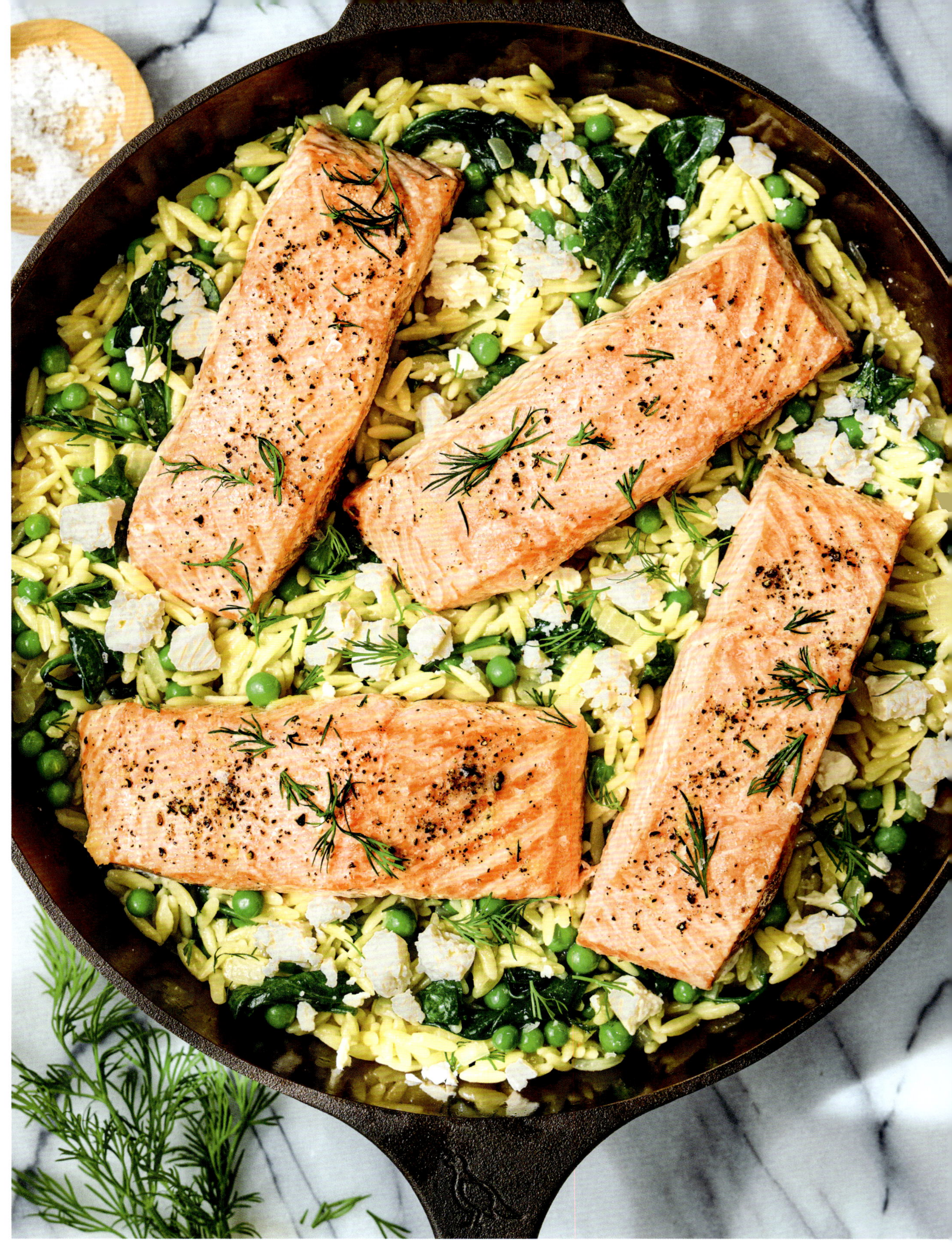

Lemony Salmon Orzo

SERVES 4
PREP TIME: 10 to 15 minutes
COOK TIME: 30 to 35 minutes

PER SERVING:	CALORIES 492 kcal	PROTEIN 34g	FAT 26g	CARBOHYDRATE 30g	FIBER 5g

2 tablespoons extra-virgin olive oil

1 yellow onion, diced

1½ cups orzo

3½ cups chicken broth (or preferred broth)

4 salmon fillets (6 ounces each)

½ teaspoon kosher salt, divided

2½ cups lightly packed spinach, chopped

1½ cups frozen peas

5 tablespoons minced fresh dill, divided

¼ cup fresh lemon juice (about 1 lemon)

½ cup crumbled feta cheese

Freshly ground black pepper (optional)

Looking for a new family favorite? This light and lemony, chock-full of flavor, color, vitamins, and minerals dish is for you. It's so good that even Katie Couric loves it and *loves* talking about it. Added bonus: It's perfectly balanced with carbs, protein, healthy fats, and veggies.

What makes this dish shine even brighter is the fact that even though the flavors are layered and complex, like something you'd expect from a fancy pants restaurant, it's one of the easiest dishes to make in the book. I love that. My fiancé is obsessed with this recipe, so we cook it on a regular basis. Sometimes weekly, which is good, since it's recommended to consume fatty fish at least twice a week.

Preheat the oven to 450°F.

In a large pan, heat the olive oil over medium heat until hot. Add the onion and cook, stirring occasionally, until it begins to soften, 5 to 7 minutes. Add the orzo and cook, stirring occasionally, until it is lightly toasted, 2 to 3 minutes. Add the chicken broth and bring to a boil. Decrease the heat to low, cover, and simmer until the orzo is tender and has absorbed most of the broth, about 10 minutes.

Meanwhile, line a sheet pan with aluminum foil, extending it a few extra inches on both ends. Place the salmon (skin-side down if there is skin) on the foil and sprinkle with ¼ teaspoon of the salt. Pull up the ends of the foil and lightly crimp and close the foil over the fillets so they are covered but with some gaps for steam to escape. Bake until it is fully cooked (check the middle) and flakes easily, 12 to 14 minutes. Set aside.

Once the orzo is cooked, add the spinach, peas, ¼ cup of the dill, lemon juice, and the remaining ¼ teaspoon salt to the pan and stir well to combine. Cook, nudging everything around in the pan, until the spinach has wilted and the peas are cooked, 2 to 3 minutes.

Use a spoon or spatula to create small wells in the orzo for the salmon fillets. Place the fillets into the wells. Sprinkle the feta evenly over everything. Cover the pan for 1 to 2 minutes so the feta slightly melts and the salmon warms. Garnish with the remaining 1 tablespoon of dill and pepper, if desired, and serve immediately.

STORAGE + REHEAT

Once cooled, store airtight in the refrigerator for up to 3 days. To reheat, warm in a pan over medium heat until heated through, or microwave.

Crispy Roasted Chicken Thighs *with* Buttery Hot Sauce

SERVES 4 TO 6
PREP TIME: 10 minutes
COOK TIME: 30 minutes

PER SERVING:	**CALORIES** 325 kcal	**PROTEIN** 32g	**FAT** 22g	**CARBOHYDRATE** 1g	**FIBER** 0g

6 bone-in, skin-on chicken thighs (6 to 8 ounces each), trimmed

1 tablespoon sweet paprika

1¼ teaspoons kosher salt

1 teaspoon freshly ground black pepper

2 tablespoons extra-virgin olive oil

Buttery Hot Sauce (recipe follows), for serving

I can't tell you how perfect and easy this roasting technique is for bone-in chicken thighs. The skin gets nice and crispy, and the meat is super tender and juicy. If you want to throw something else in the oven, as the thighs roast, most veggies chopped into 1- to 3-inch pieces, oiled and seasoned, will cook in roughly the same amount of time.

Did you know that dark meat (thighs and drumsticks) contains a lot more iron and zinc than white meat? Yep! And those minerals are great for energy production and immune function.

Position oven racks in the middle and in the lowest spot in the oven. Place a sheet pan, large enough to hold all the chicken thighs, on the lower rack. Preheat the oven to 450°F. You want to heat up the sheet pan so that when you put the chicken on it prior to roasting, it sears and sizzles the skin.

Place the chicken on a large plate and use a fork to poke the skin side of each thigh several times. In a small bowl, combine the paprika, salt, and pepper. Lightly coat both sides of each chicken thigh with the olive oil. Evenly season both sides of each oiled thigh with the paprika/salt/pepper mix.

Once the oven has preheated, remove the preheated sheet pan. Carefully place the oiled and seasoned thighs skin-side down on the hot sheet pan. The skin should sizzle a bit as you do. Transfer the sheet pan back to the lower rack of the oven. Roast the chicken until the skin side of the thighs begins to brown, 20 to 25 minutes, rotating the sheet pan front to back about halfway through. Remove the sheet pan from the oven and turn on the broiler.

Carefully flip the chicken to skin-side up. Discard any drippings from the pan (or reserve them for another use). Transfer the chicken to the middle oven rack and broil until the skin is nicely crisped and browned and an instant-read thermometer inserted into the thickest part of each thigh reads 160°F or more, 7 to 10 minutes, rotating the pan front to back halfway through.

Transfer the roasted chicken to a platter, let it rest for at least 5 minutes, and then enjoy with a small dish of the buttery hot sauce on the side!

NUTRITION PSA

Pair with Garlicky Blistered Green Beans & Cherry Tomatoes (page 207) to increase your fiber intake.

STORAGE + REHEAT

Once cooled, store airtight in the refrigerator for up to 3 days. To reheat, warm in a covered pan over medium heat until heated through, or heat in a covered baking dish in the oven at 350°F for 10 to 15 minutes.

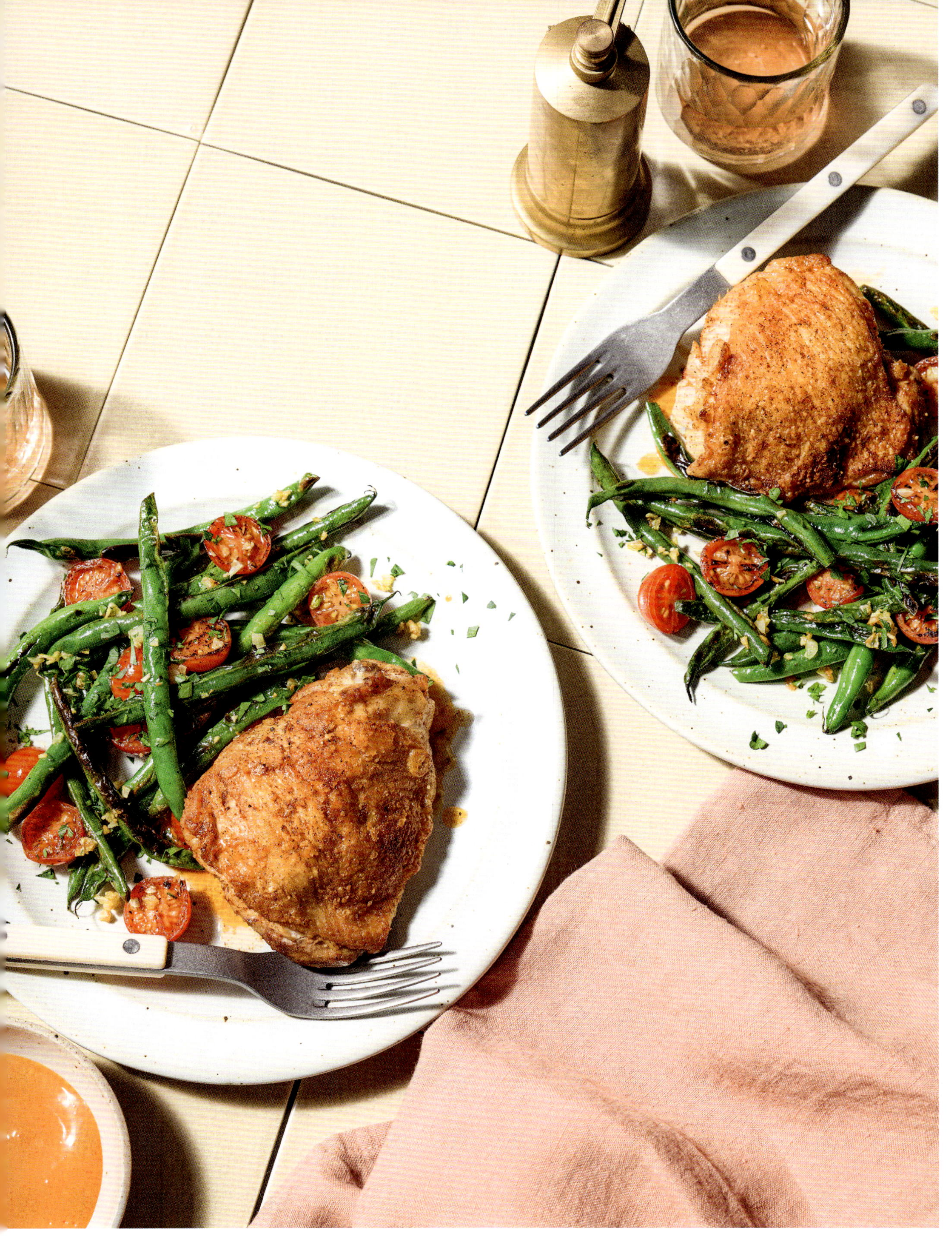

Buttery Hot Sauce

MAKES ½ CUP

PER 2 TABLESPOONS:	**CALORIES** 84 kcal	**PROTEIN** 0g	**FAT** 9g	**CARBOHYDRATE** 1g	**FIBER** 0g

¼ cup hot sauce

1¼ teaspoons cornstarch

4 tablespoons (2 ounces/½ stick) cold butter, cut into 4 pieces

Use whatever hot sauce you love the most for this buttery yumminess. If you want to go Buffalo-style, then use a hot sauce that works well for that such as Frank's.

In a small pot, whisk the hot sauce and cornstarch together until smooth and combined. Cook over medium-low heat, whisking constantly, until the sauce is bubbling and thick, about 2 minutes. Remove the pan from the heat and whisk in the butter, one piece at a time, until fully melted.

Serve the sauce warm for dipping and dunking the roasted chicken. Leftover sauce can be cooled, stored in an airtight container, and refrigerated for up to 1 week. To reheat, warm in a pot over medium heat until heated through, or microwave.

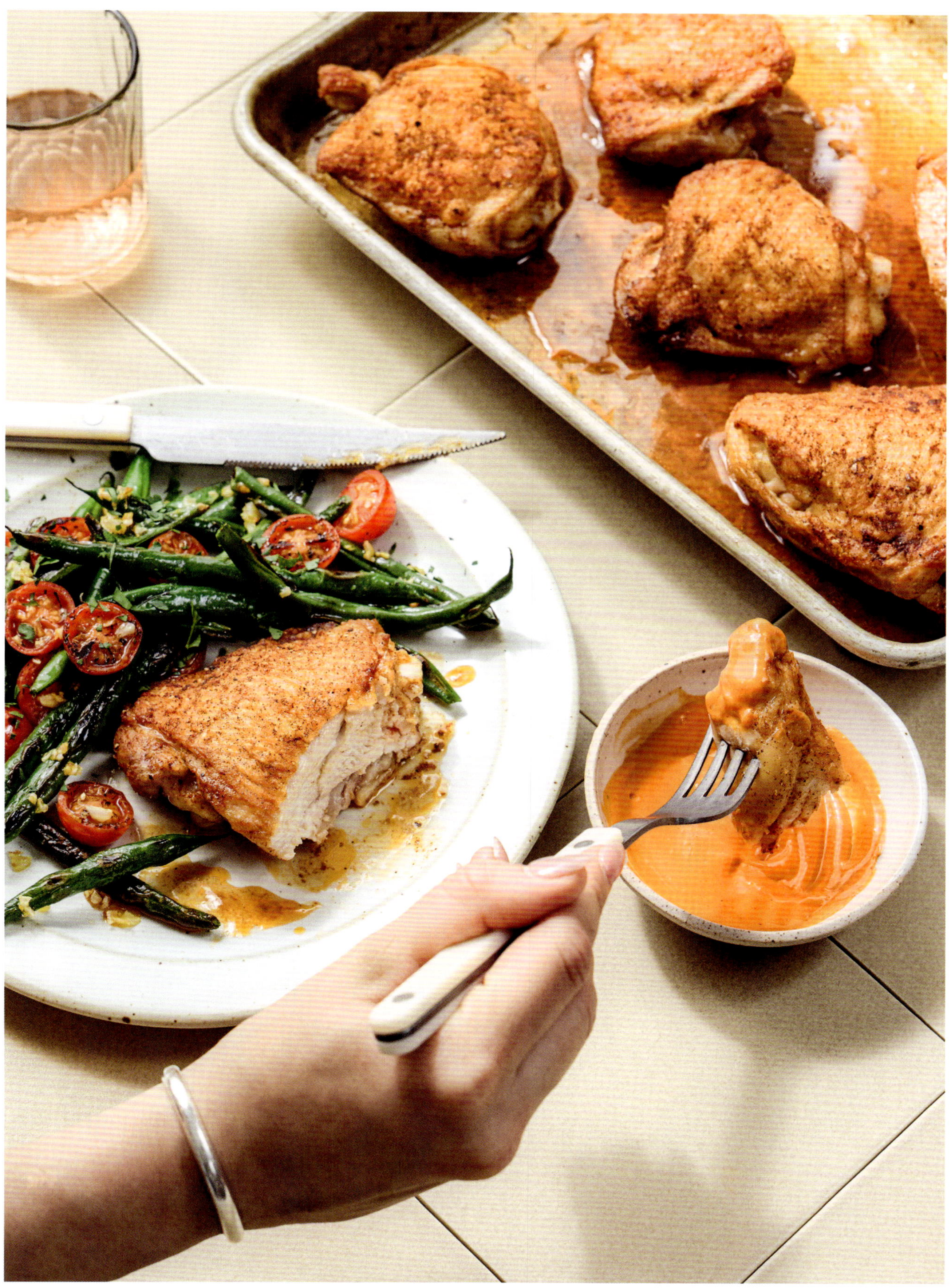

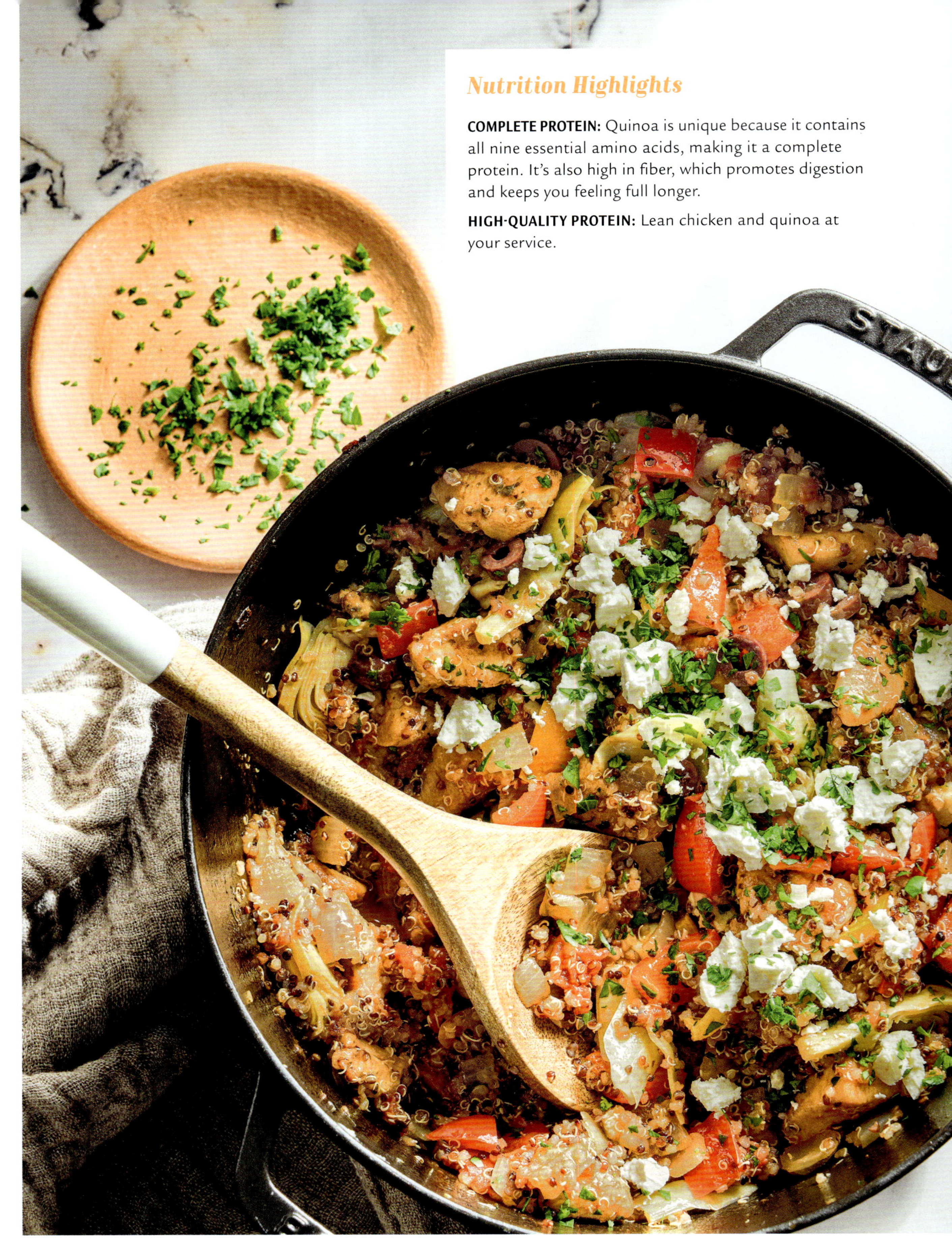

Nutrition Highlights

COMPLETE PROTEIN: Quinoa is unique because it contains all nine essential amino acids, making it a complete protein. It's also high in fiber, which promotes digestion and keeps you feeling full longer.

HIGH-QUALITY PROTEIN: Lean chicken and quinoa at your service.

Chicken & Quinoa Pilaf

SERVES 4 TO 6
PREP TIME: 10 minutes
COOK TIME: 40 minutes

PER SERVING:	CALORIES 426 kcal	PROTEIN 36g	FAT 14g	CARBOHYDRATE 37g	FIBER 7g

1 tablespoon extra-virgin olive oil

1 white onion, diced

2 red, yellow, or orange bell peppers, diced

1½ pounds boneless, skinless chicken breasts (about 3 large), cut into roughly 1-inch cubes

1 teaspoon sweet paprika

1 teaspoon dried oregano

½ teaspoon kosher salt, divided

¼ teaspoon freshly ground black pepper

1 cup quinoa, rinsed

2 cups chicken broth or water

One 14.5-ounce can diced tomatoes, undrained

½ cup sliced Kalamata olives

One 13- to 14-ounce can whole or quartered artichoke hearts in water or brine, drained and chopped

¼ cup fresh lemon juice (about 1 lemon)

Crumbled goat or feta cheese, for garnish

3 tablespoons finely chopped fresh flat-leaf parsley leaves (optional), as garnish

One-pot meals are a lifesaver on busy weeknights. From searing the chicken to simmering the quinoa and veggies, everything happens in the same pot or Dutch oven. That means fewer dishes to wash and more time to relax after dinner. Win-win. I especially love the flavor and texture of the Kalamata olives and artichoke hearts in this one. They're delicious, and they're also loaded with healthy fats, fiber, and antioxidants. Lucky you.

In a large wide pot or Dutch oven, heat the olive oil over medium heat until hot. Add the onion and cook until it begins to soften, about 3 minutes. Add the bell peppers and cook, stirring occasionally, until they begin to soften, about 3 minutes.

On a cutting board or in a medium bowl, season the chicken evenly with the paprika, oregano, ¼ teaspoon of the salt, and the pepper. Using a spoon or spatula, push the vegetables to the sides of the pot and add the cubed chicken to the middle. Cook the chicken, stirring occasionally and keeping the vegetables largely to the perimeter of the pot, until it's no longer pink and is very lightly browned, about 5 minutes.

Add the quinoa, broth, tomatoes with their juices, olives, artichoke hearts, lemon juice, and the remaining ¼ teaspoon salt. Stir to combine and make sure that the chicken is mostly submerged.

Bring everything to a boil, then decrease the heat to medium-low and simmer, covered, stirring occasionally and keeping the chicken submerged, until the quinoa is fluffy and the chicken is cooked through, 25 to 30 minutes.

Remove the pot from heat and enjoy right away. When serving, sprinkle 1 to 2 tablespoons of crumbled goat cheese over the top of each serving, and garnish evenly with the parsley, if desired.

STORAGE + REHEAT

Once cooled, store airtight in the refrigerator for up to 3 days. To reheat, warm in a pan over medium heat until heated through, or microwave.

Veggie-Loaded Chicken Tikka Masala

SERVES 4 TO 6
PREP TIME: 10 minutes
COOK TIME: 30 minutes

PER SERVING:	CALORIES 594 kcal	PROTEIN 40g	FAT 23g	CARBOHYDRATE 58g	FIBER 7g

1½ pounds boneless, skinless chicken breasts (about 3 large), cut into bite-size pieces

2½ teaspoons kosher salt, divided

¼ teaspoon freshly ground black pepper

3 tablespoons extra-virgin olive oil, divided

1 large yellow onion, finely chopped

2 tablespoons tomato paste

3 garlic cloves, minced

1-inch piece fresh ginger, peeled and finely grated or minced

1 tablespoon garam masala

1 teaspoon sweet paprika

½ teaspoon cayenne pepper

1 teaspoon ground turmeric

1 teaspoon ground cumin

4 cups cauliflower florets

1 large zucchini, diced

1 cup canned or cooked chickpeas, drained and rinsed if canned

One 14.5-ounce can diced tomatoes, undrained

½ cup whole-milk or 2% Greek yogurt

½ cup heavy cream

4 cups cooked rice (I prefer basmati)

½ cup chopped fresh cilantro leaves

My veggie-packed version of this spicy, creamy Indian classic is loaded with zucchini, cauliflower, and chickpeas, so it wins the protein plus fiber competitions. I recommend serving it with steamy, just-cooked basmati rice. Add a side of naan if you'd like (I love it) and a simple cucumber salad for some crisp, crunchy brightness. If you don't have zucchini or cauliflower on hand, don't worry, use other vegetables like bell peppers, carrots, or spinach.

Season the chicken evenly with 2 teaspoons of the salt and the pepper. In a large pot or Dutch oven, heat 1 tablespoon of the olive oil over medium heat until hot. Add the chicken and cook, stirring occasionally, until it is lightly browned on all sides, but not fully cooked, 5 to 6 minutes. Transfer the chicken to a bowl, along with its juices.

In the same pot (no need to wipe it out or wash it), add the remaining 2 tablespoons oil and the onion and cook, stirring occasionally, until the onion has softened, 4 to 5 minutes. Stir in the tomato paste, garlic, and ginger and cook until fragrant, 1 minute. Add the garam masala, paprika, cayenne, turmeric, cumin, and the remaining ½ teaspoon salt and cook, stirring to coat the onion and warm the spices, for about 1 minute, until fragrant.

Add the cauliflower, zucchini, and chickpeas (the pan will be quite full!). Cook, stirring and nudging everything around, until the veggies begin to soften, 3 to 4 minutes. Add the diced tomatoes with their juices and return the partially cooked chicken to the pan. Stir well, decrease the heat to medium-low, cover, and simmer, stirring occasionally, until the chicken is fully cooked and the vegetables are tender, about 10 minutes.

Remove the lid and decrease the heat to low. In a small bowl, stir together the yogurt and heavy cream. Add that mixture to the pot and cook for another 2 to 3 minutes, stirring regularly. Be careful not to let it boil, because the yogurt-cream mixture will separate if you do. Once heated through, serve over rice and garnish with cilantro.

STORAGE + REHEAT

Once cooled, store airtight in the refrigerator for up to 3 days, or in the freezer for up to 3 months. If freezing, add the yogurt/cream mixture once the dish has thawed and you are reheating it. To reheat, warm in a pan over medium heat until heated through, or microwave. For best results, garnish with the cilantro right before serving.

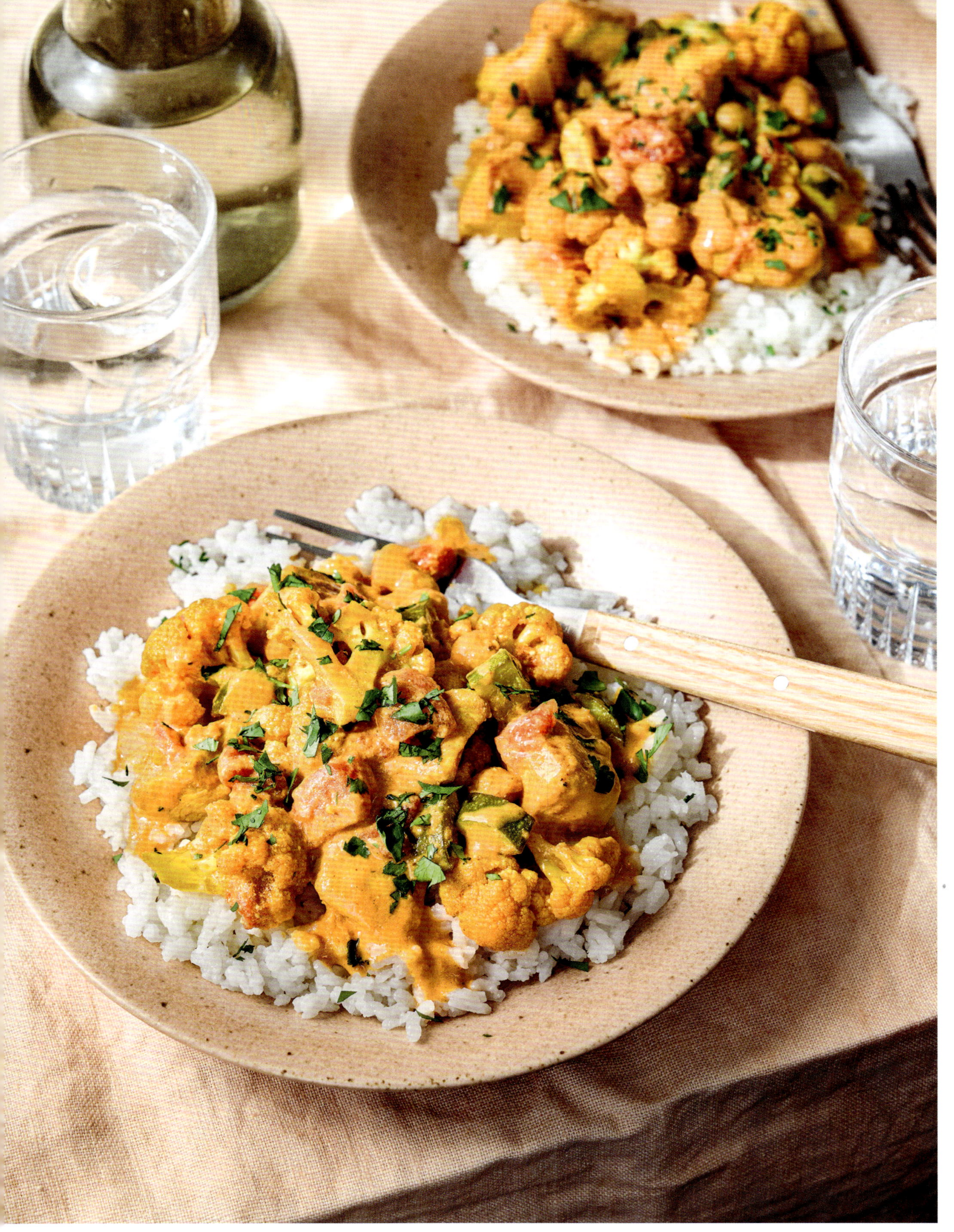

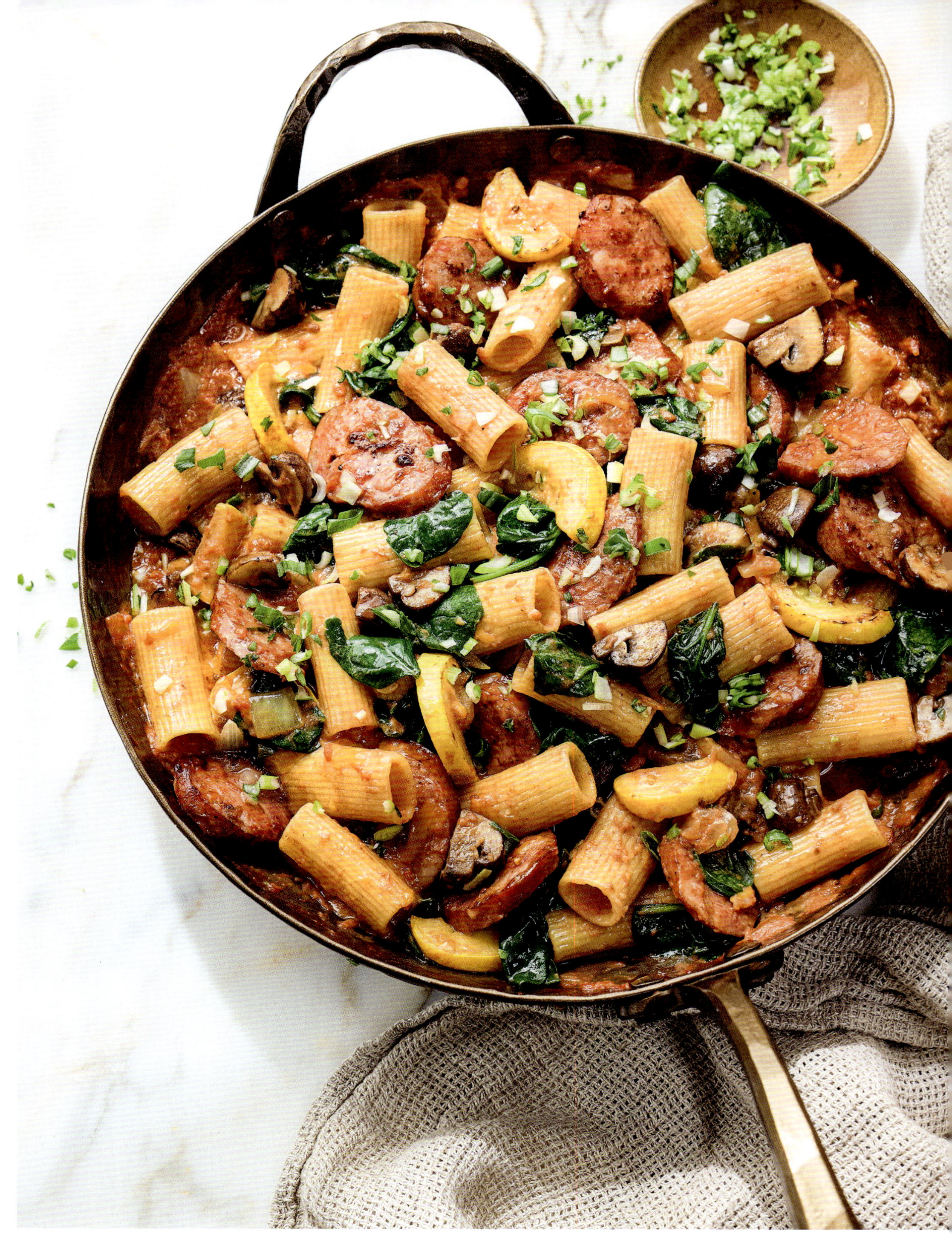

Cheesy Kielbasa Skillet

SERVES 3 OR 4
PREP TIME: 10 minutes
COOK TIME: 25 minutes

PER SERVING:	**CALORIES** 688 kcal	**PROTEIN** 31g	**FAT** 41g	**CARBOHYDRATE** 39g	**FIBER** 4g

2 tablespoons extra-virgin olive oil

14 ounces kielbasa, cut into ¼-inch-thick slices

1 small yellow onion, diced

3 cups sliced white or cremini mushrooms (or 8-ounce package sliced mushrooms)

½ yellow squash, halved lengthwise and sliced

1 cup chicken broth (or preferred broth)

One 14.5-ounce can diced tomatoes, undrained

⅓ cup whole or 2% milk

1½ cups farfalle (bow tie) or another preferred pasta (about 4 ounces)

2 cups lightly packed fresh spinach or 1 cup frozen

1 cup grated sharp Cheddar cheese

Finely chopped green onion (optional), white and green parts, for garnish

This is one of my absolute favorite dishes. It's 100 percent nutritious comfort food, and I'm sure that's a big part of why it went viral on TikTok and became a huge hit in the summer of 2021. Katie Couric also really likes this one. Swoon. The recipe is all about cozy, cheesy goodness with a powerful dose of vital veggie nutrients. It's one of my signature dishes because it strikes that perfect balance between comfort, nutrition, balance, and fun. I think you're going to love it.

Did you know that canned tomatoes have more antioxidants, particularly lycopene, than fresh tomatoes? Lycopene helps protect cells from damage caused by harmful molecules called free radicals, and it's linked to various health benefits, including reducing the risk of certain cancers and supporting heart health. The canning process also breaks down the cell walls of the tomato, making lycopene more bioavailable and easier to absorb.

In a large deep pan, heat the olive oil over medium-high heat until hot. Add the kielbasa and onion and cook, stirring occasionally, until the kielbasa begins browning, 2 to 3 minutes. Add the mushrooms and squash (the pan will be quite full) and continue cooking, stirring occasionally, until the vegetables are tender and the kielbasa has browned, 3 to 5 minutes.

Add the chicken broth, diced tomatoes with their juices, milk, and pasta. Stir to combine and bring to a boil. Decrease the heat to low and simmer, stirring occasionally, until the pasta is fully cooked, 15 to 20 minutes. Make sure that the pasta is submerged in the liquid throughout simmering, so that it absorbs the broth and fully cooks.

Add the spinach and once it has wilted, after 1 to 2 minutes, add the Cheddar. Mix well for 1 to 2 minutes until the cheese is nice and melty and coating everything. Garnish with sliced green onions (if using) and enjoy!

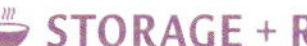

STORAGE + REHEAT

Once cooled, store airtight in the refrigerator for up to 3 days. To reheat, warm in a pan over medium heat until heated through, or microwave.

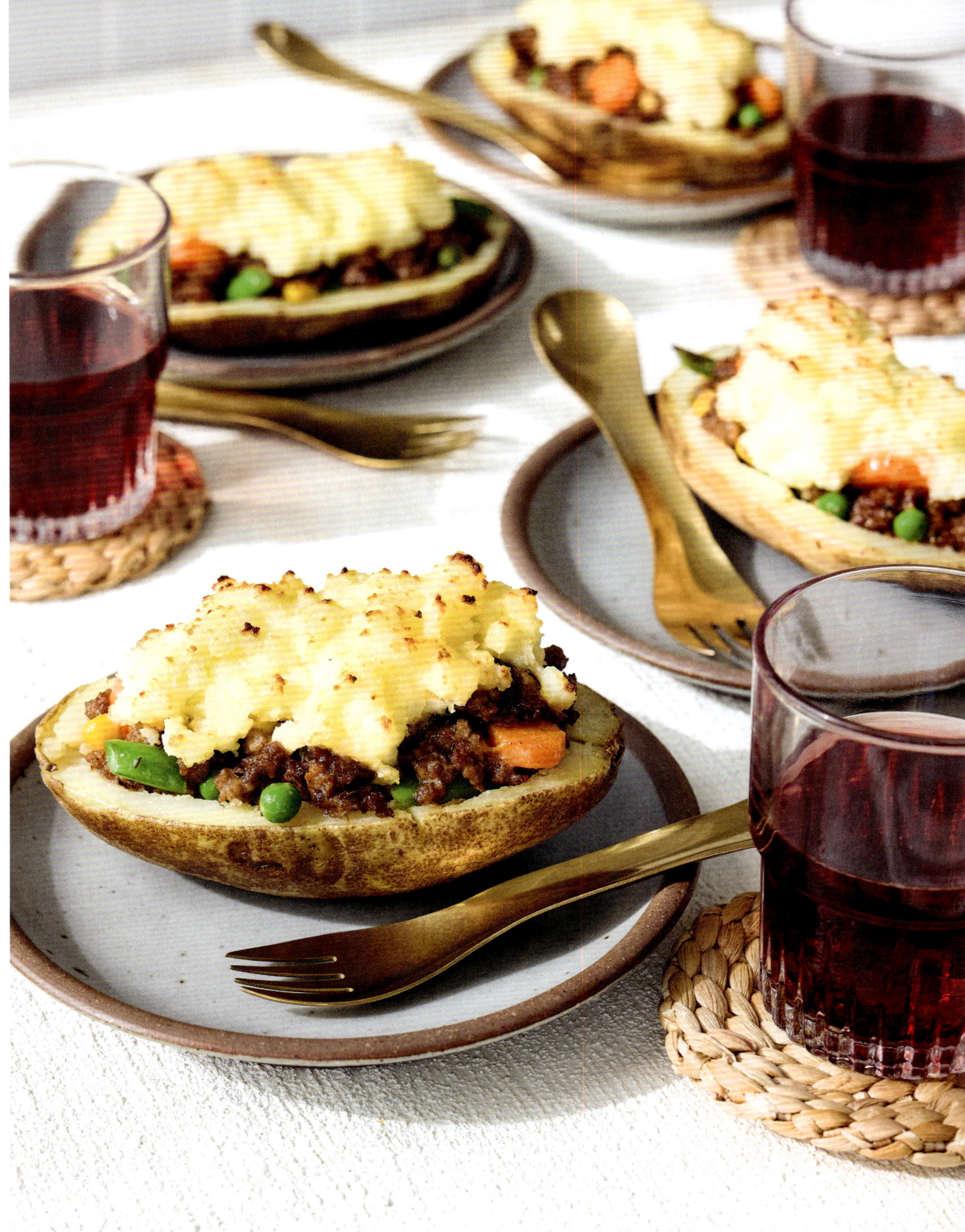

Lazy Shepherd's Pie

SERVES 4 TO 8
PREP TIME: 20 minutes
COOK TIME: 40 minutes

PER SERVING:	**CALORIES** 420 kcal	**PROTEIN** 23g	**FAT** 16g	**CARBOHYDRATE** 49g	**FIBER** 4g

4 large russet potatoes (12 ounces each), scrubbed

1 tablespoon extra-virgin olive oil

1 pound lean ground beef (10% fat or less)

1 teaspoon kosher salt, divided

½ teaspoon freshly ground black pepper, divided

2 cups (about 10 ounces) frozen vegetable mix

3 tablespoons all-purpose flour

1 tablespoon tomato paste

½ teaspoon dried thyme

½ teaspoon dried rosemary

1 cup beef broth (or preferred broth)

½ cup nonfat or low-fat Greek yogurt

4 tablespoons (2 ounces/½ stick) unsalted butter, divided

One of my family's favorite comfort foods is shepherd's pie. It's obviously very meat-and-potato-heavy, and it's also typically quite labor-intensive. I've added veg and nutrients and simplified it into a weeknight meal. These lil pies are broiled right in their potato skins. So cute! FYI, they're a great appetizer or party snack food.

Most people think that sweet potatoes and yams are more nutritious than russets, but that's false. *All* potatoes are quite nutritious, just in different ways. Russets contain a huge amount of potassium, more than a banana!

Pierce the potatoes 10 to 12 times with a fork. Place them on a large microwave-safe plate and microwave on high, turning once halfway through, until they are tender and easily fork-pierced all the way to the center, 14 to 20 minutes (microwave power varies widely). Slice the potatoes in half lengthwise and set them aside for about 15 minutes, until they are cool enough to handle.

Meanwhile, in a large pan, heat the olive oil over medium-high heat until hot. Add the ground beef, season evenly with ½ teaspoon of the salt and ¼ teaspoon of the pepper and cook, stirring occasionally, breaking up the meat as you do, until it is nicely browned, 6 to 8 minutes.

Add the frozen vegetables and cook, stirring occasionally, until thawed, about 2 minutes. Stir in the flour and cook for about 1 minute until fully incorporated. Stir in the tomato paste, thyme, and rosemary. Gradually add the beef broth, stirring as you do, until everything is incorporated. Simmer for 2 to 3 minutes to thicken the mixture into a chunky meat sauce. Season with more salt to taste. Set aside.

Once the potatoes are cool enough to handle, carefully scoop the potato flesh into a medium bowl, leaving about a ¼- to ½-inch layer of potato flesh all around the skins so that they remain intact and don't collapse. To the bowl, add the yogurt, 2 tablespoons of the butter, the remaining ½ teaspoon of salt, and the remaining ¼ teaspoon of pepper. Using a potato masher, hand mixer, or wooden spoon, mash the potatoes until they are smooth and creamy.

STEPH'S TIP

Use whatever mix of vegetables you like. I prefer a classic green beans/peas/corn/carrot mix for this.

Continued

Lazy Shepherd's Pie, continued

Preheat the broiler.

Line a sheet pan with aluminum foil (you'll thank yourself when you clean up after!).

Spoon the ground beef mixture (about ½ cup per potato half) evenly into the potato skins. Using your hands, top them evenly with the mashed potatoes (about ½ cup per potato half). Try packing the mashed potato in your hands before pressing it onto the top of each of the potato halves—this helps them stay together better. Place the stuffed-and-topped potatoes onto the sheet pan. Melt the remaining 2 tablespoons of butter and evenly brush it over the mashed potato topping.

Broil until the tops are golden brown, 4 to 6 minutes.

STORAGE + REHEAT

Once cooled, store airtight in the refrigerator for up to 3 days. To reheat, warm in a pan over medium heat until heated through, or heat in a covered baking dish in the oven at 350°F for 10 to 15 minutes.

Sheet-Pan Beef Fajitas

SERVES 4 TO 6
PREP TIME: 20 minutes
COOK TIME: 20 minutes

PER SERVING:	**CALORIES** 421 kcal	**PROTEIN** 25g	**FAT** 22g	**CARBOHYDRATE** 41g	**FIBER** 5g

3 red bell peppers, sliced

1 large red onion, sliced

2 portobello mushrooms, sliced

3 tablespoons avocado oil

2 teaspoons kosher salt, divided

½ teaspoon freshly ground black pepper, divided

1 tablespoon chili powder

1 teaspoon ground cumin

1 teaspoon smoked paprika

1 pound flank steak, sliced with the grain into three equal pieces

Six to twelve 6-inch taco-size flour tortillas

For Serving

¼ cup Jalapeño-Cream Sauce (recipe follows)

1 avocado, sliced

One 15-ounce can black beans (or 1½ cups cooked black beans), drained and rinsed

Chopped fresh cilantro leaves

With my sheet-pan meals, I shoot for the rainbow and try to get as many different colors onto the pan as possible. In general, more color equals more nutrients. These fajitas are super colorful and wonderfully balanced with protein, fiber, and essential nutrients.

I often slice and fridge-store my veggies ahead of time so that I can cook and serve dinner quickly. I also often double this recipe and use the leftovers for salads, grain bowls, and wraps throughout the week.

Preheat the oven to 475°F. Line a sheet pan with parchment paper, a silicone baking mat, or aluminum foil (you'll thank yourself when you clean up after!).

In a large bowl, toss the bell peppers, onion, and mushrooms with the avocado oil, 1½ teaspoons of the salt, and ¼ teaspoon of the pepper. Arrange everything in an even layer on the sheet pan. Roast the veggies until they have softened, about 10 minutes.

Meanwhile, in a small bowl, stir together the chili powder, cumin, smoked paprika, and the remaining ½ teaspoon salt and ¼ teaspoon pepper. Sprinkle the spice mixture evenly over both sides of the steak pieces. Wrap the tortillas in aluminum foil and set aside.

Remove the vegetables from the oven and push them to the sides of the sheet pan, making space in the middle for the steak. Add the steak and return the sheet pan to the oven. Roast until the steak is nicely browned and has reached an internal temperature of 135°F for medium-rare, 8 to 12 minutes.

Remove the pan from the oven and allow the steak and roasted veggies to rest for about 5 minutes.

Meanwhile, warm your tortillas. Place the foil-wrapped tortillas in the still-hot (but turned off) oven to warm for 5 to 10 minutes.

Slice the rested steak against the grain into thin strips. Serve the steak and vegetables with the warm tortillas, jalapeño-cream sauce, avocado, black beans, and cilantro. Assemble according to taste, and enjoy!

YOU DO YOU

To make these fajitas vegetarian or vegan, simply substitute portobello mushrooms, tofu, or tempeh for the steak.

STORAGE + REHEAT

Once cooled, store the meat and veggies airtight in the refrigerator up to 3 days. Store the tortillas, jalapeño-cream sauce, avocado, beans, and cilantro in separate airtight containers in the refrigerator up to 3 days. To reheat, warm the steak and veggies in a pan over medium heat until heated through, or heat in the oven at 350°F for 10 to 15 minutes.

Jalapeño-Cream Sauce

MAKES ABOUT 1¼ CUPS

PER 4 TABLESPOONS: | **CALORIES** 51 kcal | **PROTEIN** 3g | **FAT** 3g | **CARBOHYDRATE** 3g | **FIBER** 0g |

2 jalapeños, halved and seeded (keep the seeds if you want it extra spicy!)

4 garlic cloves, peeled

1 teaspoon avocado oil

1 cup nonfat or low-fat Greek yogurt

2 tablespoons fresh lime juice

⅛ teaspoon kosher salt

If you're making this for the Sheet-Pan Beef Fajitas (page 189), you can roast the jalapeños and garlic along with the other vegetables for the same amount of time.

Preheat the oven to 475°F. Line a small sheet pan with parchment paper, a silicone baking mat, or aluminum foil (you'll thank yourself later when you clean up after!).

Toss the jalapeños and garlic with the avocado oil. Spread on the sheet pan and roast until tender and lightly browned in spots, for about 20 minutes.

In a blender, combine the yogurt, lime juice, roasted jalapeños, roasted garlic, and salt. Blend on low speed, gradually increasing the speed to high, for 2 to 3 minutes until smooth. Use right away or store in an airtight container and refrigerate for up to 3 days.

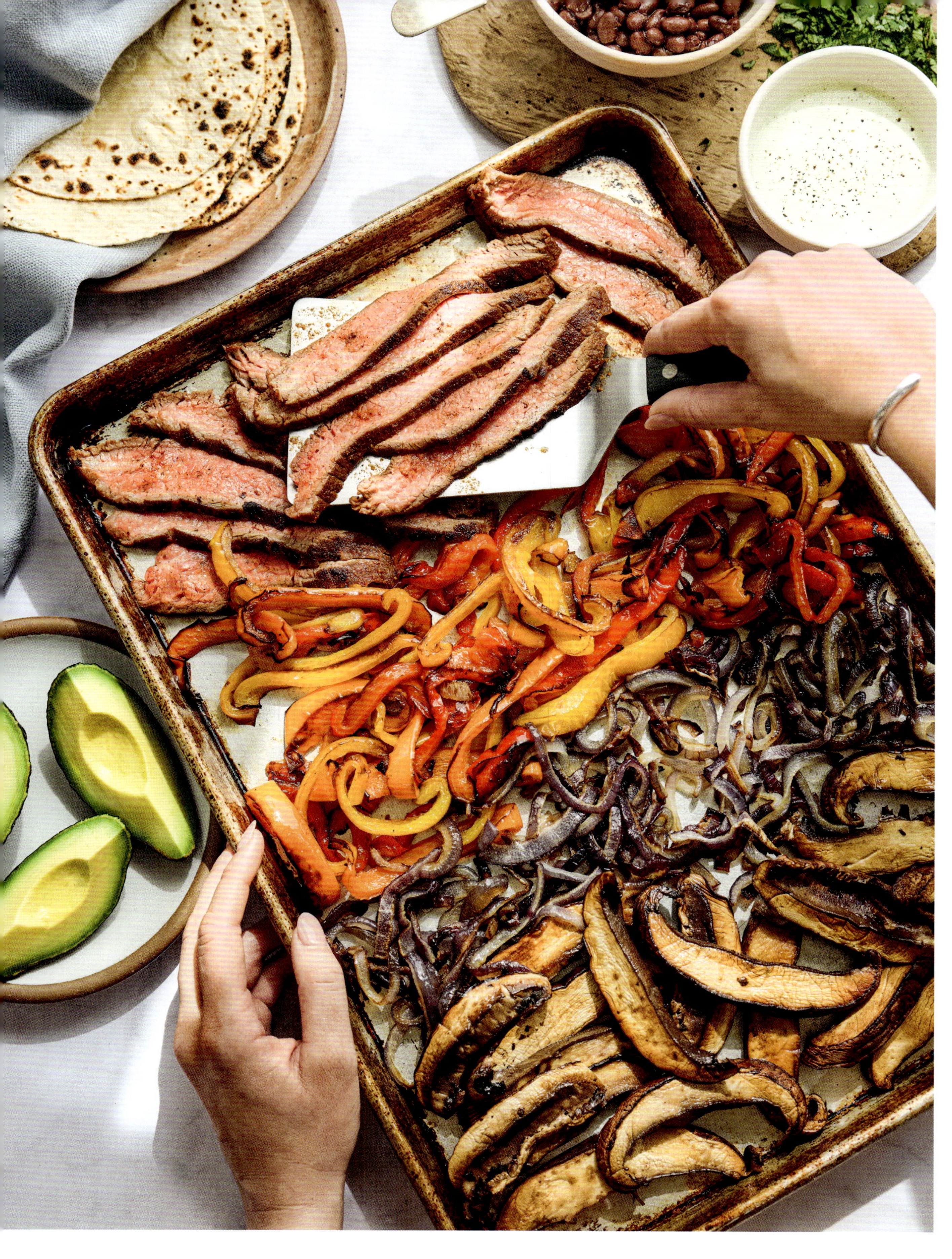

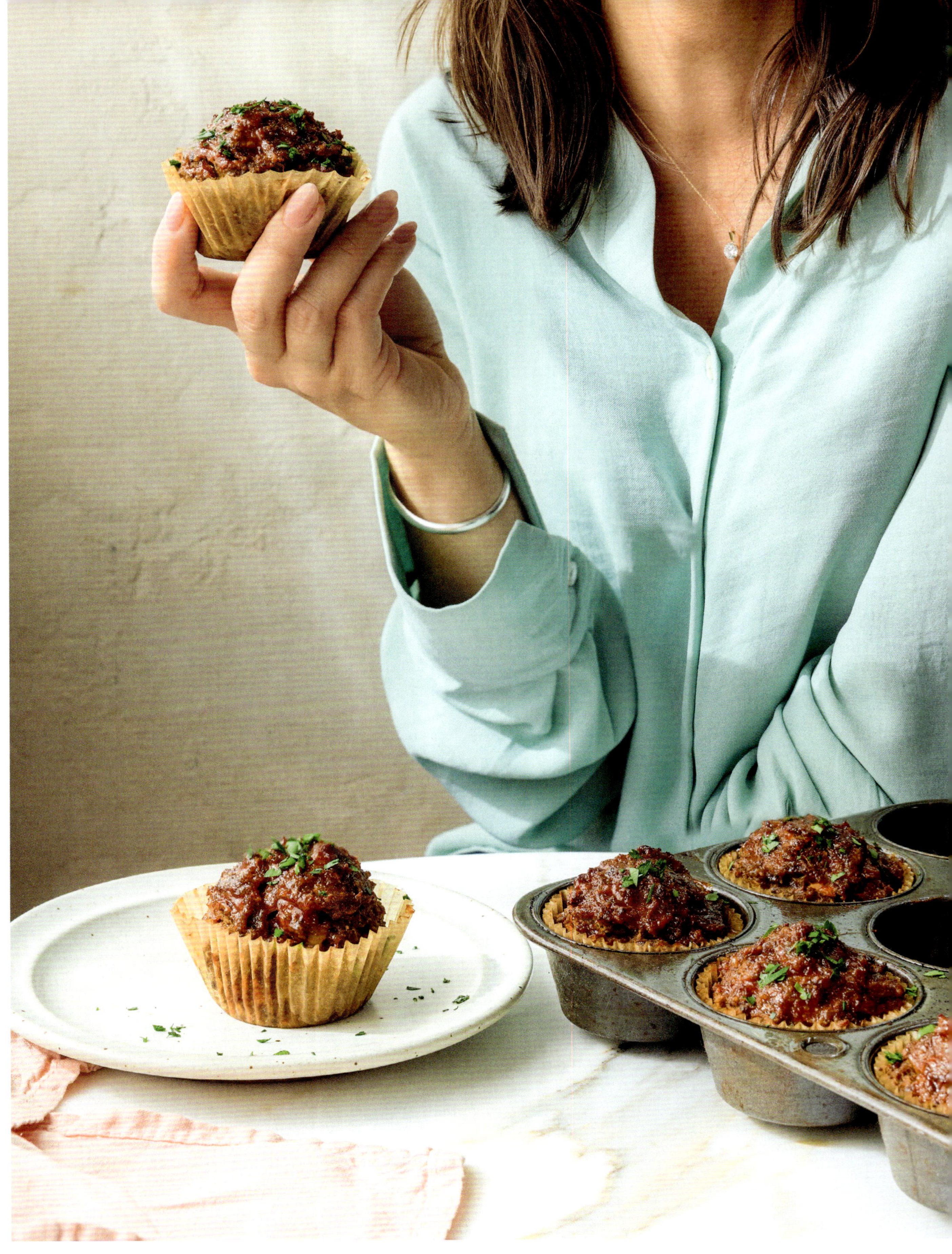

Veggie-Loaded Meatloaf Minis

MAKES 12 MINI MEATLOAVES
SERVES 4 TO 6
PREP TIME: 25 minutes
COOK TIME: 45 minutes

PER SERVING:	CALORIES 381 kcal	PROTEIN 24g	FAT 10g	CARBOHYDRATE 47g	FIBER 4g

1½ pounds sweet potatoes (about 2), cooked (see page 121)

1 pound ground beef (10% to 15% fat)

3 cups (about 10 ounces) finely chopped white or cremini mushrooms

1 cup Italian seasoned bread crumbs

¾ cup ketchup, divided

¼ cup grated Parmesan cheese

1 large egg

3 garlic cloves, minced

3 tablespoons Worcestershire sauce, divided

1½ teaspoons garlic powder

1¼ teaspoons kosher salt

½ teaspoon freshly ground black pepper

Cooking spray or neutral oil, for greasing

2 tablespoons chopped fresh flat-leaf parsley leaves (optional), as garnish

STEPH'S TIP

If you don't have, or can't source, seasoned bread crumbs, simply toss unseasoned dry bread crumbs with ½ teaspoon Italian seasoning plus ¼ teaspoon kosher salt.

I really like making these mini sweet potato- and mushroom-loaded meatloaves. They're so cute and fun baked in a standard muffin tin, and they cook way faster than a traditional hefty meatloaf! They're great for dinner, a quick lunch, or a protein-rich snack. In general, I don't like to eat too much red meat, so these baby meatloaves are just right for me.

It's pretty cool how the veggies truly feel hidden here—the finely chopped mushroom (loaded with potassium and selenium for the win!) and the mashed and blended-in sweet potato both mimic the color and texture of the beef. If you were playing veggie hide-and-seek, you'd never find them! Keep in mind that because of all the tasty and juicy veggies, they can fall apart a bit after baking as you remove them from the muffin tin. If you don't want this to happen, simply use muffin liners. I often do.

Preheat the oven to 350°F.

In a large bowl, using your hands or a spoon, scoop out the cooked sweet potato and discard the skin (or save for another use). Some parts of the potato might be significantly softer than other parts. Using a fork or potato masher, mash the potato until it is fairly smooth.

Add the ground beef, mushrooms, bread crumbs, ¼ cup of the ketchup, the Parmesan, egg, garlic, 1 tablespoon of the Worcestershire sauce, the garlic powder, salt, and pepper. Using your hands (I highly recommend doing this by hand so that you fully incorporate the mashed potato) or a large spoon, mix until well combined.

Lightly spray or oil 12 cups of a standard muffin tin or line with muffin liners. Fill the muffin cups evenly with about ½ cup of meatloaf mixture per cup, pressing down lightly to form them so that they don't fall apart and shaping the tops to look like rounded muffin tops. Transfer the muffin tin to the oven and bake until the meatloaf minis are lightly browned, about 30 minutes.

Meanwhile, in a small bowl, mix together the remaining ½ cup ketchup and remaining 2 tablespoons Worcestershire sauce until fully combined. It will look very similar to a classic red BBQ sauce.

Remove the meatloaf minis from the oven and top each evenly with a scant tablespoon of the ketchup-Worcestershire mix. Return to the oven and bake until the sauce topper has warmed and an instant-read

Continued

thermometer registers at least 160°F in the middle of the mini meatloaves, 5 more minutes. They will likely be close to 200°F.

Set them aside to cool for 5 minutes before carefully removing them from the muffin tin. If you are not using muffin liners, use a small rubber spatula, or table knife, along with a small spoon to carefully scoop them out. Garnish with chopped fresh parsley (if using) and serve.

STORAGE + REHEAT

Once cooled, store airtight in the refrigerator for up to 3 days. To reheat, warm in a pan over medium heat until heated through, or microwave. For best results, garnish with the parsley right before serving.

SIMPATICA

If you like cooking these meatloaf minis, I highly recommend my baked Eggy Quinoa Cups (page 61), which you also bake in a muffin tin. Long live the muffin tin!

Spaghetti Oh-Ohs *with* Mini Meatballs

SERVES 4 TO 6
PREP TIME: 20 minutes
COOK TIME: 1 hour

PER SERVING:	CALORIES 507 kcal	PROTEIN 28g	FAT 28g	CARBOHYDRATE 39g	FIBER 4g

Meatballs

½ cup Italian seasoned bread crumbs

⅓ cup milk (dairy or nondairy)

1 pound lean ground beef (10% fat or less)

½ small yellow onion, finely minced (about 1 scant cup)

1 large egg

1 teaspoon kosher salt

½ teaspoon freshly ground black pepper

Sauce & Pasta

½ small yellow onion, sliced

2 large red bell peppers, stemmed, seeded, and quartered

3 tablespoons extra-virgin olive oil, divided

1 teaspoon kosher salt, divided

¼ teaspoon freshly ground black pepper

4 cups chicken broth, divided, plus more broth or water as needed

¼ cup tomato paste

1 teaspoon dried oregano

1 teaspoon Italian seasoning

½ cup heavy cream

2 cups ditalini pasta or another small pasta

¼ cup grated Parmesan cheese, plus more for serving

1 tablespoon sugar (optional), for a classic SpaghettiOs sweetness

One of my favorite after-school snacks in elementary school was SpaghettiOs with meatballs. For my *Crave, Cook, Nourish* version, I took all the canned favorite's smooth and velvety textures, sweet tomato flavors, and pasta goodness, and infused them with bright, fresh nutrition. You get protein (meatballs), carbohydrates (pasta), and vegetables (roasted red peppers and onions) for a well-rounded, satisfying meal. Pair it with a side salad, and you get even more fiber and nutrients.

This is another great hidden veggie dish, like my Veggie-Loaded Meatloaf Minis (page 193) and Hidden Veggie Smoothies (page 83). Feel free to add carrots or yellow squash to the roasting pan as well. They have the same level of sweetness, and you'll keep that orange-red classic color. I always add the tablespoon of sugar at the end because it gets to that nostalgic taste for me.

Preheat the oven to 400°F. Line two sheet pans with parchment paper, a silicone baking mat, or aluminum foil (you'll thank yourself when you clean up after!).

Make the meatballs: In a small bowl, stir together the bread crumbs and milk until fully incorporated. In a large bowl, stir together the ground beef, soaked bread crumbs, minced onion, egg, salt, and pepper. I like to do this mixing by hand (clean hands!) and then move directly into hand forming the meatballs. Form the beef mixture into small meatballs (roughly 1 heaping tablespoon of mixture; about 25 meatballs) and place them on one of the prepared sheet pans.

Prepare the sauce: On the second sheet pan, arrange the sliced onion and bell peppers. Drizzle with 2 tablespoons of the olive oil, season with ½ teaspoon of the salt, and the pepper, and toss with tongs to coat.

Roast the meatballs and the veggies at the same time. Roast the meatballs until cooked through, with a slight tinge of pinkness, and not overdone (slice one to check), 12 to 14 minutes. Set aside. Roast the veggies for 25 to 30 minutes, flipping about halfway through (when you remove the meatballs from the oven!), until fairly tender. Set aside to cool for about 5 minutes.

Transfer the roasted veggies to a blender or food processor and add ½ cup of the broth. Blend, starting at low and slowly increasing to high, for 2 to 3 minutes until smooth. Set aside.

Continued

Spaghetti Oh-Ohs with Mini Meatballs, continued

In your largest pan or Dutch oven (at least 10-cup capacity), heat the remaining 1 tablespoon olive oil over medium heat. Stir in tomato paste, oregano, and Italian seasoning. Cook for 1 minute, breaking up the tomato paste a bit, until fragrant. Add the remaining 3½ cups broth, the heavy cream, blended roasted veggie sauce, and the remaining ½ teaspoon salt. Stir well to combine.

Add the pasta to the sauce, increase the heat to medium-high, and bring it to a gentle simmer while stirring. Cook uncovered, stirring regularly so that the pasta doesn't stick together or to the bottom of the pan, until the pasta is al dente, 12 to 16 minutes.

Add the baked meatballs, Parmesan, and sugar (if using) and cook until the pasta is tender and the meatballs are warmed through, 2 to 3 more minutes.

Serve warm with additional Parmesan, if desired.

STEPH'S TIPS

If you don't have, or can't source, seasoned bread crumbs, simply toss unseasoned dry bread crumbs with ¼ teaspoon Italian seasoning plus ⅛ teaspoon kosher salt.

Depending on who you're cooking for—littles, bigs, or both—you can use pasta rings (just like SpaghettiOs!), alphabet pasta, animal-shaped pasta, macaroni, orecchiette (means "little ears"), or whatever you'd like, in place of the ditalini.

STORAGE + REHEAT

Once cooled, store airtight in the refrigerator for up to 3 days. To reheat, warm in a pan over medium heat until heated through, or microwave.

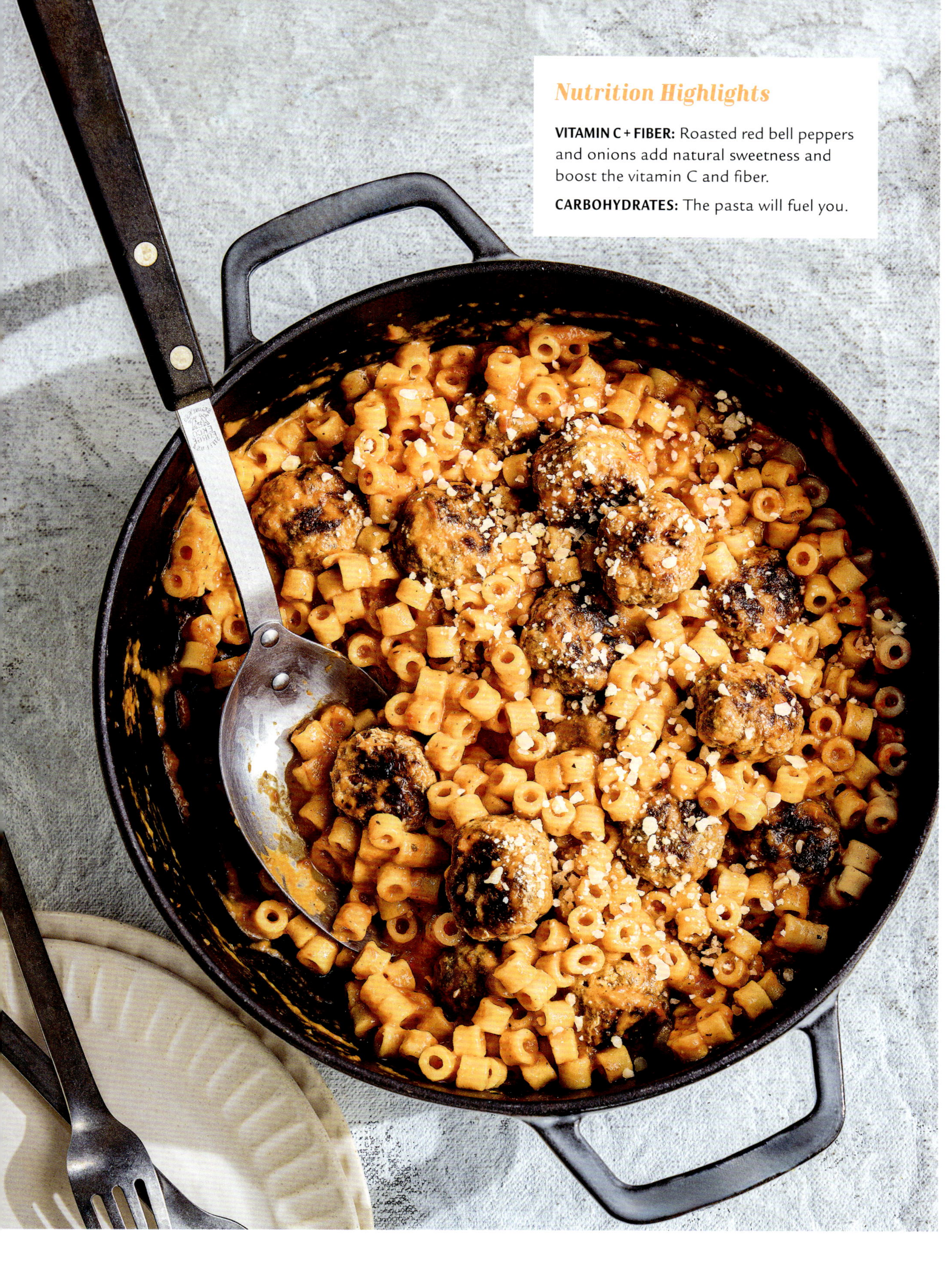

Nutrition Highlights

VITAMIN C + FIBER: Roasted red bell peppers and onions add natural sweetness and boost the vitamin C and fiber.

CARBOHYDRATES: The pasta will fuel you.

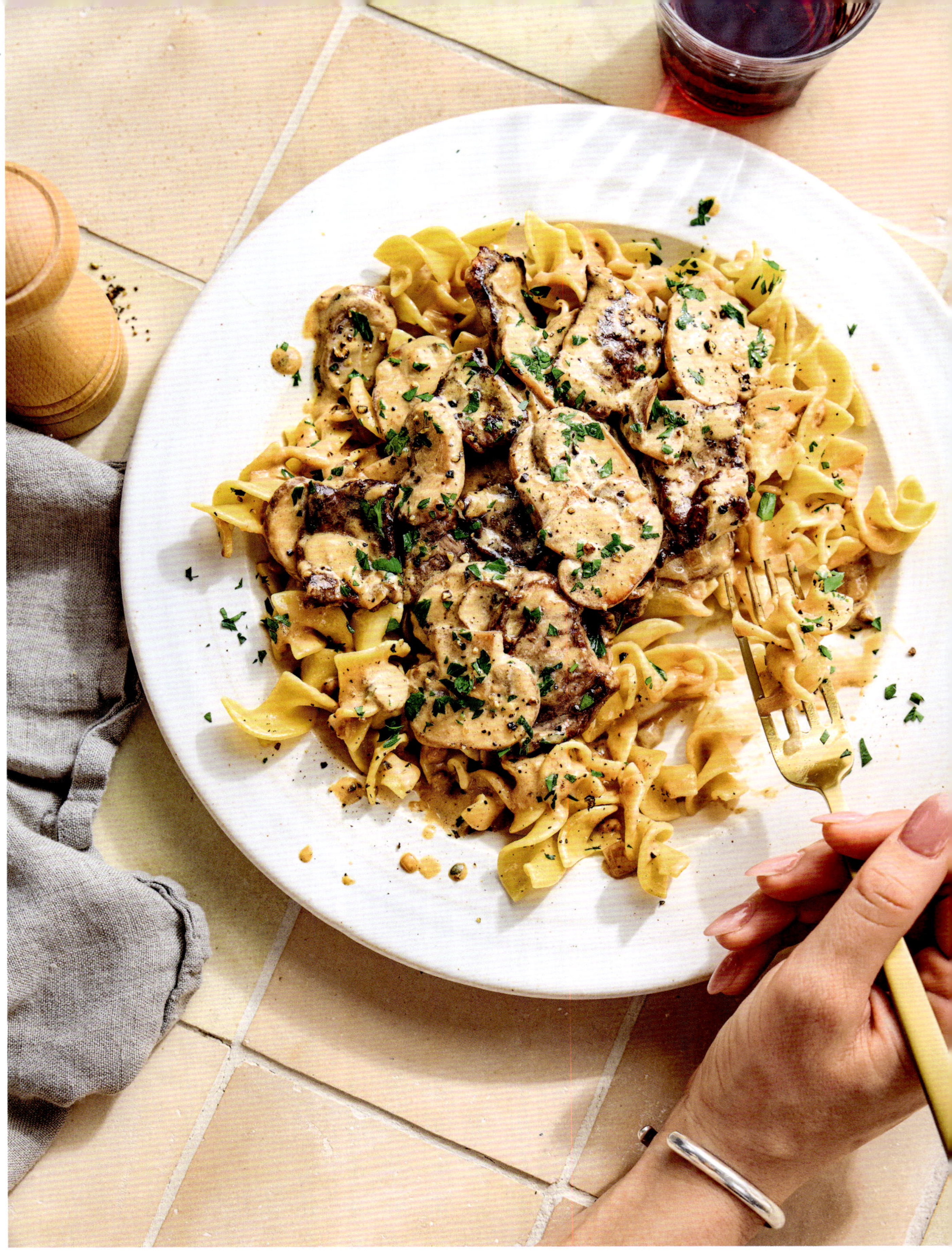

Beef Stroganoff

SERVES 4
PREP TIME: 10 minutes
COOK TIME: 30 minutes

PER SERVING:	**CALORIES** 535 kcal	**PROTEIN** 31g	**FAT** 25g	**CARBOHYDRATE** 36g	**FIBER** 3g

½ teaspoon kosher salt, plus more for boiling the noodles

3 cups egg noodles

1 pound lean beef sirloin

⅛ teaspoon freshly ground black pepper

1 tablespoon cornstarch or flour, plus more for thickening if desired

2 tablespoons extra-virgin olive oil, divided

1 small white onion, finely chopped

4 cups sliced white or cremini mushrooms (or 8-ounce package sliced mushrooms)

1½ cups beef broth

2 teaspoons Dijon mustard

2 teaspoons Worcestershire sauce

½ teaspoon dried thyme

½ cup whole-milk or 2% Greek yogurt

½ cup heavy cream

Chopped fresh parsley leaves (optional), for garnish

Beef stroganoff was another family favorite in my house growing up. It was such a treat when my mom made it. My version has all the classic components including that rich, creamy sauce. I lighten it up a bit, but no flavor is sacrificed!

Bring a large pot of lightly salted water to a boil over high heat. Add the egg noodles and cook to your desired firmness, 6 to 8 minutes. Drain and set aside.

Meanwhile, slice the sirloin against the grain into pieces roughly 2 inches long and ¼ to ½ inch thick. In a medium bowl, season the beef with ½ teaspoon of the salt and the pepper, then sprinkle on the cornstarch and toss to coat.

In a large pan, heat 1 tablespoon of the olive oil over medium-high heat until hot. Add the beef and cook, stirring occasionally, until lightly browned but not fully cooked, 3 to 4 minutes. Transfer to a bowl (with the juices!) and set aside.

In the same pan (no need to wipe it off or wash it), add the remaining 1 tablespoon olive oil, the onion, and mushrooms and cook over medium-high heat until they begin to soften, about 5 minutes. Stir in the beef broth, mustard, Worcestershire sauce, and thyme. Bring to a boil, then decrease the heat to low and simmer for about 5 minutes for the sauce to come together.

Remove the pan from the heat and let it cool for 5 minutes. In a small bowl, stir together the yogurt and heavy cream. Add that mixture to the pan and whisk to combine. If desired, sprinkle in an additional 1 tablespoon cornstarch to thicken and thoroughly whisk out any clumps.

Return the pan to medium-low heat and stir in the beef and its juices. Simmer for about 5 minutes, until the sauce has thickened to your desired consistency. I like my sauce to be like a light gravy, the longer you cook it, the thicker it gets.

Enjoy the beef stroganoff right away on a plate or in a bowl over the cooked egg noodles garnished with fresh parsley, if desired.

STORAGE + REHEAT

Once cooled, store the noodles and stroganoff in separate airtight containers for up to 3 days. To reheat, gently warm both in a pan over medium-low heat until heated through, or microwave. Add a little water or broth if needed.

Hearty Beef & Bean Chili

SERVES 8
PREP TIME: 10 minutes
COOK TIME: 1 hour 30 minutes

PER SERVING:	**CALORIES** 643 kcal	**PROTEIN** 45g	**FAT** 36g	**CARBOHYDRATE** 38g	**FIBER** 9g

2 tablespoons extra-virgin olive oil, divided

1 large white onion, diced

1 red bell pepper, diced

¼ cup chili powder

2 tablespoons smoked paprika

2 tablespoons ground cumin

1 teaspoon garlic powder

1 teaspoon dried oregano

4 cups beef broth (or preferred broth)

One 28-ounce can crushed tomatoes, undrained

½ cup freshly brewed coffee

One 6-ounce can tomato paste

1 tablespoon brown sugar

¼ ounce unsweetened chocolate, chopped

2 teaspoons kosher salt, plus more to taste

2½ pounds lean ground beef (10% fat or less)

Four 15-ounce cans red kidney beans (or 6 cups cooked red kidney beans), drained and rinsed

2 cups sour cream

2 cups grated cheese (whatever cheese you prefer)

4 green onions (white and green parts), thinly sliced

This recipe is largely based on my fiancé's, Miles's, dad's recipe. His dad, Chris, is a fantastic cook, and this rich, well-spiced chili—that gets almost velvety from the mid-simmer blending—is a favorite. It's the best chili I've ever had. The secret ingredients: coffee and unsweetened baking chocolate. Both are great for you. Coffee contains polyphenols, and chocolate is loaded with magnesium and antioxidants.

In a large pot, heat 1 tablespoon of the olive oil over medium heat until hot. Add the onion and bell pepper and cook, stirring occasionally, until they have softened, about 5 minutes. Stir in the chili powder, smoked paprika, cumin, garlic powder, and oregano and cook until fragrant, 1 minute.

Add the broth, crushed tomatoes, coffee, tomato paste, brown sugar, chocolate, and salt and stir to combine. Simmer uncovered, stirring occasionally, until the chili has slightly reduced, about 45 minutes.

Remove the pot from heat. Use an immersion blender (or countertop blender) to blend until fairly smooth, 1 to 2 minutes.

In a large pan (🍲), heat the remaining 1 tablespoon olive oil over medium-high heat until hot. Add the ground beef and cook, stirring occasionally, breaking up the meat as you do, until it is nicely browned, 8 to 10 minutes. Drain and discard any excess fat.

Add the kidney beans and browned ground beef to the chili pot, stir to combine, and return to medium heat to bring to a boil. Decrease the heat to low and simmer uncovered, stirring occasionally, until everything is tender, about 30 minutes. Season with additional salt to taste.

Portion into bowls and serve! Top each serving of chili with ¼ cup sour cream, ¼ cup grated cheese, and 1 to 2 tablespoons sliced green onions.

STEPH'S TIP

You may need to brown the ground beef in batches to avoid overcrowding. If you do, simply divide the olive oil.

STORAGE + REHEAT

Once cooled, store airtight in the refrigerator for up to 4 days, or in the freezer for up to 3 months. To reheat, gently warm in a pot over medium-low heat until heated through, or microwave.

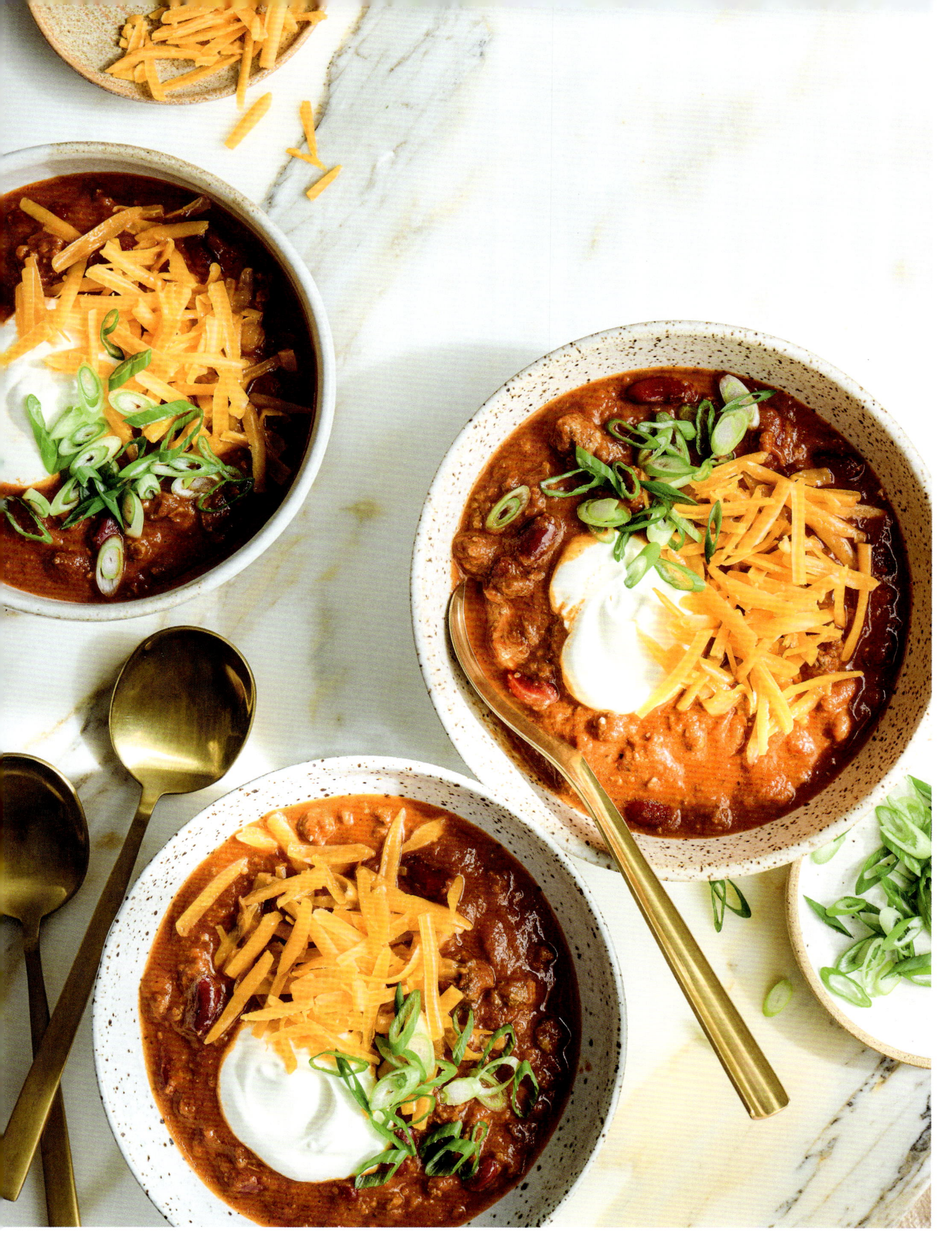

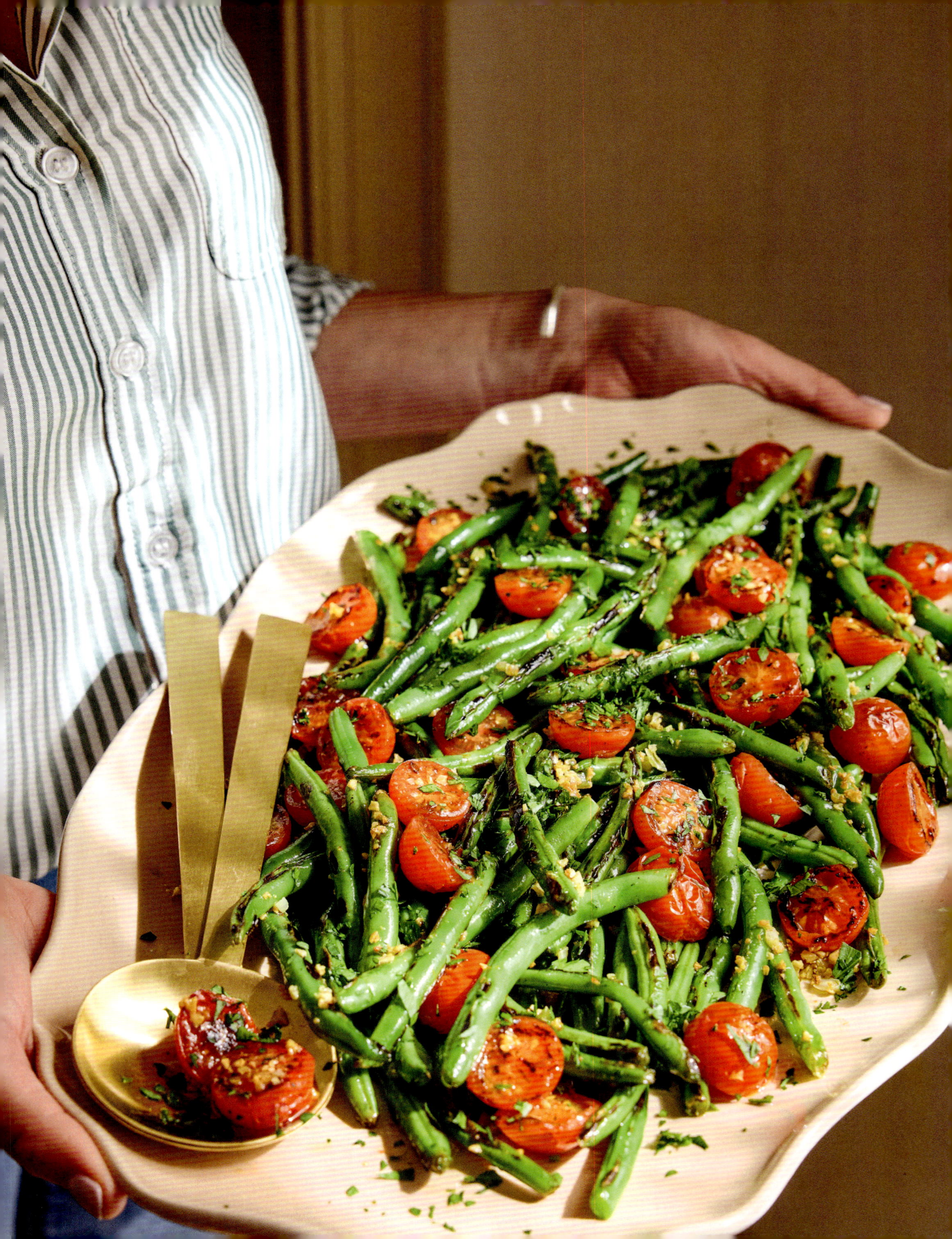

Nutrition-Boosting Sides

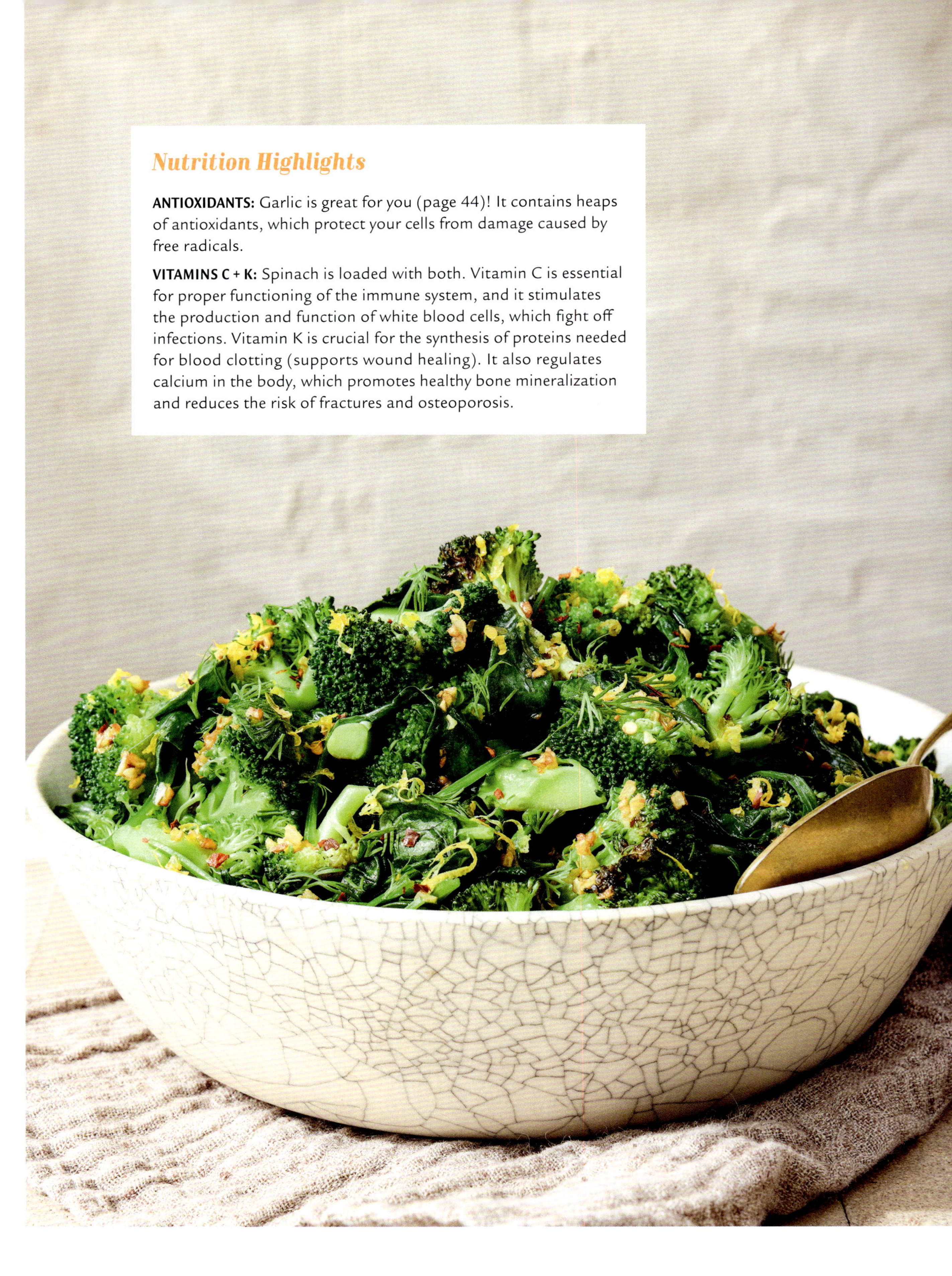

Nutrition Highlights

ANTIOXIDANTS: Garlic is great for you (page 44)! It contains heaps of antioxidants, which protect your cells from damage caused by free radicals.

VITAMINS C + K: Spinach is loaded with both. Vitamin C is essential for proper functioning of the immune system, and it stimulates the production and function of white blood cells, which fight off infections. Vitamin K is crucial for the synthesis of proteins needed for blood clotting (supports wound healing). It also regulates calcium in the body, which promotes healthy bone mineralization and reduces the risk of fractures and osteoporosis.

Zesty Spinach & Broccoli

SERVES 4
PREP TIME: 5 minutes
COOK TIME: 6 minutes

PER SERVING:	**CALORIES** 142 kcal	**PROTEIN** 5g	**FAT** 11g	**CARBOHYDRATE** 10g	**FIBER** 4g

3 tablespoons extra-virgin olive oil

4 garlic cloves, minced

1 pound baby spinach

3 cups 1-inch pieces broccoli (about 1 small head, 8 ounces)

½ teaspoon kosher salt

½ teaspoon red pepper flakes

1 tablespoon finely grated lemon zest (about ½ small lemon)

1 tablespoon fresh lemon juice (about ½ small lemon)

1 tablespoon fresh dill, finely chopped

When I was little, I was not a fan of spinach and other greens. It wasn't until my mom tuned me into Popeye (the old-school cartoon sailor who got all his strength from canned spinach), and his obsession with spinach, that I changed my tune. I imagined how much stronger it would make me (just like Popeye!), and my taste buds caught up. I've adored all greens ever since.

My biggest piece of advice: Don't overcook the spinach and broccoli! You want both to stay bright green, which equals nutrients, and go for just-tender, no mush. Prep everything in advance, so that your ingredients are ready and waiting. It goes fast.

In a large pan, heat the olive oil over medium heat until hot. Add the garlic and sauté until it is golden and fragrant, about 2 minutes. Stir in the spinach and broccoli and cook until both are coated in oil and garlic and the spinach is slightly wilted, 2 to 3 minutes. The pan will be very full! Use tongs or a heatproof spatula to carefully turn and nudge the spinach and broccoli and move them around the pan until it all fits.

Cover the pan for about 1 minute, to steam the spinach and broccoli. Uncover and stir. Once the spinach has completely wilted, remove the pan from the heat. Add the salt, pepper flakes, lemon zest, lemon juice, and dill and stir to fully incorporate. Serve immediately. This dish is best enjoyed day of.

NUTRITION PSA

For a fiber boost, add 1 tablespoon of chia seeds or flaxseeds after cooking!

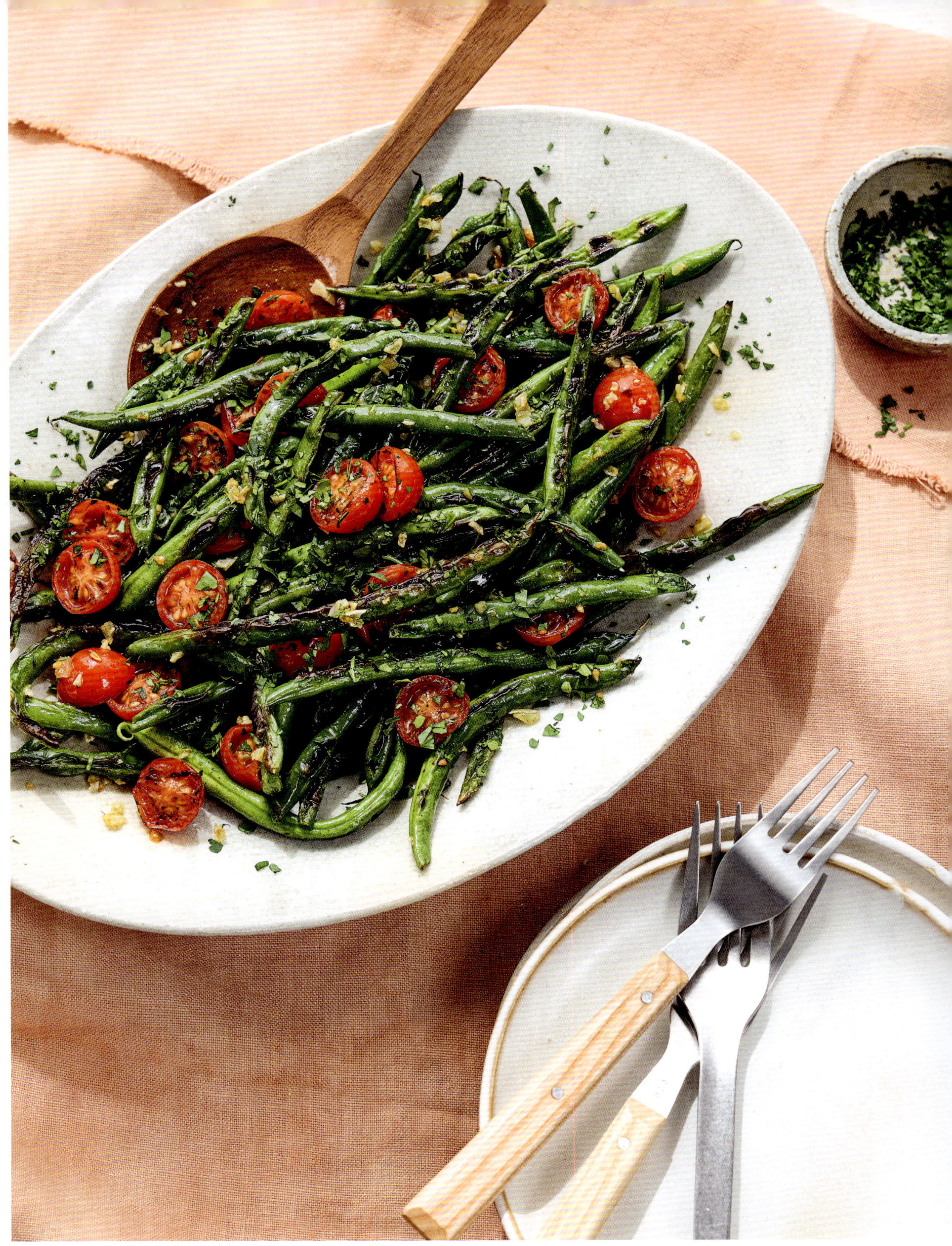

Garlicky Blistered Green Beans & Cherry Tomatoes

SERVES 2 TO 4
PREP TIME: 5 minutes
COOK TIME: 10 minutes

PER SERVING:	CALORIES 116 kcal	PROTEIN 3g	FAT 5g	CARBOHYDRATE 17g	FIBER 5g

1 pound green beans, trimmed

1 tablespoon extra-virgin olive oil

½ teaspoon kosher salt, divided

1 pint cherry tomatoes, halved

5 garlic cloves, minced

¼ cup plus 1 tablespoon finely chopped fresh parsley leaves, divided

You can thank my fiancé, Miles, for this weeknight dinner recipe favorite. We usually pair it with some sort of protein like grilled fish or roasted chicken—it's great with the Crispy Roasted Chicken Thighs with Buttery Hot Sauce (page 176). I really like how colorful it is and the olive oil-coated sweet blistered tomatoes are a treat.

Growing up, my family rarely ate green beans, but as a dietitian I fell hard for them. I love the texture and flavor!

Bring water to a boil in a steamer pot, allowing at least 2 inches between the water and where the steamer basket will be. Evenly spread the green beans in the steamer basket. Once the water is boiling, with oven mitts or a kitchen towel, carefully place the steamer basket on or in the pot. Cover and steam until the green beans are bright green and crisp-tender, 3 to 4 minutes. Remove from the heat.

In a large pan, heat the olive oil over medium-high heat until hot. Add the green beans and ¼ teaspoon of the salt. Cook, shaking the pan and flipping the beans occasionally, until the beans have slightly blistered and softened, about 3 minutes.

Add the tomatoes and the remaining ¼ teaspoon salt. Toss everything together and continue cooking until the beans are nicely blistered and the tomatoes are warmed through and just starting to break up a bit, about 3 minutes.

Decrease the heat to low and add the garlic. Cook everything stirring frequently to avoid burning, for about 1 minute, until fragrant. Stir in ¼ cup of the parsley. Remove from the heat, serve warm garnished with the remaining 1 tablespoon of parsley, and enjoy!

STORAGE + REHEAT

Once cooled, store airtight in the refrigerator for up to 4 days. To reheat, warm in a pan over medium heat until heated through, or microwave.

Sheet-Pan Honey-Glazed Carrots & Parsnips

SERVES 4
PREP TIME: 10 minutes
COOK TIME: 25 minutes

PER SERVING:	**CALORIES** 299 kcal	**PROTEIN** 2g	**FAT** 15g	**CARBOHYDRATE** 42g	**FIBER** 5g

1 pound carrots, peeled and cut on the bias into ¼-inch-thick slices

1 pound parsnips, peeled and cut on the bias into ¼-inch-thick slices

5 tablespoons (2½ ounces) unsalted butter

4 garlic cloves, minced

1 tablespoon minced fresh rosemary, plus more for garnish

3 tablespoons honey

½ teaspoon kosher salt, plus more to taste

⅛ teaspoon freshly ground black pepper, plus more to taste

It took me a bit to come around to parsnips and their slightly sweet and earthy flavor, but I sure do love them now. My favorite way to cook them is to roast them in a honey glaze with carrots, rosemary, and garlic. Roasting brings out the natural sweetness of both root veggies, and I love how crispy and browned they become on the outside while the insides get steamy and tender. Your kitchen and home will smell amazing before (while preparing the glaze) and after you roast this dish.

Carrots and parsnips have a lot in common nutritionally. They're both loaded with vitamin C (antioxidant support), vitamin K (crucial for blood clotting and bone health), potassium (blood pressure regulation), and fiber. Carrots are also known for their high levels of vitamin A thanks to the beta-carotene, which is key for eye health and immunity.

Preheat the oven to 425°F. Line a sheet pan with parchment paper, a silicone baking mat, or aluminum foil (you'll thank yourself when you clean up after!).

In a large bowl, combine the carrots and parsnips.

In a large nonstick pan, melt the butter over medium-low heat. Add the garlic and rosemary and cook, stirring frequently until the garlic is golden and fragrant, about 2 minutes. Remove the pan from the heat and stir in the honey until well combined.

Pour the honey-butter mixture over the carrots and parsnips. Season with the salt and pepper and toss until well coated. Transfer the veggies to the sheet pan and spread them in an even layer.

Roast for 10 minutes. Remove the sheet pan from the oven and flip, toss, and move the carrots and parsnips around in the pan. Continue to roast until they are tender and just starting to brown, about 10 minutes. For more caramelization, broil on high for the last 3 to 4 minutes.

Remove the sheet pan from the oven, season with additional salt and pepper to taste, garnish with additional fresh rosemary, and serve.

STORAGE + REHEAT

Once cooled, store airtight in the refrigerator for up to 4 days. To reheat, warm in a pan over medium heat until heated through, or microwave.

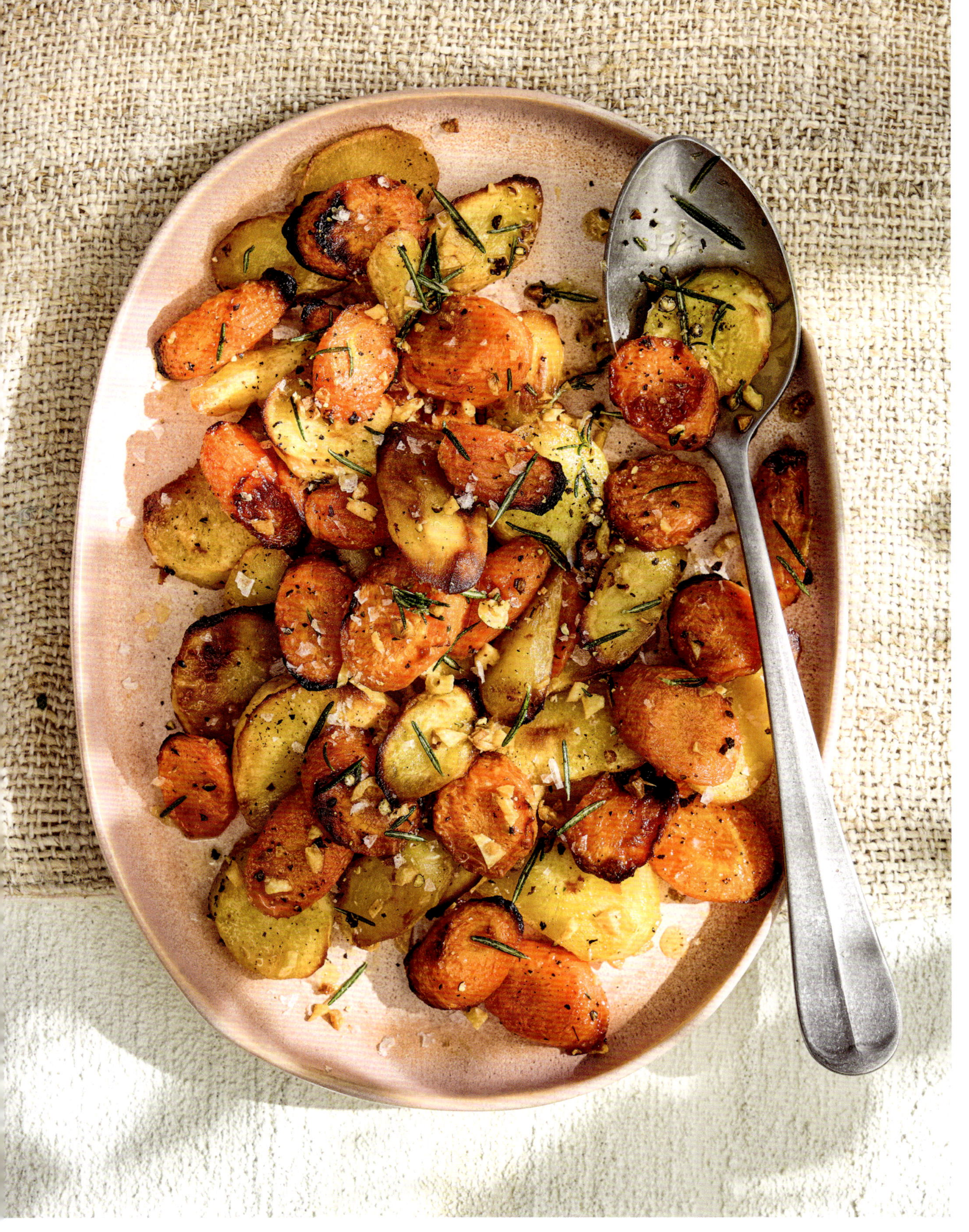

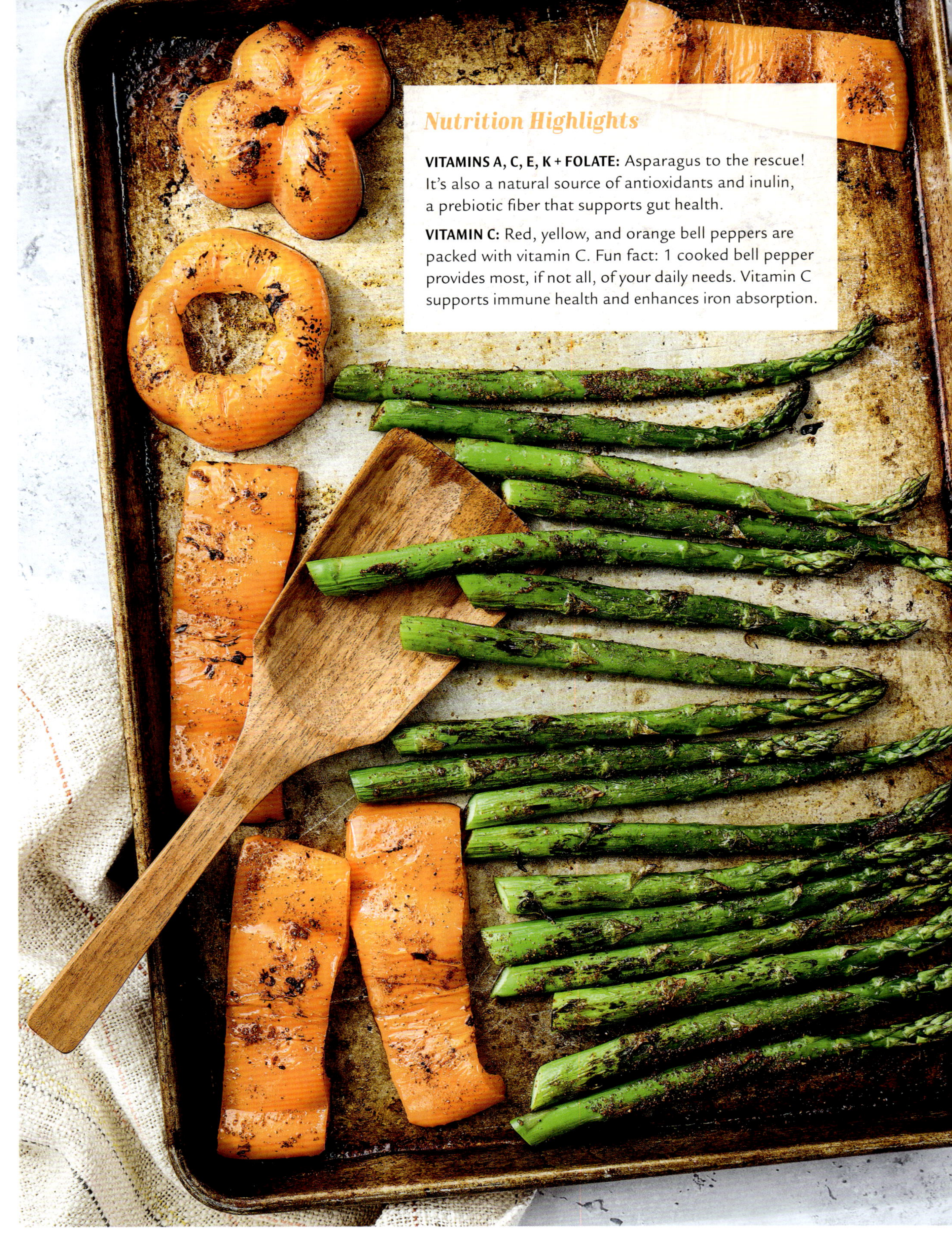

Nutrition Highlights

VITAMINS A, C, E, K + FOLATE: Asparagus to the rescue! It's also a natural source of antioxidants and inulin, a prebiotic fiber that supports gut health.

VITAMIN C: Red, yellow, and orange bell peppers are packed with vitamin C. Fun fact: 1 cooked bell pepper provides most, if not all, of your daily needs. Vitamin C supports immune health and enhances iron absorption.

Sheet-Pan Asparagus & Bell Peppers

SERVES 4
PREP TIME: 5 minutes
COOK TIME: 15 minutes

PER SERVING:	CALORIES 102 kcal	PROTEIN 6g	FAT 6g	CARBOHYDRATE 10g	FIBER 3g

1 bunch of asparagus (about 1 pound), trimmed

2 bell peppers (red, yellow, or orange), sliced into four parts (top, bottom, and two halves), stems and seeds removed

1 tablespoon extra-virgin olive oil

1 teaspoon garlic powder

½ teaspoon smoked paprika

¼ teaspoon kosher salt

¼ teaspoon freshly ground black pepper

¼ to ⅓ cup grated Parmesan cheese, for garnish

When I want to add some vibrant, fresh veggies to my plate, this sheet-pan asparagus and bell pepper dish always delivers. It practically cooks itself while I work on the main course, which for me is often Veggie-Loaded Meatloaf Minis (page 193) or Beef Stroganoff (page 199). To prep the bell peppers, I start by cutting a small circle around the stem and then pull out the stem and seeds. Then I slice off the top, the bottom, and finally I halve the main body and flatten the halves. This keeps all four pieces of each pepper fairly flat for roasting and broiling, so that they cook evenly.

Place an oven rack 6 to 8 inches below the broiler and another rack in the middle. Preheat the oven to 425°F. Line a sheet pan with aluminum foil (you'll thank yourself when you clean up after!).

Place the asparagus and bell peppers on the prepared baking sheet. Drizzle with the olive oil and evenly sprinkle with the garlic powder, smoked paprika, salt, and pepper. Toss with tongs and spread everything in a single layer.

Roast on the middle rack for 12 to 14 minutes, flipping the vegetables about halfway through, until they are crisp-tender. Remove from the oven and turn the broiler to high. Broil on the upper rack for about 3 minutes, until the vegetables are slightly charred.

Remove from the oven and sprinkle evenly with the Parmesan, depending on how cheesy you'd like them.

STORAGE + REHEAT

Once cooled, store airtight in the refrigerator for up to 2 days. Reheat in the oven or stovetop in a pan to retain the best texture.

Sheet-Pan Smashed Brussels Sprouts

SERVES 2 TO 4
PREP TIME: 5 minutes
COOK TIME: 20 minutes

PER SERVING:	**CALORIES** 148 kcal	**PROTEIN** 6g	**FAT** 7g	**CARBOHYDRATE** 15g	**FIBER** 3g

One 12-ounce bag frozen Brussels sprouts (do not thaw!)

1 tablespoon extra-virgin olive oil

½ teaspoon garlic powder

½ teaspoon sweet paprika

¼ teaspoon kosher salt

¼ cup grated Parmesan cheese

1 to 2 tablespoons Balsamic Glaze, homemade (page 172) or store-bought

I'm regularly asked for ways to prepare frozen veggies, since they are easy to store, affordable, and a quick way to add color and nutrition to a plate. This technique—preheat a sheet pan, add the frozen veg to the pan when it's ripping hot, and then roast—is foolproof for most frozen veggies.

Think of these Brussels sprouts as a bit like a roasted and then smashed potato. They get nice and crispy thanks to the roasting and the Parm, but they're softer than most roasted-from-fresh veggies.

Place an oven rack 6 to 8 inches below the broiler and another rack in the middle. Preheat the oven to 400°F. Place a sheet pan on the upper rack in the oven to heat while you prepare the Brussels sprouts. You want to heat up the sheet pan, so that when you put the sprouts on it they sear and sizzle.

In a large bowl, toss the frozen Brussels sprouts with the olive oil, garlic powder, paprika, and salt. Once the oven has preheated, remove the hot sheet pan. Carefully (it will be hot) place the Brussels sprouts on it evenly in a single layer.

Roast on the middle rack until cooked through, 10 minutes.

Remove the Brussels sprouts from the oven. Using a canning jar or a sturdy cup and an oven mitt (be careful not to burn yourself!), carefully smash each sprout flat. Sprinkle them evenly with the Parmesan. It's okay if some of the cheese falls onto the pan, just scrape up the crispy lacy Parm at the end and serve it over the sprouts. Make sure that there is a bit of space between the sprouts (so that they brown properly) before returning them to the oven.

Bake on the middle rack until the cheese has melted and the sprouts have started to brown, 10 minutes longer. Turn on the broiler to high, move the sheet pan to the upper rack, and broil until crispy and golden brown, 2 to 3 minutes.

Remove from the oven, transfer to a serving dish, and drizzle with balsamic glaze. I like to use the full 2 tablespoons, but that may be too sweet for some. Serve immediately.

STORAGE + REHEAT

Once cooled, store airtight in the refrigerator for up to 3 days. To reheat, warm in a pan over medium heat until heated through, or heat in the oven at 350°F for 5 to 10 minutes until warmed through and crispy. Do not microwave, because they will end up quite soggy.

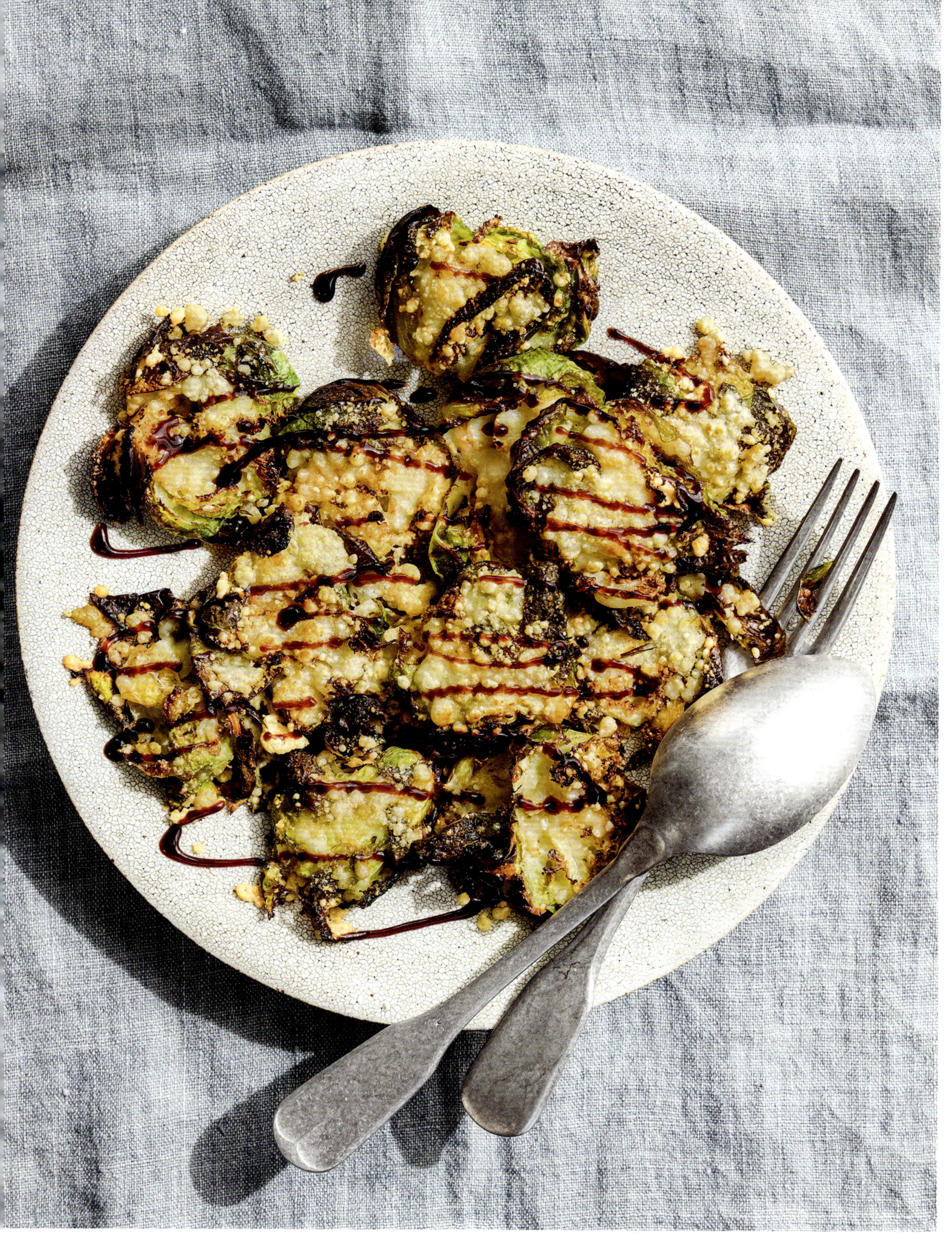

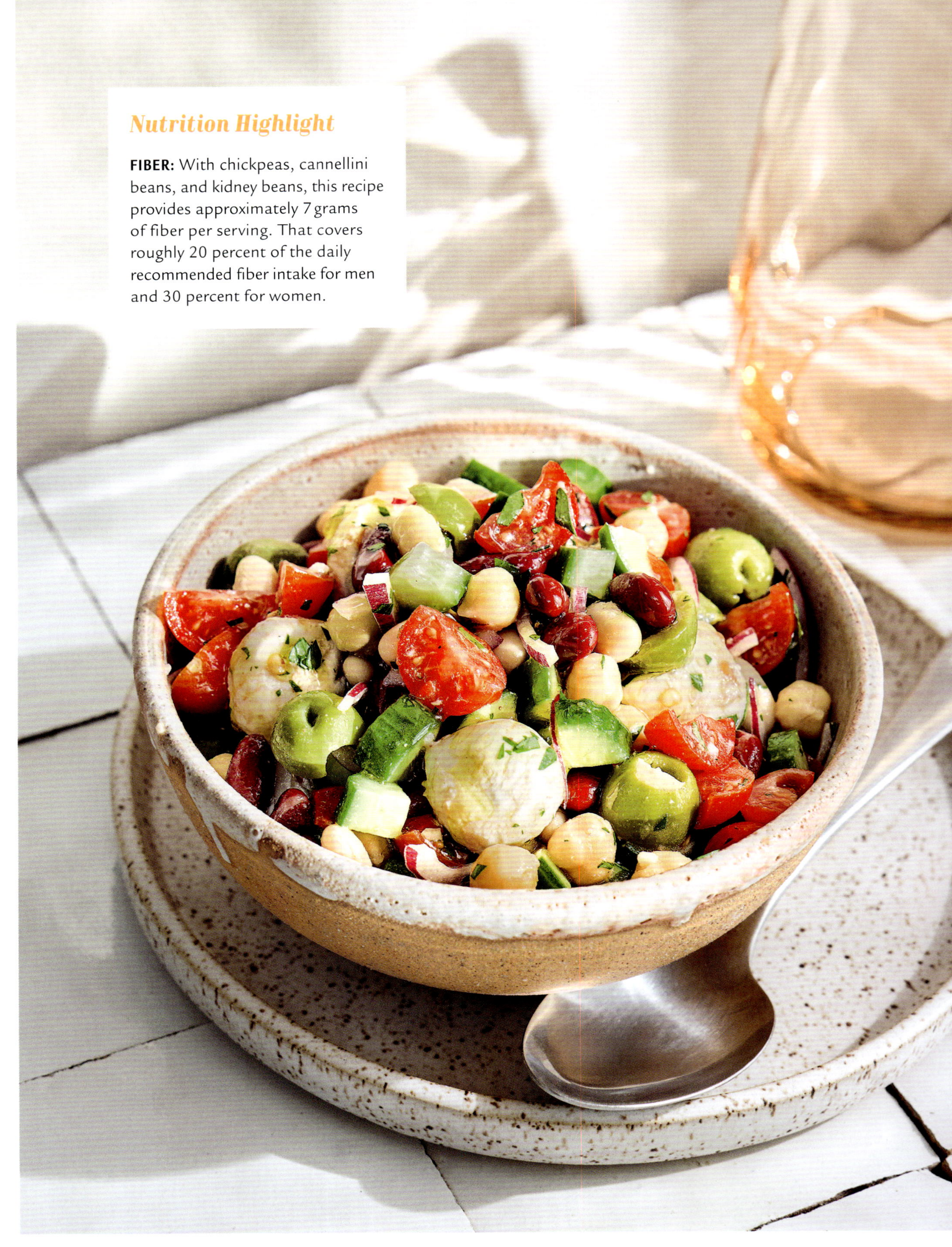

Nutrition Highlight

FIBER: With chickpeas, cannellini beans, and kidney beans, this recipe provides approximately 7 grams of fiber per serving. That covers roughly 20 percent of the daily recommended fiber intake for men and 30 percent for women.

Three-Bean Salad *with* Fresh Mozzarella & Olives

SERVES 6 TO 8
PREP TIME: 15 minutes

PER SERVING SALAD:	**CALORIES** 198 kcal	**PROTEIN** 12g	**FAT** 5g	**CARBOHYDRATE** 26g	**FIBER** 7g
VINAIGRETTE (PER 2 TBSP):	**CALORIES** 75 kcal	**PROTEIN** 0g	**FAT** 8g	**CARBOHYDRATE** 1g	**FIBER** 0g

Garlicky Red Wine Vinaigrette

¼ cup extra-virgin olive oil

¼ cup fresh lemon juice (about 1 lemon)

3 tablespoons red wine vinegar

1 tablespoon Dijon mustard

2 garlic cloves, minced

½ teaspoon red pepper flakes

1 teaspoon kosher salt

¼ teaspoon freshly ground black pepper

Salad

One 15-ounce can chickpeas (or 1½ cups cooked chickpeas), drained and rinsed

One 15-ounce can cannellini beans (or 1½ cups cooked cannellini beans), drained and rinsed

One 15-ounce can kidney beans (or 1½ cups cooked kidney beans), drained and rinsed

1 English or large salad cucumber, diced

1 cup quartered cherry tomatoes

1 cup small fresh mozzarella balls

½ red onion, thinly sliced

½ cup pitted and halved green olives

½ cup canned or jarred roasted red peppers, chopped

¼ cup chopped fresh parsley leaves

¼ cup chopped fresh cilantro leaves

I often add this salad to the plate when my main needs a little extra protein. It's also a really nice high-protein snack, especially post-workout. The three-bean mix is packed with plant-based protein and fiber, which together help with muscle repair, digestion, and satiety. And I adore the little fresh and creamy mozzarella pearls! They're bite-size, super convenient, adorable, and they make this salad feel a little fancy.

Growing up, our salads were usually super simple—lettuce, cucumbers, and some ranch dressing. That's why salads like this one, with beans, fresh herbs, homemade vinaigrette, etc., feel like such a treat to me. I almost always make my own dressing at home now, by the way. It's so easy, tastes much better, and I get to control exactly what goes into it.

Make the garlicky red wine vinaigrette: In a large bowl, big enough to hold all the salad, whisk together the olive oil, lemon juice, vinegar, mustard, garlic, pepper flakes, salt, and pepper until well combined.

Assemble the salad: Add the chickpeas, cannellini beans, kidney beans, cucumber, tomatoes, mozzarella, onion, olives, roasted red pepper, parsley, and cilantro and toss to combine.

Enjoy right away!

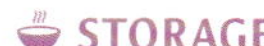

STORAGE

Store airtight in the refrigerator for up to 3 days.

Saucy Farro *with* Blistered Tomatoes

SERVES 4 TO 6
PREP TIME: 10 minutes
COOK TIME: 40 minutes

PER SERVING:	**CALORIES** 249 kcal	**PROTEIN** 8g	**FAT** 14g	**CARBOHYDRATE** 23g	**FIBER** 4g

4 tablespoons extra-virgin olive oil, divided

1 small white onion, finely diced

1 cup farro

1¾ cups chicken broth (or preferred broth)

One 14.5-ounce can fire-roasted diced tomatoes or another variety of diced canned tomato, undrained

1 pint cherry tomatoes

2 tablespoons chopped fresh flat-leaf parsley leaves (from 3 to 4 sprigs), plus more for garnish

1 teaspoon garlic powder

½ teaspoon kosher salt

½ cup grated Parmesan cheese

Farro, a close kin to whole-wheat berries, is one of my favorite grains. If you've never cooked with it, it's nutty and chewy and so tasty in salads, soups, and in this saucy dish. Aside from its delicious qualities, farro is also nutritious. It's primarily composed of complex carbohydrates, providing a good deal of fiber per serving. And, it's a great source of protein.

In a medium pot, heat 1 tablespoon of the olive oil over medium heat until hot. Add the onion and cook, stirring occasionally, until it begins to soften, about 3 minutes. Add the farro and stir for about 1 minute until everything is evenly coated in oil.

Pour in the broth and canned tomatoes with their juices. Bring the mixture to a boil, then decrease the heat to low, cover, and simmer, stirring occasionally, until the farro is tender, has a slight bite, and has absorbed most of the liquid, 25 to 45 minutes ( ).

While the farro cooks, preheat a large nonstick pan over medium heat for 3 to 4 minutes. Carefully add the remaining 3 tablespoons olive oil, swirling to coat the entire pan. Carefully add the cherry tomatoes to the pan, turning them quickly with a spatula to coat them in oil. Cover and cook the tomatoes for 3 minutes, undisturbed. Carefully flip and move them around and cook, covered, until they deflate and get nicely blistered and browned in spots, 2 to 3 more minutes.

Remove the pan from the heat and let cool for 2 to 3 minutes. Once the oil has stopped splattering, stir in the parsley, garlic powder, and salt. Add the farro and stir to combine. Stir in the Parmesan. Garnish with parsley and serve.

STORAGE + REHEAT

Once cooled, store airtight in the refrigerator for up to 5 days. To reheat, warm in a pan over medium heat until heated through, or microwave. Add a little water or broth if needed to loosen the mixture. For best results, garnish with the parsley right before serving.

STEPH'S TIP

Farro has a wide-range in terms of cooking time, depending on whether you are using whole-grain, semi-pearled, or pearled (the latter two cook faster), so taste it at 25 minutes, and in 5-minute increments after that if you need to cook it longer.

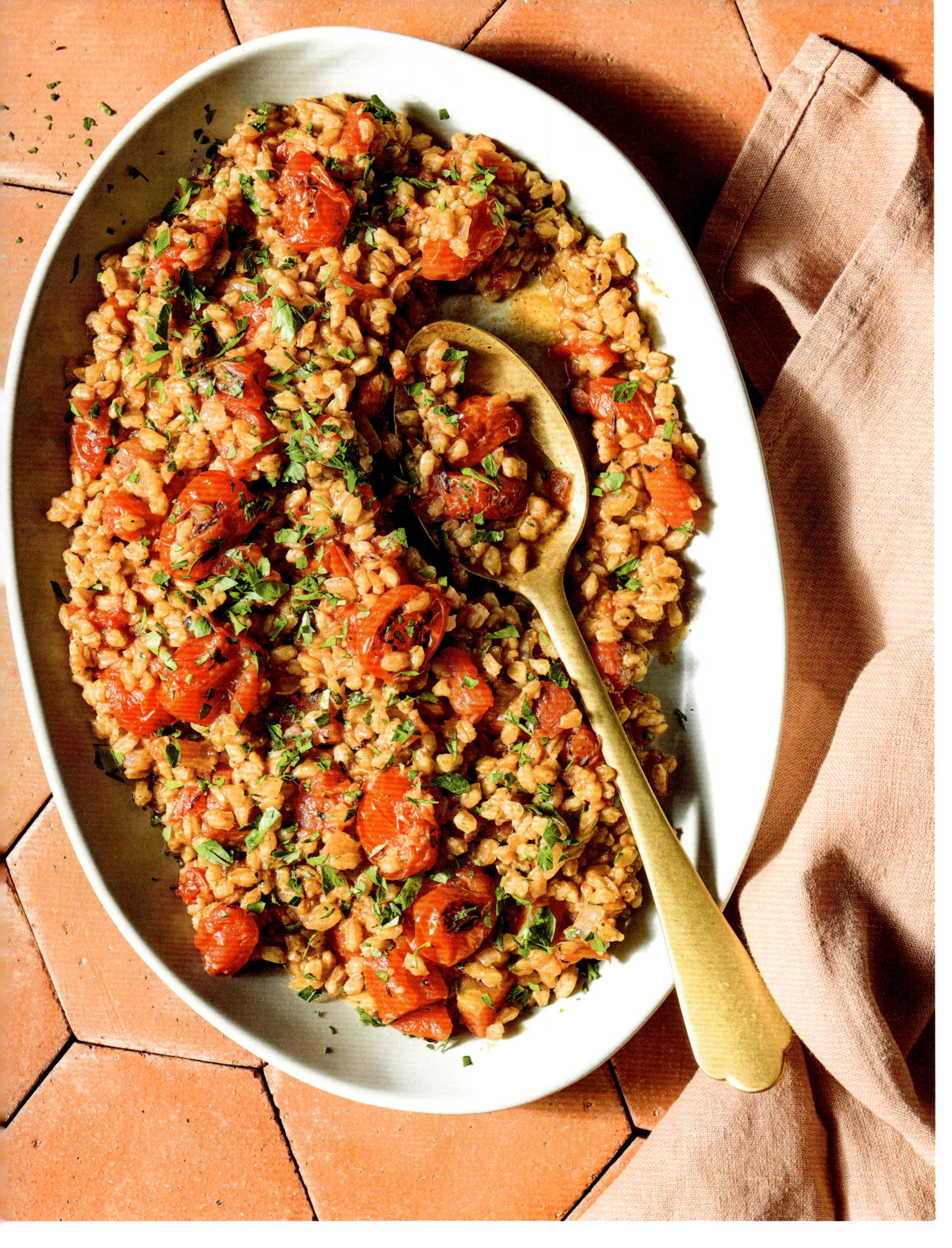

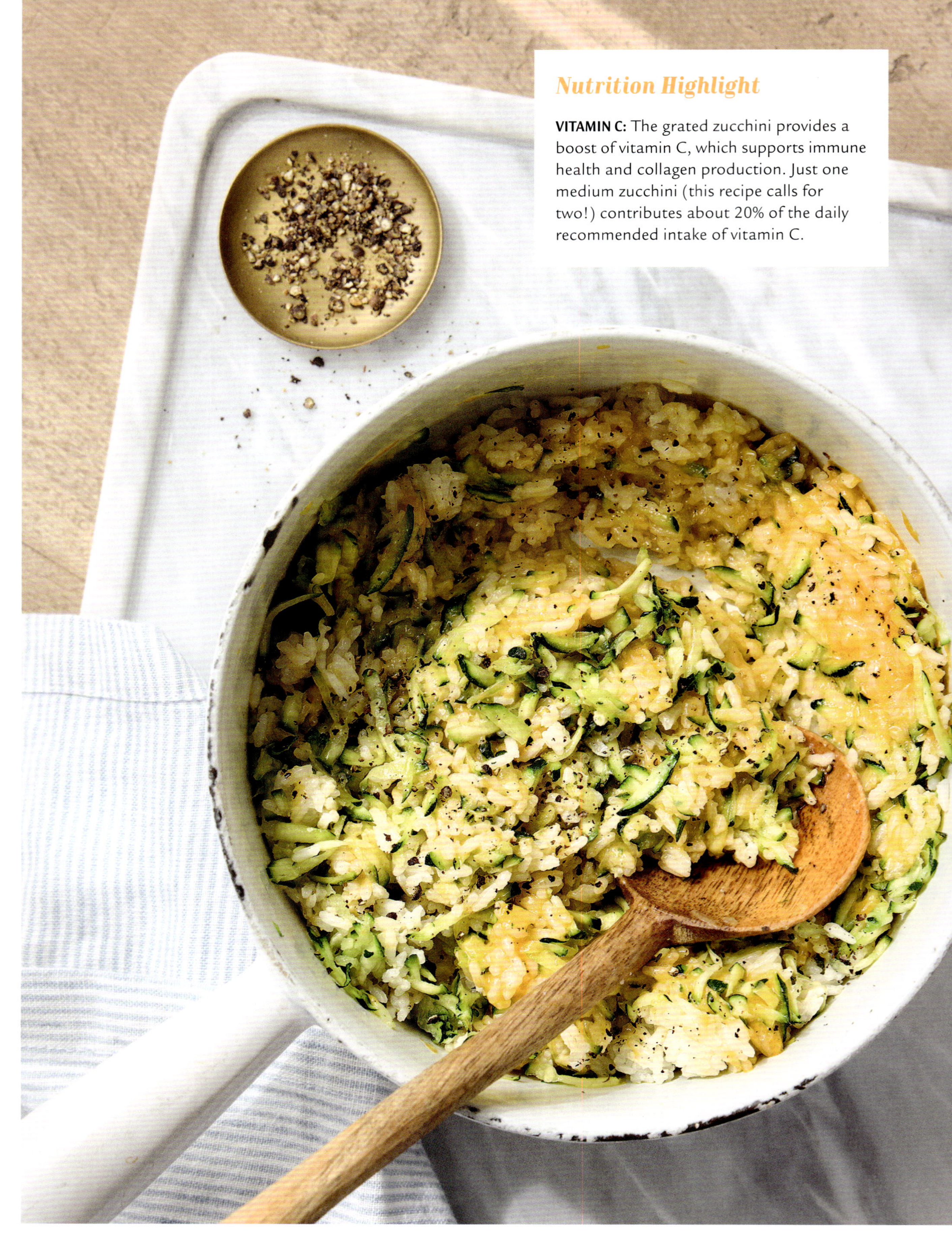

Nutrition Highlight

VITAMIN C: The grated zucchini provides a boost of vitamin C, which supports immune health and collagen production. Just one medium zucchini (this recipe calls for two!) contributes about 20% of the daily recommended intake of vitamin C.

Cheesy Zuke Rice

SERVES 4 TO 6
PREP TIME: 15 minutes
COOK TIME: 20 minutes

PER SERVING:	**CALORIES** 347 kcal	**PROTEIN** 10g	**FAT** 19g	**CARBOHYDRATE** 34g	**FIBER** 2g

1 pound zucchini (about 2)

¼ teaspoon kosher salt

1 cup long-grain white rice

2 cups chicken broth (or preferred broth)

2 tablespoons extra-virgin olive oil, divided

1 cup grated sharp Cheddar cheese

Freshly ground black pepper (optional)

I love a slow-cooked, veg-plus-broth, cheesy, savory rice. It's comfort food made healthy. It has that throwback feeling of Rice-A-Roni, made extra good for you by adding fresh ingredients.

Comfort = cooking up a pot of steamy white rice. Nourish = adding zucchini, chicken broth, and sharp Cheddar (the sharper the better!). The bite of the salted and grated zuke is so good here. And zucchini is packed with vitamin C, potassium, and antioxidants, which is lovely for immune health. I really like the combo of soft and steamy from the rice along with crunchy and bright in this one. So good!

Grate the zucchini (don't peel it) on the large holes of a box grater. Place it in a colander, sprinkle it with the salt, and stir to incorporate. Set it aside for about 10 minutes, so that the salt pulls out moisture (see Steph's Tip).

Meanwhile, in a fine-mesh sieve, rinse the rice until the water runs almost clear. In a medium pot, bring the broth, 1 tablespoon of the olive oil, and the rice to a boil. Once boiling, give it a quick stir, and then decrease the heat to low. Cover the pot and simmer until the rice is fairly tender and the broth is absorbed, 12 to 15 minutes.

After the zucchini has drained for 10 minutes, grab handfuls of it and tightly squeeze out and discard as much of the excess moisture as possible.

Once the rice is fairly tender, remove the pot from the heat. Stir in the remaining 1 tablespoon olive oil, the zucchini, and Cheddar and stir until well combined. Return the pot to low heat and cook, stirring occasionally, until the cheese has melted and the zucchini is heated through, 3 to 4 minutes. Season with pepper, if desired, and enjoy!

STORAGE + REHEAT

Once cooled, store airtight in the refrigerator for up to 4 days. To reheat, warm in a pan over medium heat until heated through, or microwave.

STEPH'S TIP

I recommend batch grating, salting, squeezing, and keeping the zucchini in the fridge for a few days for this recipe and for quick stir-fries, scrambles, melts, and more. Feel free to swap in different veggies (or cheeses!), like grated butternut squash, yellow squash, carrot, or cauliflower florets. No need to salt and squeeze those except for the yellow squash.

Freezer-Feed Cheesy Veggies

SERVES 3 OR 4
PREP TIME: 5 minutes
COOK TIME: 10 minutes

PER SERVING:	**CALORIES** 181 kcal	**PROTEIN** 10g	**FAT** 9g	**CARBOHYDRATE** 16g	**FIBER** 6g

One 10-ounce bag frozen chopped spinach

Half 14-ounce bag frozen white pearl onions

½ cup frozen peas

One 13- to 14-ounce can quartered artichoke hearts in water or brine, drained

¼ cup heavy cream

¼ cup nonfat or low-fat Greek yogurt

1 teaspoon garlic powder

½ teaspoon kosher salt

⅓ cup grated Parmesan cheese

I'm here to tell you that frozen veggies can be just as nutritious as fresh ones. My freezer is *full* of them year-round. Frozen veggies are typically flash-frozen shortly after harvest, which locks in all the good essential nutrients like vitamins, minerals, and antioxidants. Plus, they are cheaper and lead to less food waste (nothing wilting, getting slimy, or dying in the fridge), which is a win for both your wallet and the planet. This creamy cheesy veg-loaded dish proves beyond doubt that frozen veggies can be just as delicious as fresh. Cook it up and see for yourself!

In a medium pan, combine the spinach (breaking it up a bit as you do), pearl onions, and peas. Do not thaw first! Cover and cook over medium-high heat, stirring occasionally, until the vegetables are heated through and tender, 5 to 7 minutes.

Carefully tilt the pan over your sink to drain and discard any excess liquid, then return to low heat. Add the artichoke hearts, heavy cream, yogurt, garlic powder, and salt and stir to combine. Sprinkle in the Parmesan and stir to incorporate. Simmer for about 5 minutes to slightly thicken the sauce.

Serve as a side with your favorite protein or main.

STORAGE + REHEAT

Once cooled, store airtight in the refrigerator for up to 3 days. To reheat, warm in a pan over medium heat until heated through, or microwave.

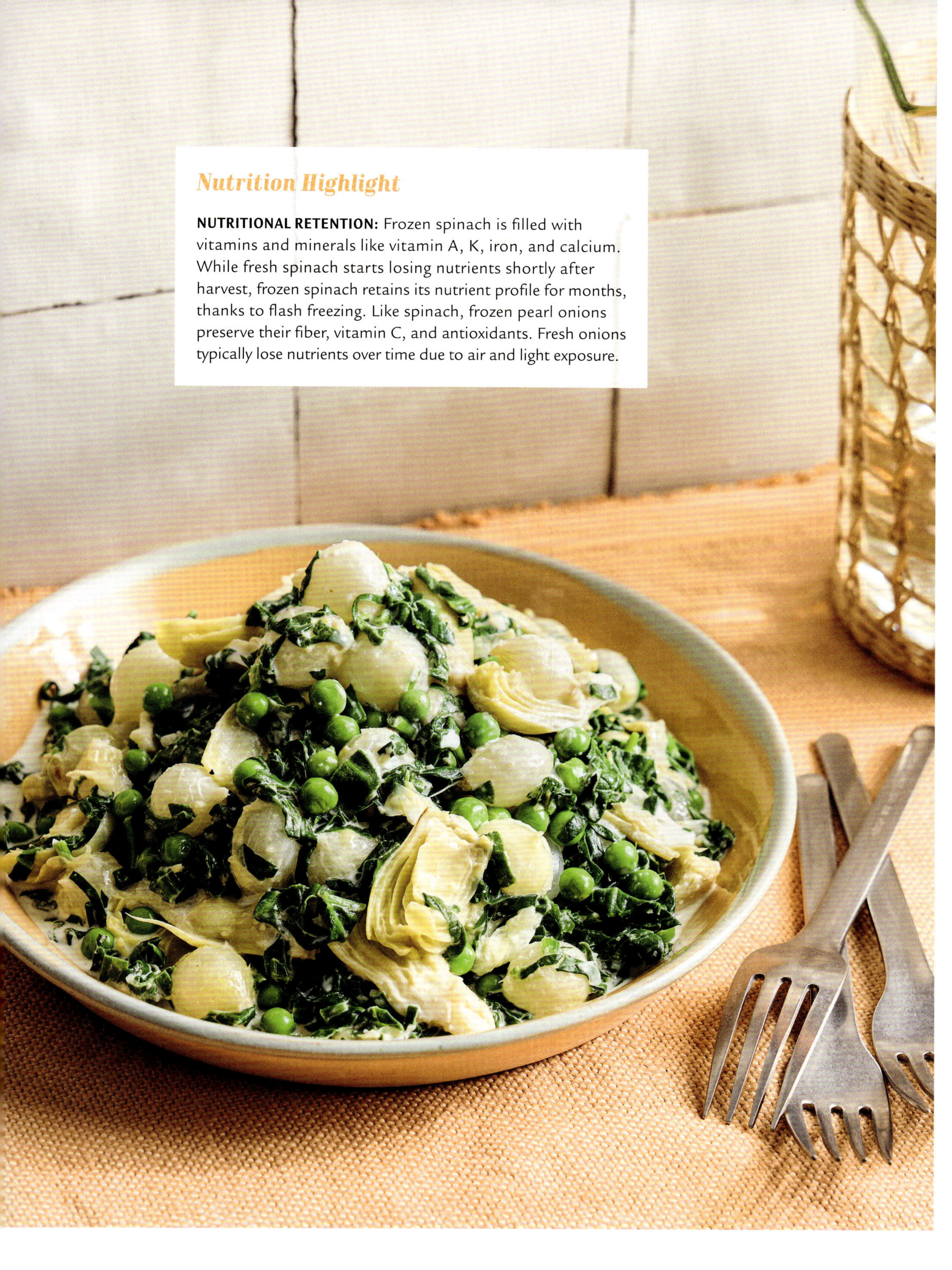

Nutrition Highlight

NUTRITIONAL RETENTION: Frozen spinach is filled with vitamins and minerals like vitamin A, K, iron, and calcium. While fresh spinach starts losing nutrients shortly after harvest, frozen spinach retains its nutrient profile for months, thanks to flash freezing. Like spinach, frozen pearl onions preserve their fiber, vitamin C, and antioxidants. Fresh onions typically lose nutrients over time due to air and light exposure.

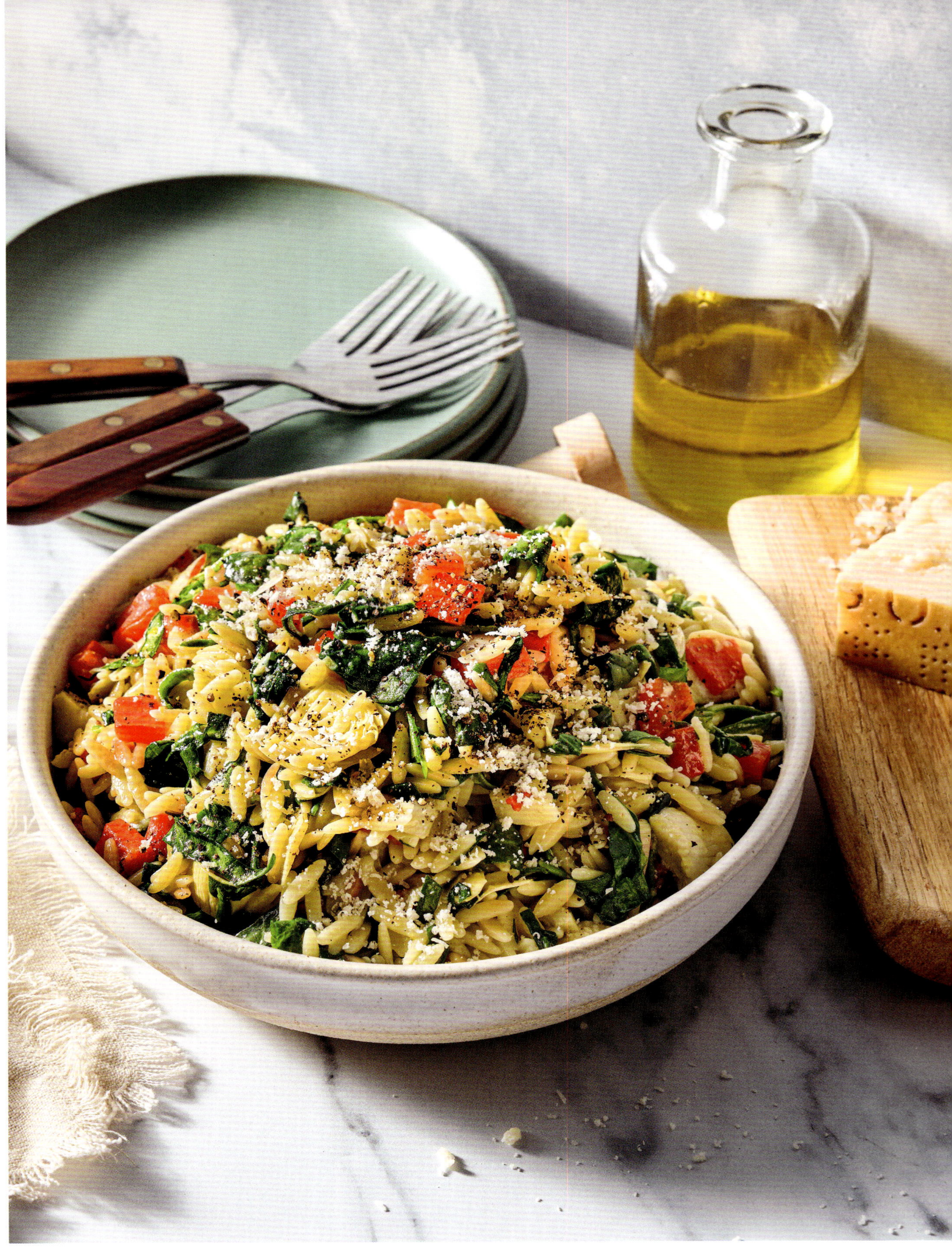

Spinach & Artichoke Orzo

SERVES 4
PREP TIME: 10 minutes
COOK TIME: 15 minutes

PER SERVING:	**CALORIES** 268 kcal	**PROTEIN** 11g	**FAT** 6g	**CARBOHYDRATE** 40g	**FIBER** 5g

1 tablespoon extra-virgin olive oil

1 cup orzo

2 cups chicken broth

4 cups lightly packed spinach, coarsely chopped

One 13- to 14-ounce can whole or quartered artichoke hearts in water or brine, drained and chopped

1 cup canned or jarred roasted red peppers or sun-dried tomatoes, sliced

1 tablespoon fresh lemon juice (about ½ small lemon)

1 teaspoon finely grated lemon zest

¼ teaspoon kosher salt

¼ cup grated Parmesan cheese, plus more for garnish

I cook and eat a lot of orzo year-round. It's tasty at any temperature, and great as a pasta salad, side, main, or in soups. I think this orzo dish is best served warm with the melted Parm and the lemon juice and zest just added. You're going to love it. As far as nutrition goes, the artichoke hearts are the real star. Canned artichoke hearts are so convenient and affordable, while also low in calories and high in fiber.

In a large pan, heat the olive oil over medium heat until hot. Add the orzo and stir for about 2 minutes, until it is coated in oil and slightly toasted. Add the broth, increase the heat to high, and bring it to a boil. Once boiling, decrease the heat to low and simmer covered, stirring occasionally, until the orzo is almost tender and a lot of the broth has been absorbed, 8 to 10 minutes.

Add the spinach, artichoke hearts, roasted peppers, lemon juice, lemon zest, and salt. Continue cooking, stirring occasionally, until the spinach has wilted, the orzo is fully cooked, and only a bit of broth remains, 3 to 5 more minutes.

Remove from the heat and stir in the Parmesan. Sprinkle additional grated Parmesan over the top when serving.

STORAGE + REHEAT

Once cooled, store airtight in the refrigerator for up to 3 days. To reheat, gently warm in a pan over medium heat until heated through, or microwave. Add a splash of broth or water if the mixture seems dry.

Creole-Style Rice & Beans

SERVES 8 TO 10
PREP TIME: 15 minutes
COOK TIME: 50 minutes

PER SERVING:	**CALORIES** 255 kcal	**PROTEIN** 9g	**FAT** 12g	**CARBOHYDRATE** 26g	**FIBER** 3g

- 1 cup long-grain white rice
- 3½ cups vegetable broth (or preferred broth), divided
- 1 tablespoon extra-virgin olive oil
- 12 ounces kielbasa, cut into ½-inch-thick slices
- 1 large yellow onion, diced
- 2 green onions (white and green parts), sliced, divided
- 1 large green bell pepper, diced
- 3 to 4 celery stalks, diced
- 5 garlic cloves, minced
- 1 tablespoon salted Cajun or Creole seasoning, such as Tony Chachere's or Cajun's Choice
- One 15-ounce can red kidney beans (or 1½ cups cooked red kidney beans), drained and rinsed
- Kosher salt and freshly ground black pepper

I fell in love with Creole food when I went to New Orleans in 2023 and got to try all sorts of dishes. I learned about Creole cuisine and the deep and diverse roots of the historic communities that settled in Louisiana. Their unique cuisine combines European techniques with bold, flavorful ingredients and dishes from the Caribbean, Africa, and South America.

That trip was unforgettable in so many ways, and it inspired me to add this tasty dish to the book. Lucky for us, it's perfectly balanced with protein, fiber, and complex carbs. So simple and so good! And, even though rice and beans is often served as a side, I've definitely made a meal out of this one on more than one occasion.

In a medium pot, rinse the rice in cold water until the water runs fairly clear. The way I like to do this is to fill the pot about one-quarter of the way with water, swish and move the rice around in the water by hand, and then slowly and carefully (so that you don't pour out any rice) tilt the pot and pour out the water. I usually repeat this once or twice until the water that I'm discarding is fairly clear.

In the same pot, combine the rinsed rice with 1½ cups of the broth. Bring to a boil over high heat. Once boiling, give it a good stir, and then decrease the heat to low. Cover and simmer until the rice is tender and the broth is absorbed, 15 to 20 minutes. Remove from the heat and let sit covered for 5 minutes. Fluff with a fork and set aside.

In a large pan or Dutch oven, heat the olive oil over medium heat until hot. Add the kielbasa and cook, stirring occasionally, until browned, 4 to 5 minutes. Remove the sausage to a clean plate and set aside.

In the same pan (no need to discard the oil, or wipe it off or wash it) over medium heat, add the yellow onion, the white parts of the green onion, the bell pepper, and celery and cook, stirring occasionally, until the vegetables have softened and the onion is starting to become translucent, 5 to 6 minutes.

Add the garlic, the green parts of the green onion, and the Cajun seasoning. Stir and cook for 1 to 2 minutes, until the garlic is fragrant.

Continued

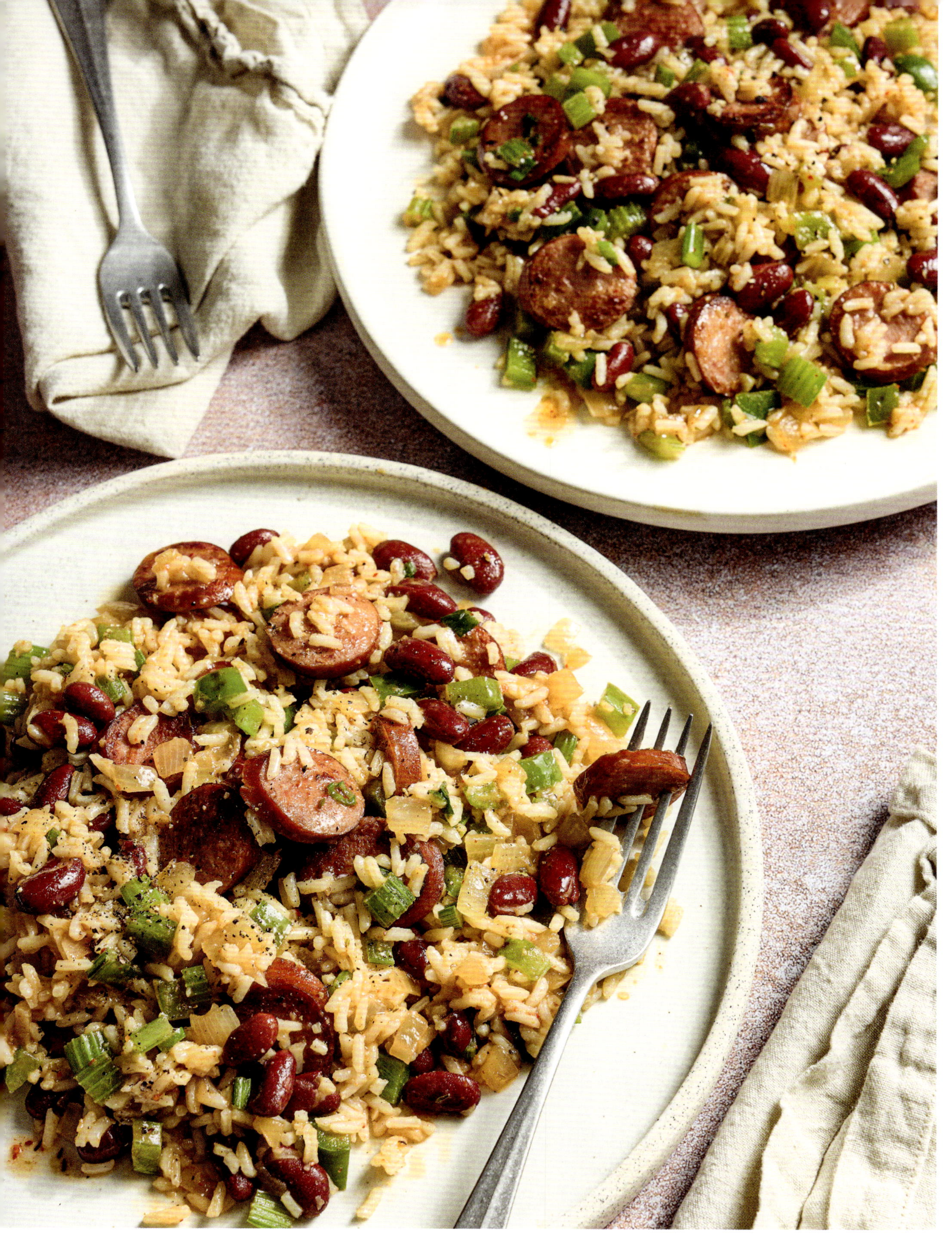

Add the beans and the remaining 2 cups broth and stir well to combine. The pan will be quite full. Increase the heat to high and bring everything to a boil, then decrease the heat to low, and simmer uncovered, stirring occasionally, until the flavors meld and the broth has slightly reduced, about 20 minutes. If the mixture becomes too thick and is sticking to the pan at any point, add a little more broth or water.

Stir in the cooked rice, mixing everything thoroughly. Return the kielbasa to the pan and stir to combine. Cook for 2 to 3 more minutes to warm the kielbasa through, stirring occasionally.

Season with salt and pepper to taste. Transfer everything to a serving dish or serve it right out of the pan.

STEPH'S TIP

If you'd prefer to use brown rice here, simply increase the broth and cook time. For 1 cup of uncooked brown rice, use 2 cups of broth and cook for about 45 minutes, then rest and fluff in the same way as for the white.

NUTRITION PSA

For a lower-sodium version, simply use a low-sodium veggie broth and don't season with salt to taste. Add greens like spinach or kale toward the end for a vitamin and mineral boost.

STORAGE + REHEAT

Once cooled, store airtight in the refrigerator for up to 4 days. To reheat, gently warm in a pan over medium heat until heated through, or microwave. Add a splash of broth or water if the mixture seems dry.

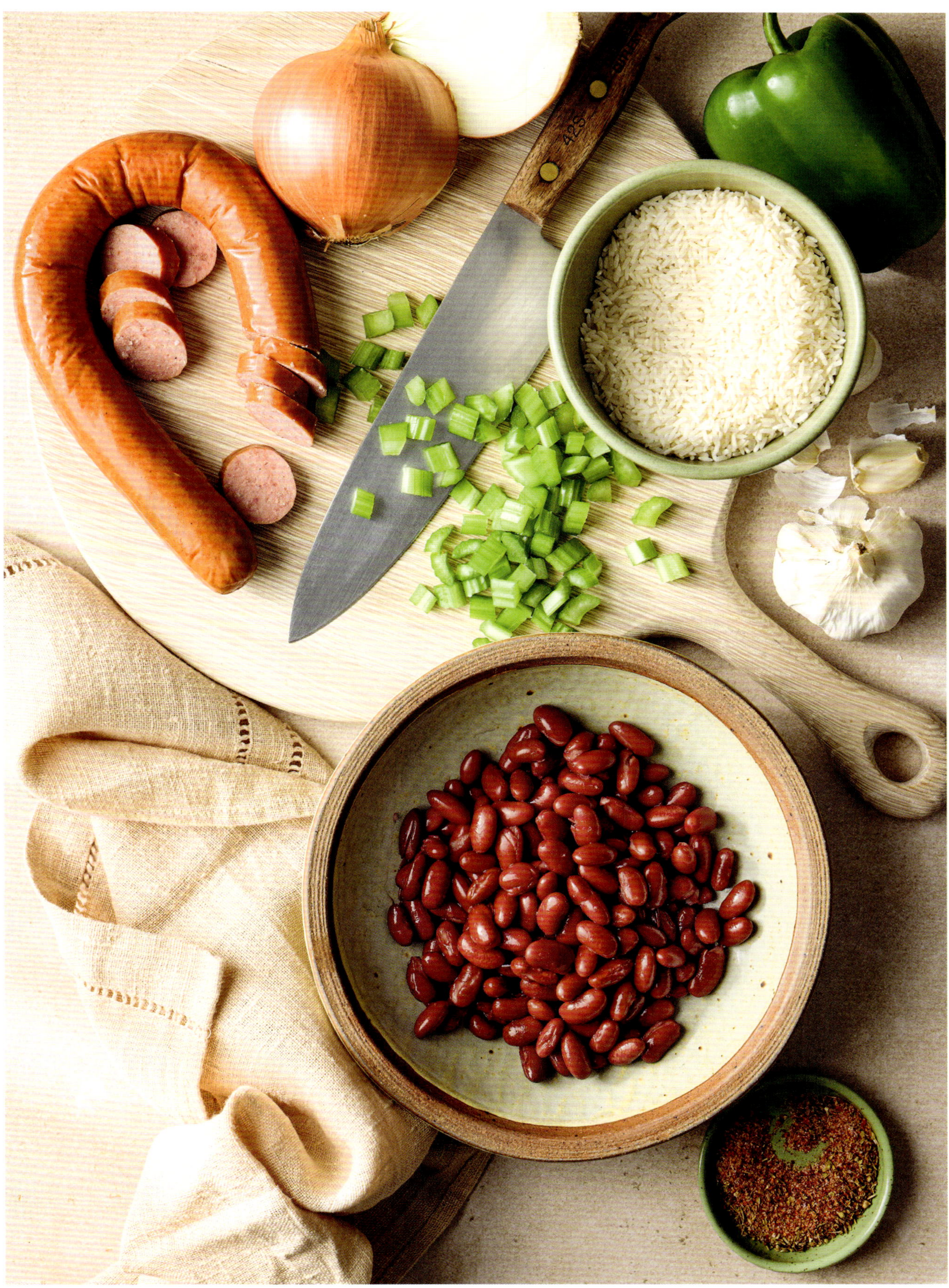

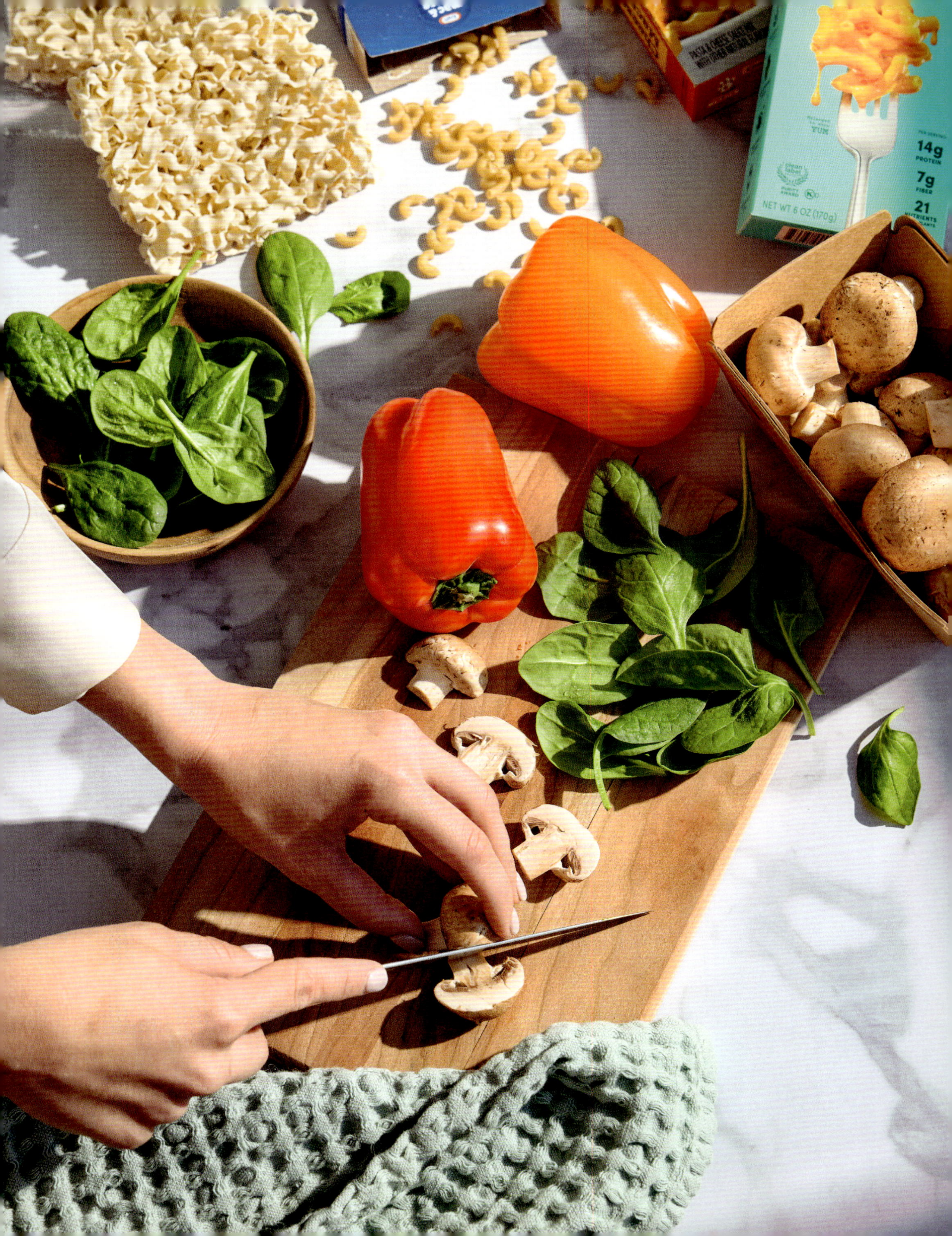
YUM
14g
PROTEIN
7g
FIBER
21
clean label
PURITY AWARD
NET WT 6 OZ (170g)

Doctored-Up

Comfort Classics

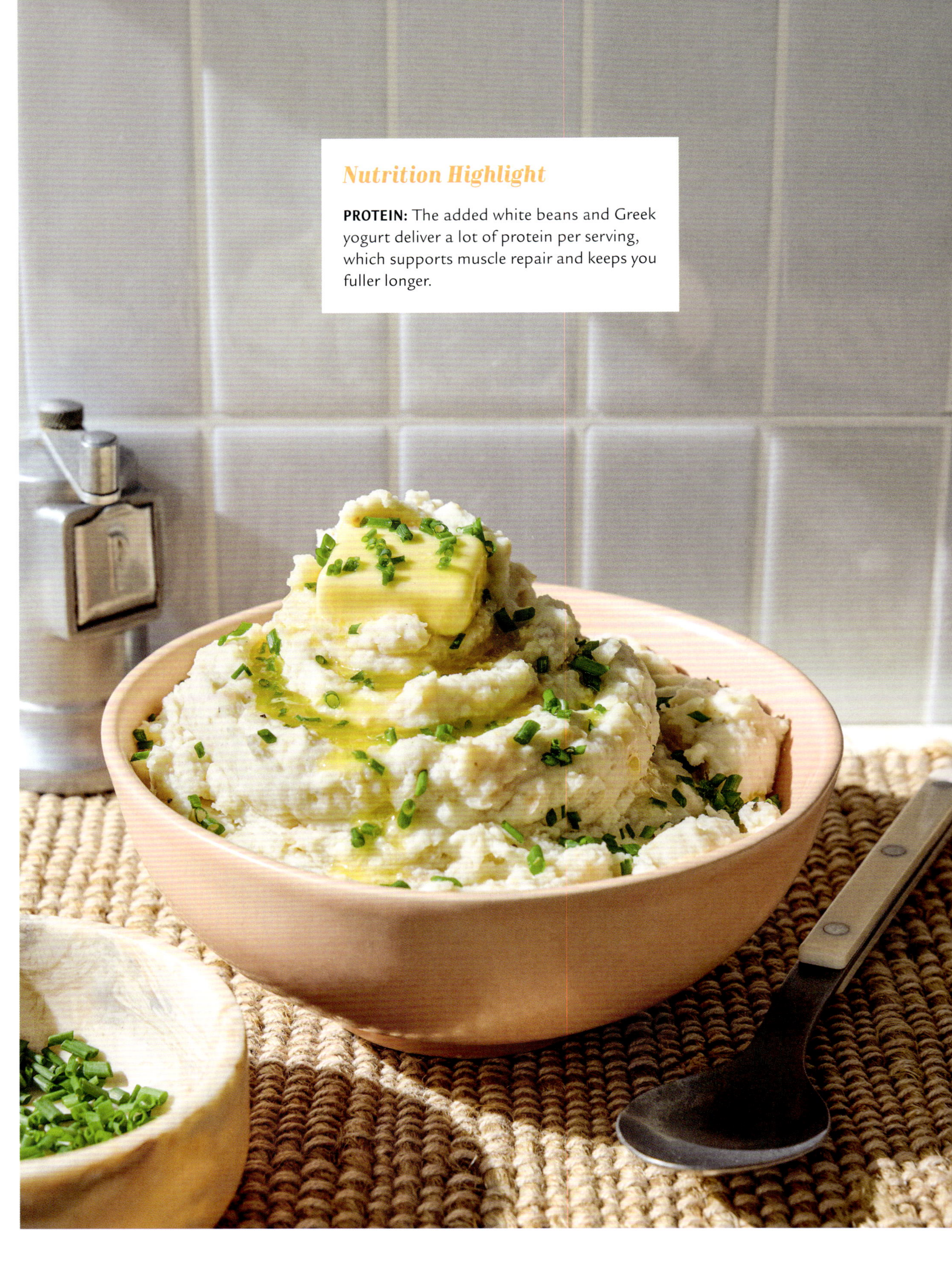

Nutrition Highlight

PROTEIN: The added white beans and Greek yogurt deliver a lot of protein per serving, which supports muscle repair and keeps you fuller longer.

Instant Spuds *Made Right*

SERVES 2 OR 3
PREP TIME: 5 minutes
COOK TIME: 10 minutes

PER SERVING:	CALORIES 302 kcal	PROTEIN 17g	FAT 2g	CARBOHYDRATE 53g	FIBER 6g

1 heaping cup canned (or cooked) Great Northern beans or any other white bean such as butter, navy, or cannellini beans (about two-thirds of a can), drained and rinsed if canned

1⅓ cups milk (dairy or nondairy) or more as needed

2 garlic cloves, minced

¼ teaspoon kosher salt, plus more to taste

⅛ teaspoon freshly ground black pepper, plus more to taste

1⅓ cups instant mashed potato flakes

½ cup nonfat or low-fat Greek yogurt

Chopped fresh herbs (optional)

These mashed potatoes, made with instant potato flakes, are my healthy twist on a comfort food favorite. By adding Greek yogurt and white beans to the mix, you get added protein plus fiber and a lovely creamy texture with zero butter or heavy cream. They're so easy to whip up, thanks to the wonders of food science and dehydration. These are perfect for a busy weeknight, but don't overlook them as a tasty holiday side dish.

In a medium bowl, mash the beans with a potato masher or a wooden spoon until fairly smooth.

In a large pan, warm the milk over medium heat for 1 to 2 minutes, making sure that it doesn't boil. Add the mashed beans, garlic, salt, and pepper. Stir well to combine and cook for 2 to 3 minutes, until hot.

Gradually add the potato flakes to the pan, stirring constantly for about 2 minutes. Fold in the yogurt and combine it with the mixture until it is heated through, about 2 minutes. If the mashed potatoes are too thick, add a bit more milk until the desired consistency is reached.

Taste and adjust seasoning with additional salt and pepper. Serve warm as a healthy side dish, garnished with fresh herbs, if desired.

STORAGE + REHEAT

Once cooled, store airtight in the refrigerator for up to 3 days. To reheat, warm in the microwave or on the stovetop until heated through. Add a splash of milk, if needed, to get to desired texture.

Veggie Crafted Beef Mac & Cheese

SERVES 3 OR 4
PREP TIME: 5 minutes
COOK TIME: 20 minutes

PER SERVING:	**CALORIES** 580 kcal	**PROTEIN** 38g	**FAT** 30g	**CARBOHYDRATE** 39g	**FIBER** 2g

One 7.25-ounce box Kraft Mac & Cheese original flavor (or another brand of boxed mac and cheese with a cheese powder packet)

¼ cup nonfat or low-fat Greek yogurt

1 tablespoon extra-virgin olive oil

1 pound lean ground beef (10% fat or less)

1 yellow squash

2 tablespoons hemp hearts (hulled hemp seeds)

Kosher salt

Boxed mac and cheese was a staple when I was growing up. I especially loved it after field hockey practice in high school when I'd be so hungry. The only problem with boxed mac is the lack of substantial fiber or protein, which your body needs, especially after a good workout. I've got you with the squash, ground beef, hemp hearts, and Greek yogurt.

Greek yogurt is such a great way to add protein without losing any dairy creaminess. In fact, I prefer the texture of Greek yogurt here to half-and-half or milk for the way it coats the noodles! One of the best things about this doctored-up classic is it's still fairly yellow-orange for any picky eaters.

Fill a medium pot three-quarters full with water and bring it to a boil over high heat. Add the macaroni and cook until tender, 6 to 7 minutes. Drain the macaroni and return it to the pot. Add the yogurt and cheese powder (from the box) and stir until well combined.

Meanwhile, in a large pan, heat the olive oil over medium-high heat until hot. Add the ground beef and cook, stirring occasionally, breaking up the meat as you do, until it is nicely browned, 8 to 10 minutes. Drain and discard any excess fat from the pan and transfer the browned beef to a plate. Set aside.

Halve the squash lengthwise, then cut each half lengthwise again. Slice all four sections crosswise into roughly ¼-inch-thick pieces. In the same pan (no need to wipe it off or wash it) over medium heat, add the squash and cook, stirring occasionally, until it has softened a bit and starts to brown, 4 to 5 minutes.

Return the browned ground beef to the pan and cook for 1 to 2 minutes to warm the beef through. Add the mac and cheese mixture to the pan. Stir to combine and cook for 1 to 2 minutes to warm the macaroni through. Remove from the heat.

Sprinkle in the hemp hearts and stir to fully incorporate. Season with salt to taste. Serve and enjoy!

NUTRITION PSA

Lower the energy: Use ground turkey (7% fat) or ground chicken instead of ground beef. Use ½ pound ground meat instead of 1 pound and add more veggies to bulk it up.

STORAGE + REHEAT

Once cooled, store airtight in the refrigerator for up to 3 days. To reheat, warm in a pan over medium heat until heated through, or microwave.

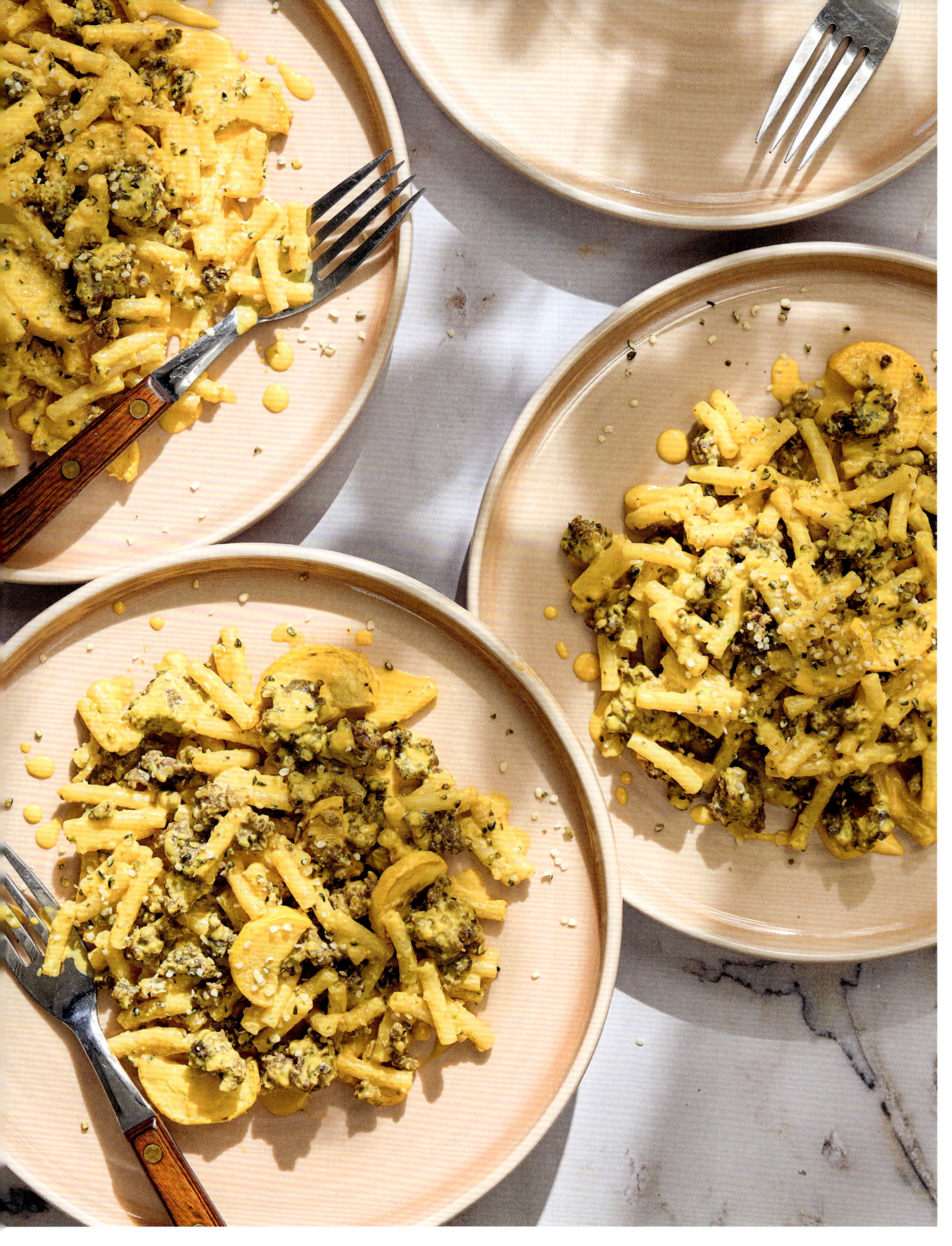

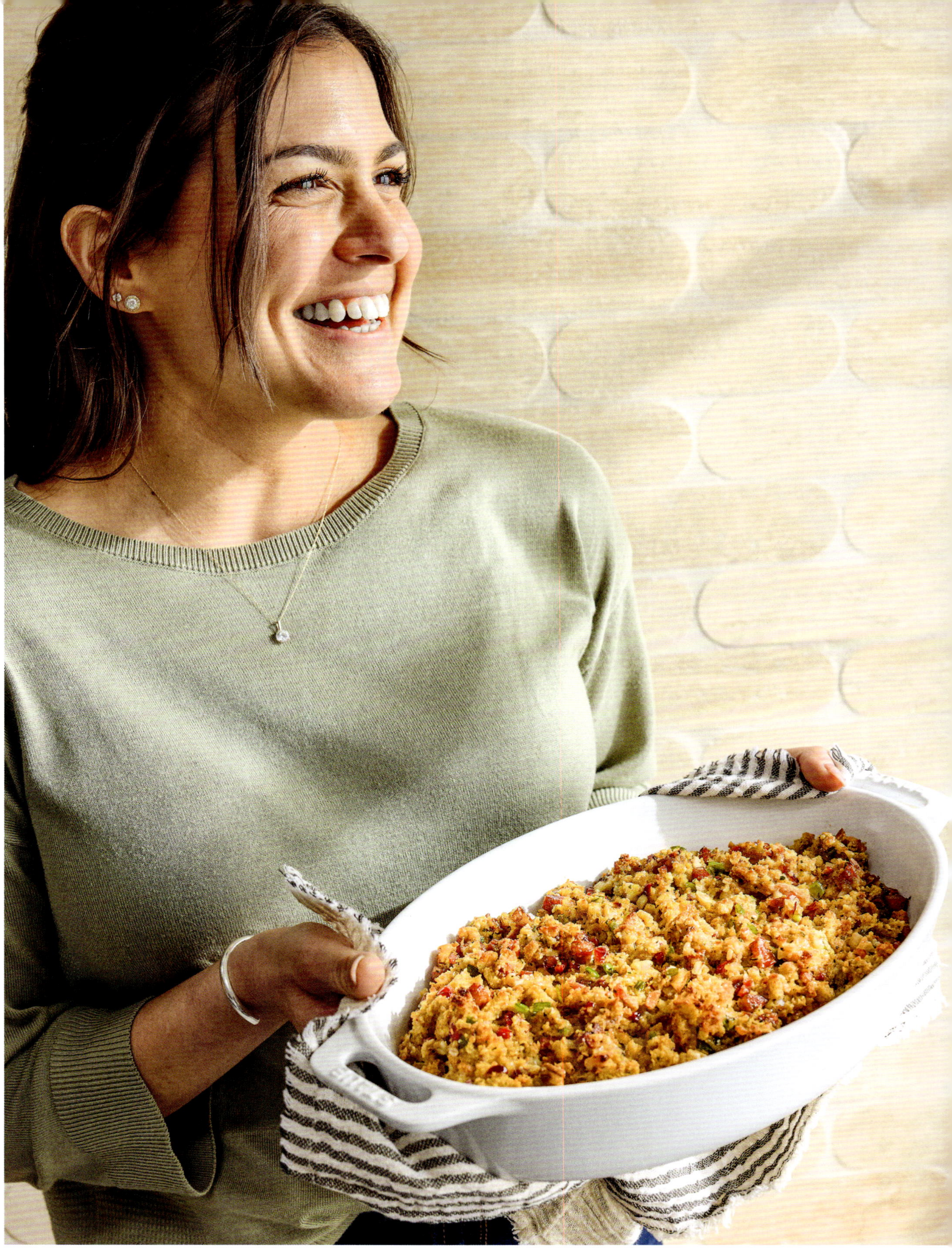

Stove Top Stuffing Remix

SERVES 6
PREP TIME: 10 minutes
COOK TIME: 40 minutes

PER SERVING:	CALORIES 281 kcal	PROTEIN 10g	FAT 16g	CARBOHYDRATE 25g	FIBER 2g

Cooking spray or neutral oil, for the baking dish

1 tablespoon unsalted butter

1 cup finely chopped precooked sausage (about one 4-ounce sausage)

½ white onion, chopped

¾ cup finely chopped celery (about 2 stalks)

2 garlic cloves, minced

¼ cup dried cranberries

¼ cup chopped walnuts

1 tablespoon finely chopped fresh rosemary

1 tablespoon finely chopped fresh sage

¼ teaspoon kosher salt

One 6-ounce box chicken Stove Top stuffing mix (or your preferred flavor)

1¼ cups chicken broth (or preferred broth)

1 large egg, beaten

½ cup grated Parmesan cheese

Why do we reserve stuffing solely for Thanksgiving? It's so good! When I smell all the roasty toasty, herby, and savory smells of stuffing, I immediately think of togetherness and cozy sweet times. I don't think that should be solely relegated to one day in late November. So, I encourage you, too, to doctor up your Stove Top stuffing like this any time the craving hits.

My family was fairly plain Jane with boxed stuffing growing up. We didn't add much to it beyond what the box called for. I've balanced it here, made it even tastier, and heaped on more nutrition, with added protein and fiber thanks to the veggies, sausage, cranberries, walnuts, and more. Walnuts, by the way, deliver a big dose of immunity-strengthening omega-3 fatty acids. We can all use more of that year-round.

Preheat the oven to 350°F. Lightly grease (with cooking spray or oil) a 9 by 13-inch baking dish and set aside.

In a large pan, melt the butter over medium heat. Add the sausage, onion, celery, and garlic. Cook, stirring occasionally, until the onion has softened, about 5 minutes. Stir in the cranberries, walnuts, rosemary, sage, and salt. Cook for another 2 minutes, stirring occasionally, then remove from the heat.

In a large bowl, combine the Stove Top stuffing mix with the cooked vegetable/sausage mixture. Pour in the chicken broth and stir well. Let the mixture sit for 3 to 4 minutes to absorb the broth.

Add the egg and Parmesan and stir until well combined. Transfer the stuffing mixture to the greased baking dish, spreading it evenly.

Bake until the top of the stuffing is golden-brown and slightly crispy, about 30 minutes. Enjoy!

STORAGE + REHEAT

Once cooled, store airtight in the refrigerator for up to 3 days. To reheat, gently warm in a pan over medium-low heat until heated through, or microwave.

Buffalo Tuna Melt Quesadilla

SERVES 1 OR 2
PREP TIME: 5 minutes
COOK TIME: 6 minutes

PER SERVING:	CALORIES 545 kcal	PROTEIN 49g	FAT 28g	CARBOHYDRATE 27g	FIBER 2g

1 tablespoon nonfat or low-fat Greek yogurt

2 tablespoons Buffalo wing sauce

One 5- to 6-ounce can solid white albacore tuna in water, drained

½ teaspoon garlic powder

1 cup grated part-skim or whole-milk mozzarella cheese, divided

1 large burrito-size flour tortilla

1 cup lightly packed spinach, chopped

1½ teaspoons extra-virgin olive oil

The crispy, cheesy gooeyness of a quesadilla is something I crave often. I make mine more balanced by adding fiber and protein. You're going to make this one again and again. Trust me.

This quesadilla is *fully loaded.* Before you put it in the pan, it will be 2 to 3 inches tall. If you want a thinner quesadilla, use the same amount of filling on one entire tortilla, topping it the same way, to 1 inch of the edge of the tortilla, and then top it with another tortilla. Slightly reduce the pan cooking time to 2 to 2½ minutes per side.

In a medium bowl, stir together the yogurt and Buffalo sauce until they are smooth and blended. Add the drained tuna and garlic powder and break up the tuna with a fork or spoon while stirring everything together so that it's fully incorporated.

Put half of the mozzarella evenly onto one half of the tortilla, leaving about 1 inch of cheese-free space from the edge to prevent overflow melting into the pan. Top the cheese evenly with the tuna mixture and then the spinach. Top the spinach with the remaining cheese. Fold the untopped half of the tortilla over the topped half so that all of the filling is covered, and lightly press down.

In a large nonstick pan, warm the olive oil over medium-low heat. Gently swirl the oil around the pan to coat. When the oil is hot, place the quesadilla spinach-filled-side down in the pan. Cook until the tortilla is golden brown on both sides and the cheese has fully melted, about 3 minutes per side.

Carefully transfer the cooked quesadilla to a cutting board. Let it cool for about 1 minute, then slice it into wedges. Serve warm and enjoy!

YOU DO YOU

Swap out the flour tortilla for a whole-wheat or low-carb one to increase fiber. And, feel free to add extra vegetables, such as bell peppers, onions, or tomatoes for added flavor and nutrition.

STORAGE + REHEAT

Once cooled, store airtight in the refrigerator for up to 3 days. To reheat, warm in a pan over medium heat until heated through, or microwave.

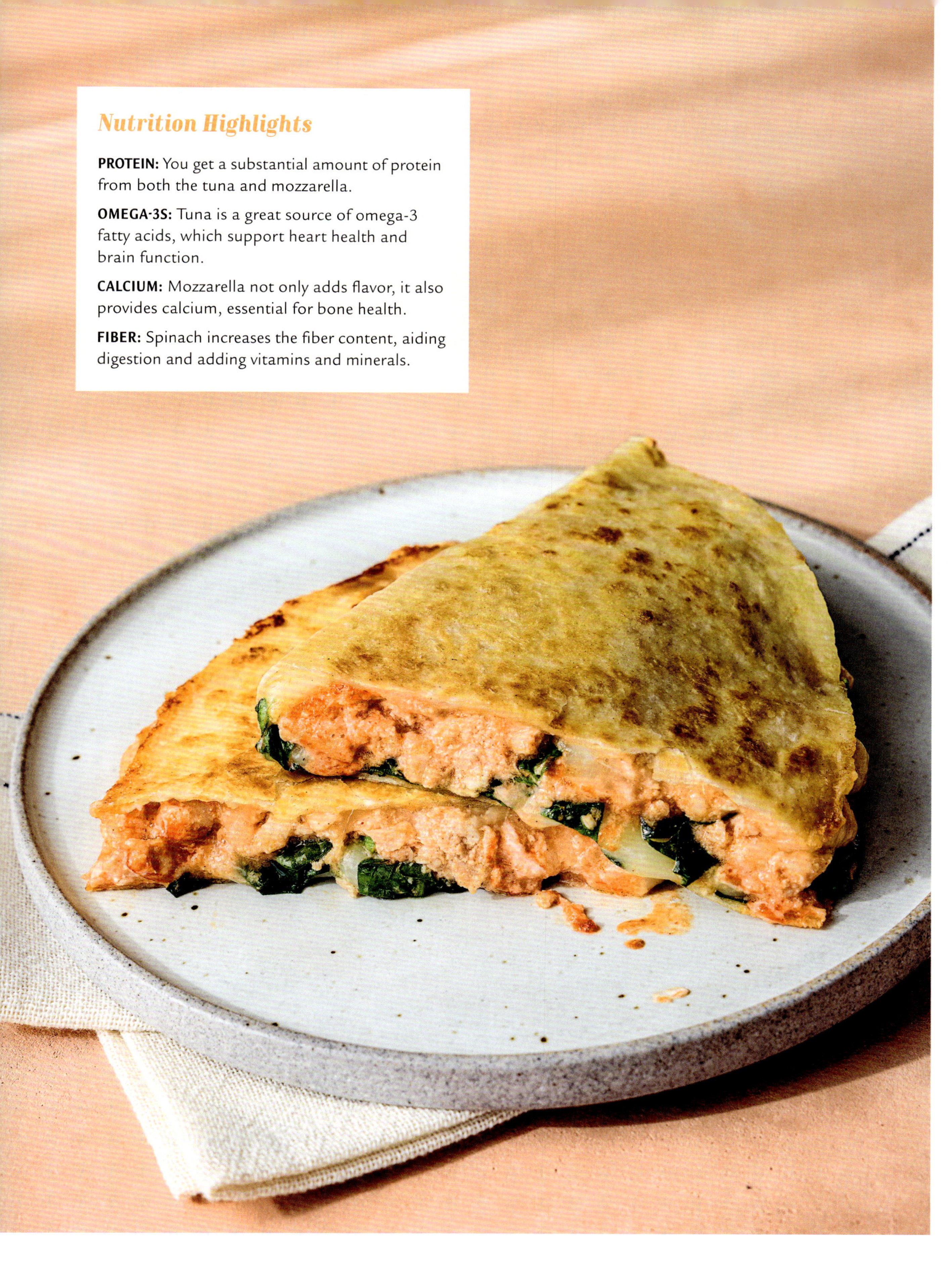

Nutrition Highlights

PROTEIN: You get a substantial amount of protein from both the tuna and mozzarella.

OMEGA-3S: Tuna is a great source of omega-3 fatty acids, which support heart health and brain function.

CALCIUM: Mozzarella not only adds flavor, it also provides calcium, essential for bone health.

FIBER: Spinach increases the fiber content, aiding digestion and adding vitamins and minerals.

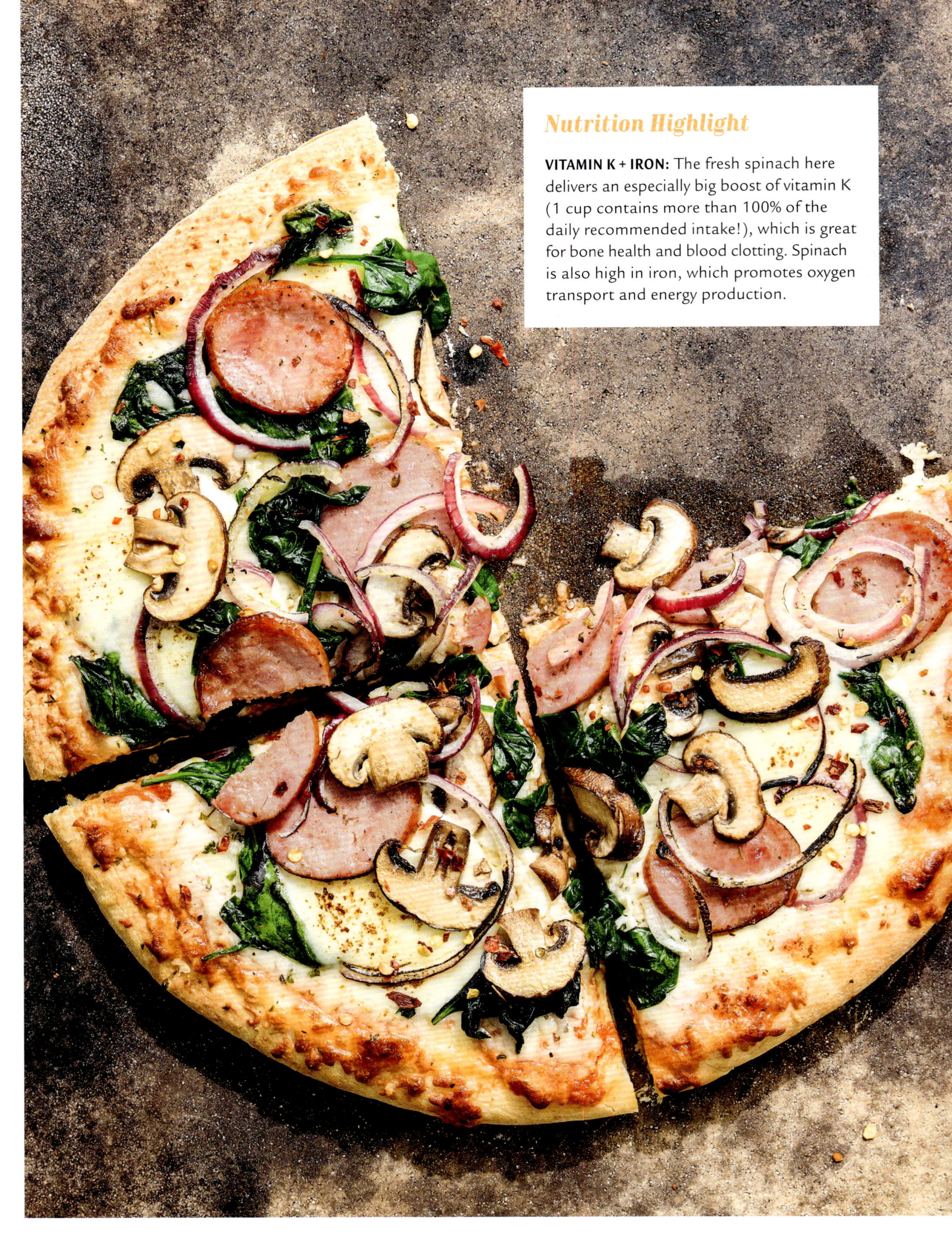

Nutrition Highlight

VITAMIN K + IRON: The fresh spinach here delivers an especially big boost of vitamin K (1 cup contains more than 100% of the daily recommended intake!), which is great for bone health and blood clotting. Spinach is also high in iron, which promotes oxygen transport and energy production.

Gardened-Up Frozen Pizza

SERVES 4
PREP TIME: 5 minutes
COOK TIME: 8 to 10 minutes

PER SERVING:	CALORIES 576 kcal	PROTEIN 25g	FAT 32g	CARBOHYDRATE 45g	FIBER 2g

One 18- to 20-ounce frozen pizza

1 cup lightly packed spinach leaves

4 or 5 thick slices fresh mozzarella cheese

1 cup thinly sliced white or cremini mushrooms

½ cup kielbasa slices (about 2 ounces), cut ¼ inch thick

⅓ cup thinly sliced red onion (about ¼ onion)

2 tablespoons extra-virgin olive oil

1 teaspoon Italian seasoning

3 tablespoons grated Parmesan cheese

When I'm craving a slice, frozen pizza is my go-to because of its endless possibilities for customization. I stack my frozen pizzas high with all sorts of added veggie and protein goodness. This recipe is so versatile, and easy to tailor to dietary preferences and nutrition goals. Just know that if you add more watery veggies than I have here, such as more leafy greens, you should cook them a bit first, to cook off those liquids, before topping the pizza. If you add zucchini or tomatoes, thinly slice them as you do the mushrooms. No one wants pizza soup!

Preheat the oven to 550°F, or the highest temperature that your oven allows if it doesn't go that high.

Remove the frozen pizza from its packaging and place it on a pizza pan or sheet pan. Top it evenly with the spinach. It will cover most of the pizza. Top the spinach with the mozzarella slices, mushrooms, and kielbasa.

In a small bowl, toss the red onion with the olive oil and Italian seasoning. Top the pizza evenly with the seasoned red onion and use a brush (or a paper towel, or drizzle with a spoon) to coat the outer edge of the crust with the leftover seasoned oil (). Sprinkle the Parmesan evenly over the pizza.

Bake the pizza, keeping an eye on it so that it doesn't burn, until the crust is golden and nicely crisped, and the cheese is bubbling and a bit browned, 8 to 10 minutes. Let it sit at room temperature for 1 to 2 minutes, then slice and eat!

STORAGE + REHEAT

Once cooled, store airtight in the refrigerator for up to 4 days.

To reheat in the oven: Preheat the oven to 375°F. Place the pizza slices on a sheet pan and cover loosely with aluminum foil. Heat for 10 to 15 minutes to warm through.

To reheat in the microwave: Place a slice of pizza on a microwave-safe plate and cover with a microwave-safe cover. Heat on high for 1 to 2 minutes, checking frequently to avoid overcooking.

To reheat on the stovetop: Heat a pan over medium heat. Place a slice or more of pizza in the pan and cover it with a lid. Heat until the crust is crispy and the cheese is melty, 2 to 3 minutes.

STEPH'S TIP

Since frozen pizza crusts are often bland, brush them with this seasoned olive oil. Consider using other crust enhancements such as Parmesan cheese, red pepper flakes, or "everything" seasoning.

Chicken Nugget Veggie Power Wrap

SERVES 1
PREP TIME: 10 minutes
COOK TIME: 10 minutes

PER SERVING:	**CALORIES** 592 kcal	**PROTEIN** 26g	**FAT** 27g	**CARBOHYDRATE** 58g	**FIBER** 10g

4 ounces frozen chicken nuggets (6 to 8 nuggets)

2 tablespoons Buffalo wing sauce

3 tablespoons nonfat or low-fat Greek yogurt

½ teaspoon ranch dip or dressing seasoning

1 burrito-size whole-wheat or flour tortilla

1 cup lightly packed mixed salad greens

¼ cup grated carrot

¼ cup thinly sliced English cucumber

¼ cup thinly sliced red bell pepper

¼ avocado, sliced

I used to *love* chicken nuggets as a kid. I still do as an adult! This wrap elevates that childhood favorite to a more balanced meal. It's a really good way to please picky eaters while getting them to eat more nutrients. The mixed greens, carrots, bell peppers, and avocado load this wrap up with vitamins A and C, fiber, and healthy fats.

If you are a parent who always has chicken nuggets in the freezer for your kiddos, this is a great way to enjoy them yourself as well. And if you're not a fan of Buffalo sauce, no problem, simply swap it out with one of your favorite sauces, such as barbecue, honey mustard, or whatever your heart desires.

Preheat the oven to 425°F.

Place the chicken nuggets on a sheet pan and bake until they are golden and crispy, 8 to 14 minutes (follow package cook time), flipping them about halfway through. In a medium bowl, toss them with the Buffalo wing sauce until fully coated.

In a small bowl, combine the yogurt and ranch seasoning. Stir until well combined. Warm the tortilla for 10 to 15 seconds in the microwave, or 10 to 20 seconds in a dry pan over a burner until warm and pliable.

Place the tortilla flat on a clean surface. You'll want to leave a 1-inch space around the edge as you fill it. Start by spreading the ranch mix evenly over the tortilla. Next arrange the greens in an even layer. Then add the carrots, cucumbers, bell peppers, and avocado. Arrange the Buffalo-coated nuggets on top of the veggies and drizzle the toppings with any leftover sauce.

To roll the wrap, carefully fold the tortilla up from the bottom over the filling, then fold in the sides, and roll the wrap up until it is snug and sealed. This is a pretty full wrap, so you'll want to squeeze it and carefully roll it so that the filling doesn't fall out.

For easier handling, and to prevent filling from falling out, wrap the wrap in parchment paper or waxed paper, tucking in the ends as you roll the same way that you rolled up the wrap. Slice the wrap in half diagonally and enjoy! This wrap is best enjoyed day of.

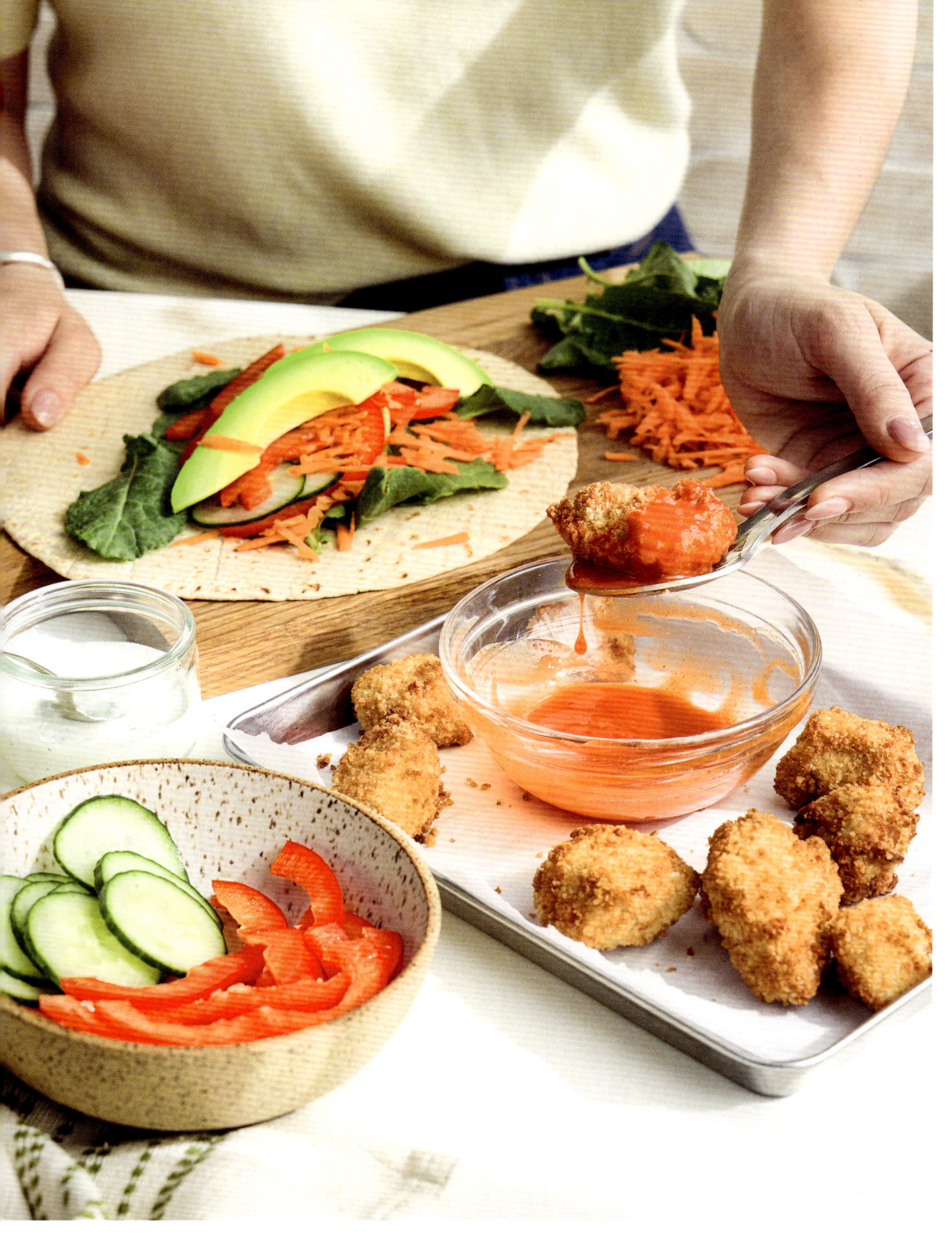

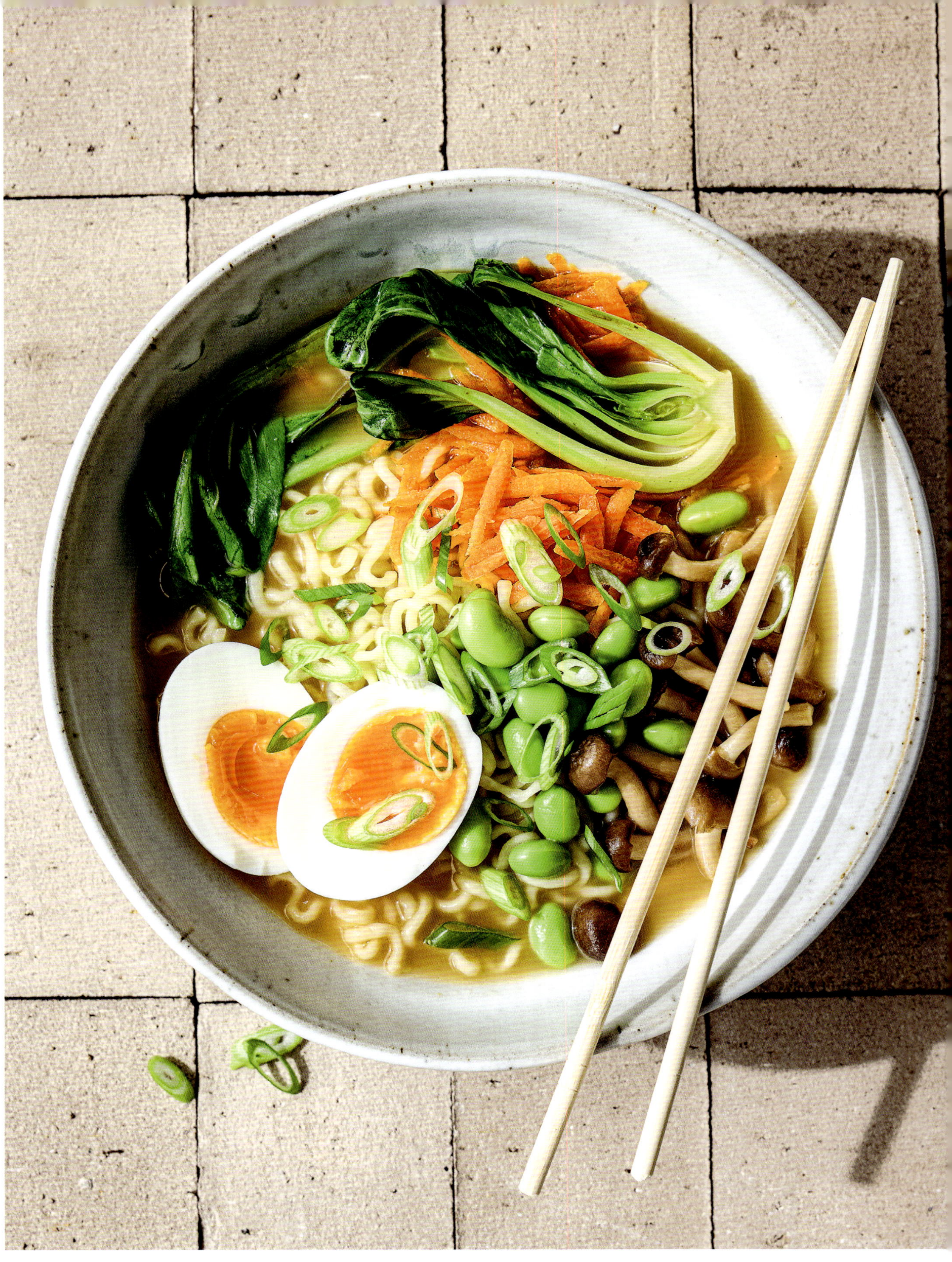

Doctored Instant Ramen

SERVES 1
PREP TIME: 5 minutes
COOK TIME: 15 minutes

PER SERVING:	**CALORIES** 689 kcal	**PROTEIN** 33g	**FAT** 28g	**CARBOHYDRATE** 76g	**FIBER** 9g

1 large egg

1½ teaspoons extra-virgin olive oil

1 cup sliced white or cremini mushrooms

¼ cup grated carrots

½ teaspoon finely grated or minced peeled fresh ginger

2 cups chicken broth (or preferred broth)

2 tablespoons reduced-sodium soy sauce

2 teaspoons Sriracha sauce

1 package instant ramen (any flavor, discard seasoning packet)

½ cup frozen shelled edamame, thawed

¼ cup milk (dairy or nondairy)

2 tablespoons thinly sliced green onion (white and green parts)

My college friends and I all went through a pretty serious instant ramen phase. You too? I'm not ashamed. Instant ramen gets a bad rap health-wise. When you think about it, it's just a bowl of carbs in broth! Repeat after me: WE LOVE CARBS. They are our bodies' preferred energy source. Please don't treat them like outcasts.

Doctoring up instant ramen is a fun and easy way to infuse a quick lunch, dinner, or late-night snack with a burst of good-for-you nutrients. The gist: Add protein, fiber-rich veggies, healthy fats, and replace the sodium-bomb seasoning packet with a wholesome broth. The goal: to pack in nutrients and stabilize the noodz so that your energy doesn't spike and crash. Feel free to add other ingredients, especially veggies, to your heart's desire. Eat what you want, add what you need. I bet you already have a bunch of these add-ons in your fridge, freezer, and pantry.

Fill a small pot three-quarters full with water and bring to a boil over high heat. Carefully add the egg to the pot, decrease the heat to medium-low, and simmer for 7 minutes. Drain the egg in a colander, rinse it with cold water until cool (or transfer it to a bowl of ice water), and set aside.

In a medium pot, heat the olive oil over medium heat until hot. Add the mushrooms and carrots and cook, stirring occasionally, until they begin to soften, 3 to 4 minutes. Add the ginger and cook until fragrant, about 1 minute.

Add the chicken broth, soy sauce, and Sriracha and bring to a boil. Once boiling, add the ramen noodles (do not use the seasoning packet!) and cook, stirring occasionally, until the noodles are cooked to your liking, about 3 minutes. Decrease the heat to low and add the edamame and milk. Cook until the edamame are heated through.

Peel and then carefully halve the soft-boiled egg (you don't want to lose any of the yummy yolk!), then float each egg half, yolk-side-up, on top of the ramen in the broth. Garnish everything with the green onions and serve hot. Instant ramen is best enjoyed day of.

Healthy Hamburger Helper

SERVES 3 OR 4
PREP TIME: 10 minutes
COOK TIME: 20 minutes

PER SERVING:	**CALORIES** 497 kcal	**PROTEIN** 37g	**FAT** 17g	**CARBOHYDRATE** 44g	**FIBER** 5g

- 1 tablespoon extra-virgin olive oil
- 1 cup finely chopped yellow onion (about ½ small onion)
- 1 pound lean ground beef (10% fat or less)
- 1 small zucchini, diced
- 2 cups chopped broccoli florets
- 1 cup snow peas
- 1½ cups chicken broth (or preferred broth)
- 1 cup milk (dairy or nondairy)
- One 5.2- to 6.6-ounce box beef flavor Hamburger Helper (or your preferred flavor)
- 1 cup lightly packed spinach, chopped
- ¼ cup chopped fresh parsley leaves (optional)

Hamburger Helper is a one-pan comfort-food classic that's a real crowd-pleaser and super easy to doctor up with fresh and nutritious additions. And this can all be done in under 30 minutes! It's a wonderfully balanced and nutrient-dense meal thanks to the lean protein of the ground beef, fiber-full veggies, and pasta carbs.

It's also endlessly adaptable. If you aren't a fan of snow peas, swap them out for a different veggie you love. If you want more veggies, load 'em up! I'll sometimes add carrots, bell peppers, and diced tomatoes. They're all great and add even more fiber and nutrients.

In a large pan, heat the olive oil over medium heat until hot. Add the onion and cook, stirring occasionally, until it starts to soften, about 3 minutes. Add the beef, increase the heat to medium-high, and cook, stirring occasionally, breaking up the meat as you do, until it is nicely browned, 6 to 8 minutes.

Add the zucchini, broccoli, and snow peas and cook, stirring occasionally, until the veggies start to soften, about 3 minutes. Stir in the chicken broth, milk, and Hamburger Helper sauce mix and pasta and bring everything to a boil. Once boiling, decrease the heat to low, cover, and simmer, stirring occasionally, until the pasta is tender, about 6 minutes.

Stir in the spinach, and cook for 1 to 2 minutes, until it has wilted. Remove from the heat, garnish with fresh parsley if desired, and enjoy.

STORAGE + REHEAT

Once cooled, store airtight in the refrigerator for up to 3 days. To reheat, warm in a pan over medium heat until heated through, or microwave.

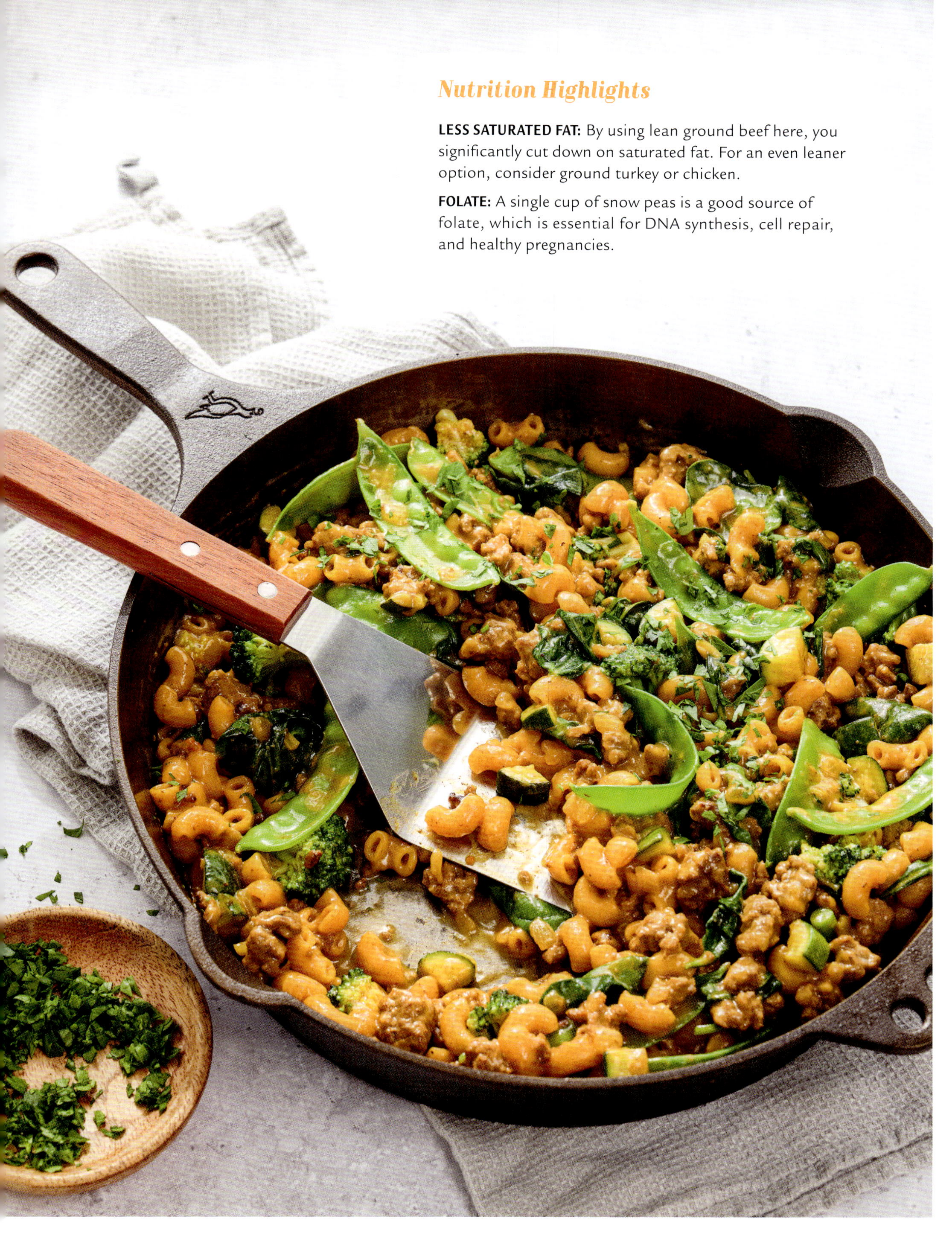

Nutrition Highlights

LESS SATURATED FAT: By using lean ground beef here, you significantly cut down on saturated fat. For an even leaner option, consider ground turkey or chicken.

FOLATE: A single cup of snow peas is a good source of folate, which is essential for DNA synthesis, cell repair, and healthy pregnancies.

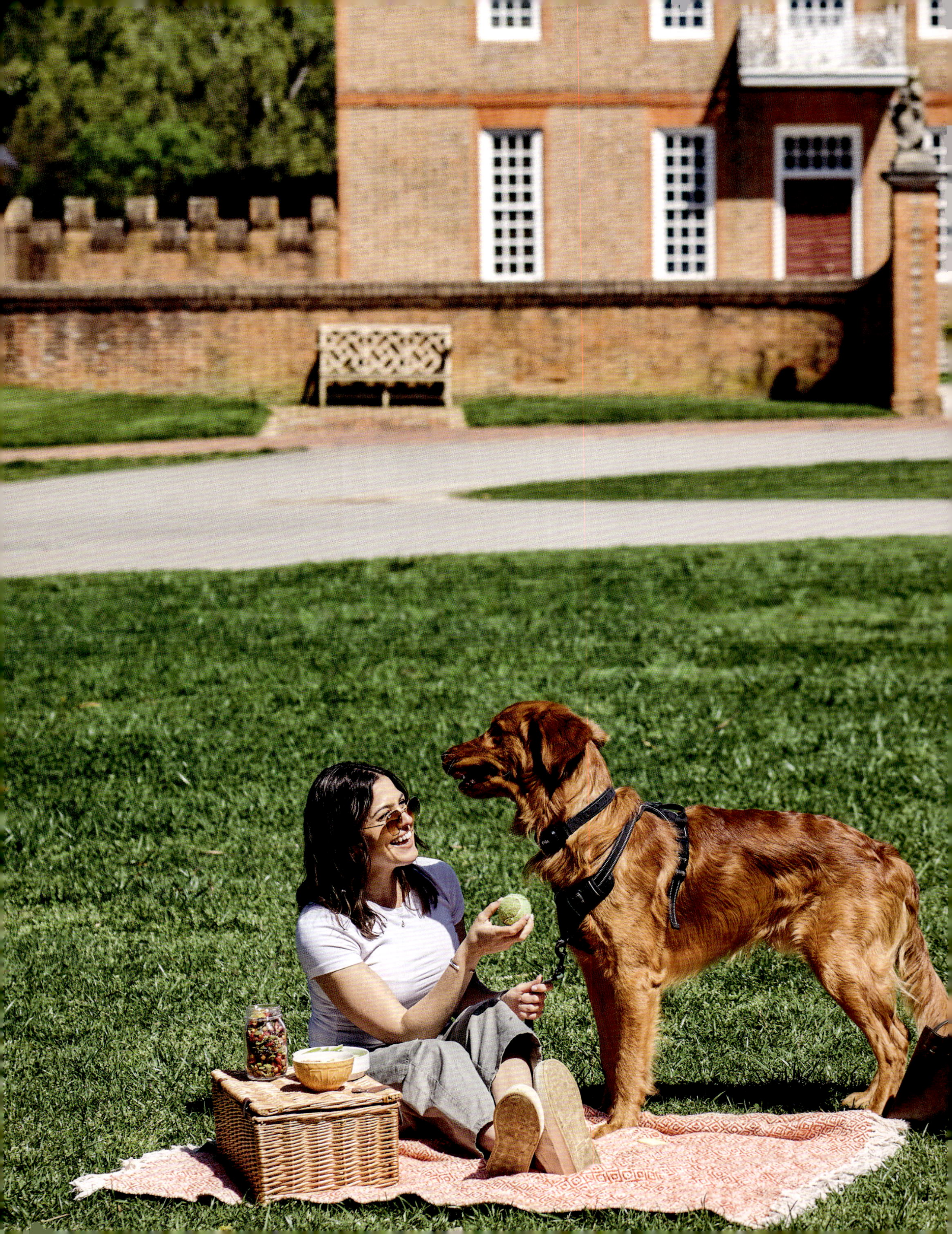

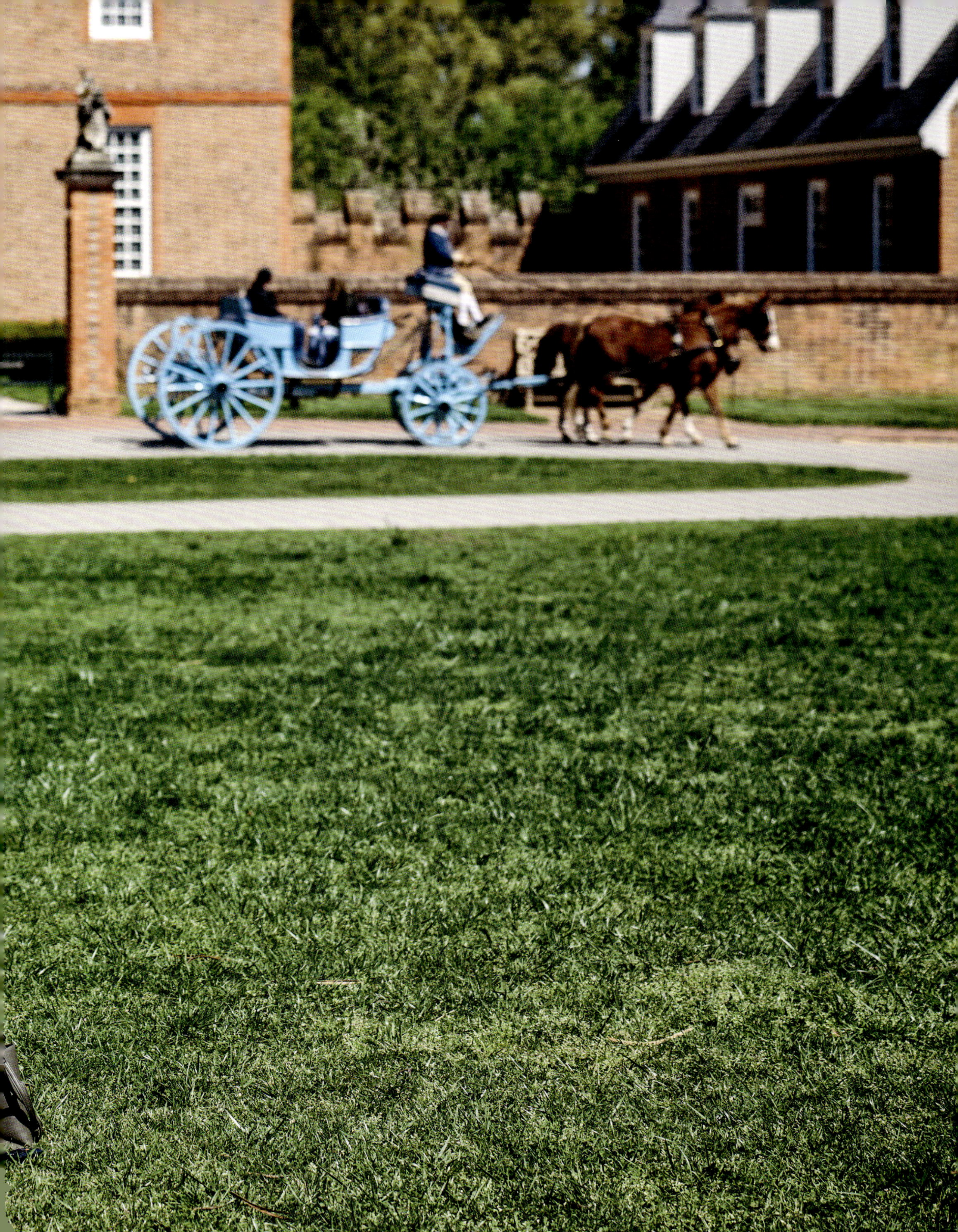

Acknowledgments

First and foremost, a heartfelt thank you to all my friends and family for your unwavering encouragement, countless taste tests, and emotional support throughout this cookbook journey. I love you. Now, some more detailed gratitude for these lovely people in my life . . .

Miles: Thank you for driving to see me every weekend, even when I was buried in recipe testing. You never complained, always had my back, and sacrificed so much to be by my side when I couldn't make it to events. Your honest (sometimes *very* honest) feedback has been invaluable, and I truly appreciate your advice and insights. You've been my number-one supporter and a huge source of recipe inspiration. I couldn't have done this without you.

Mom and Dad: Your patience and love during this process meant everything to me. Recipe testing can be so isolating, but you were always just a FaceTime call away, ready to listen or visit me when I needed it most. Dad, thank you for your suggestions . . . even if I didn't use all of them (sorry!). Mom, your enthusiasm for every little update and willingness to let me vent kept me grounded and motivated.

My sisters (Lindsay & Alessandra): Thank you for inspiring so many of the recipes in this book. Despite your busy schedules, you always checked in, keeping me connected and inspired.

Liz: I honestly don't know what I would have done without you. You made this process infinitely better than I ever imagined. I've never worked with someone who matched my energy the way you did. Your hard work, positivity, and ability to hype me up were unmatched. We had such a seamless system, and I'd write a thousand more books if I could work with you every time. Even your emails brightened my day, and you always made me feel so supported.

Jo, Olivia, the agency & the team: You all brought my dream to life. Writing a cookbook has been my goal since 2020, and you believed in me every step of the way. Thank you for never giving up on me and making this vision a reality.

Inkwell Management: Thank you for connecting me with such an incredible publisher and setting me up for success.

Ten Speed Press: A heartfelt thank you to my publisher for believing in this cookbook and bringing it to life. A special shout-out to Claire, my incredible senior editor, whose keen eye and thoughtful guidance shaped this book into what it is today. To Francesca, whose brilliant design work brought my vision to life—your creativity and attention to detail made every page shine. And to Betsy, the talented art director, thank you for your dedication and artistic vision in making this book not only informative but truly beautiful. I am so grateful to each of you.

Erin, Lillian, Paige, Mark, Andy & pup-pup Flloyd: A huge thank you to Erin and the entire photography team, who captured every recipe with such artistry and care. Your talent *exceeded* all of my expectations and had me jumping with excitement every shot. Your energy and enthusiasm made the experience truly unforgettable, and I couldn't be more grateful for the way you brought my recipes to life on the page.

Miles's dad, Chris: Your cooking tips and techniques were incredible sources of inspiration. Thank you for sharing your knowledge and encouraging my creativity in the kitchen. And thank you for always starting my week on the right note with your delicious cooking every Sunday.

Miles's mom, Victoria: A special thank you to Victoria, whose culinary legacy has deeply touched my life. Although we never had the chance to meet, cooking your recipes with Miles has brought me closer to you and filled my kitchen with your warmth and love. I can only imagine how excited you would be about this book.

Miles's family (Grannie, Granddad, Caroline & Blake): Your support has meant the world to me. Thank you for cheering me on and believing in this project.

About the Contributors

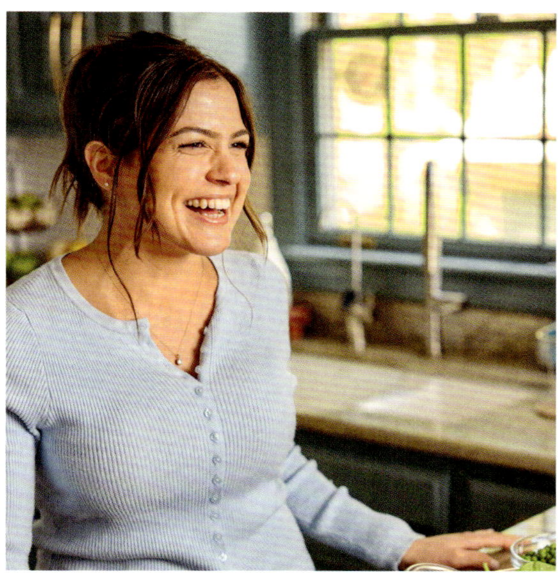

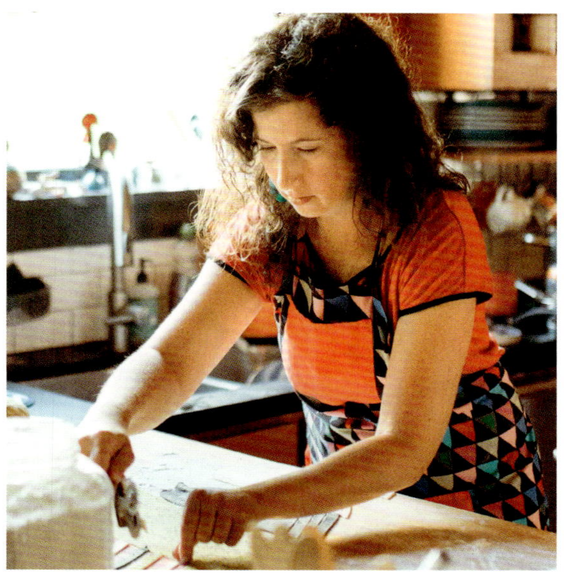

Steph Grasso is a registered dietitian and social media influencer known for making balanced eating simple, enjoyable, and accessible. By blending evidence-based nutrition with her signature charm and humor, she helps folks ditch food guilt and embrace a more sustainable, satisfying approach to eating.

With more than 2.2 million followers, Steph has been a featured dietitian on everything from *Good Morning America* and *The Rachael Ray Show* to *ABC News Live Prime* with Linsey Davis. She has also contributed to *Health Digest* and serves as a member of the U.S. News & World Report Best Diets expert panel.

Liz Crain is a longtime writer on Pacific Northwest food and drink. She is the author of *Dumplings Equal Love* and *Food Lover's Guide to Portland;* and is coauthor of *Fermenter, Toro Bravo, Hello! My Name Is Tasty,* and *Grow Your Own.* Crain is also cofounder and co-organizer of the annual Portland Fermentation Festival.

INDEX

Note: Page references in *italics* indicate photographs.

A

B

C

D

E

F

G

H

I

J

K

L

M

N

O

P

Q

R

S

T

U

V

W

Y

Z

TEN SPEED PRESS
An imprint of the Crown Publishing Group
A division of Penguin Random House LLC
1745 Broadway
New York, NY 10019
tenspeed.com
penguinrandomhouse.com

Typefaces: ITC's Legacy Sans and TypeTypes TT Moons

The plate image on pages 34–35 is Adobe Stock file #789290848 by Rawpixel.com.

Library of Congress Cataloging-in-Publication Data
Names: Grasso, Steph, 1995- author | Crain, Liz author.
Title: Crave, cook, nourish : 80+ recipes and expert guidance for healthy, happy nutrition / by Steph Grasso, MS, RD with Liz Crain.
Identifiers: LCCN 2025008828 (print) | LCCN 2025008829 (ebook) | ISBN 9780593837221 hardcover | ISBN 9780593837238 ebook.
Subjects: LCSH: Reducing diets—Recipes | Nutrition | LCGFT: Cookbooks.
Classification: LCC RM222.2 .G71695 2026 (print) | LCC RM222.2 (ebook) | DDC 641.5/63—dc23/eng/20250825
LC record available at https://lccn.loc.gov/2025008828
LC ebook record available at https://lccn.loc.gov/2025008829

Hardcover ISBN 978-0-593-83722-1
Ebook ISBN 978-0-593-83723-8

Editor: Claire Yee | Production editor: Natalie Blachere
Designer: Francesca Truman | Art director: Betsy Stromberg
Production designers: Mari Gill and Faith Hague
Production: Jane Chinn | Prepress color manager: Neil Spitkovsky
Food stylist: Lillian Kang | Food stylist assistant: Paige Arnett
Photo assistants: Mark Davis and Andy Omvik
Copy editor: Kate Slate | Proofreaders: Patricia Dailey, Andrea Connolly Peabbles, and Miriam Taveras | Indexer: Elizabeth Parson
Publicist: Natalie Yera-Campbell | Marketer: Stephanie Davis

Manufactured in China

10 9 8 7 6 5 4 3 2 1

First Edition

The authorized representative in the EU for product safety and compliance is Penguin Random House Ireland, Morrison Chambers, 32 Nassau Street, Dublin D02 YH68, Ireland, https://eu-contact.penguin.ie.